30p

D1357750

306

ITALIAN LABYRINTH

Italy in the 1980s

ITALIAN LABYRINTH

Italy in the 1980s

BY

JOHN HAYCRAFT

SECKER & WARBURG
LONDON

First published in England 1985 by
Martin Secker & Warburg Limited
54 Poland Street, London W1V 3DF

Copyright © John Haycraft 1985

British Library Cataloguing in Publication Data

Haycraft, John
Italian labyrinth : Italy in the 1980s.
1. Italy—Social conditions—1976–
I. Title
945.092'8   HN475.5

ISBN 0 436 19137 7

Typeset in 12/13 Monophoto Bembo
Printed in Great Britain by
St Edmundsbury Press, Bury St Edmunds, Suffolk

To Merlyn

"And don't ... go with that awful tourist idea that Italy's only a museum of antiquities and art. Love and understand the Italians, for the people are more marvellous than the land."

    E. M. Forster, *Where Angels Fear to Tread*

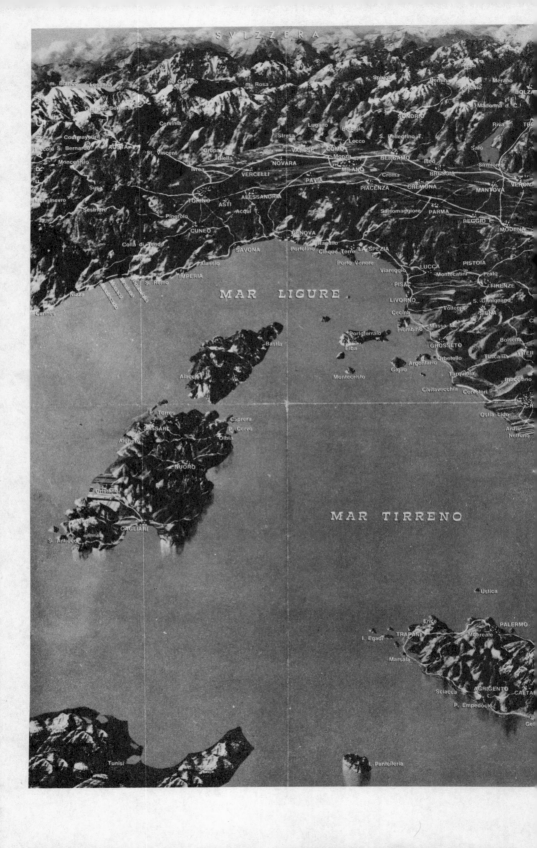

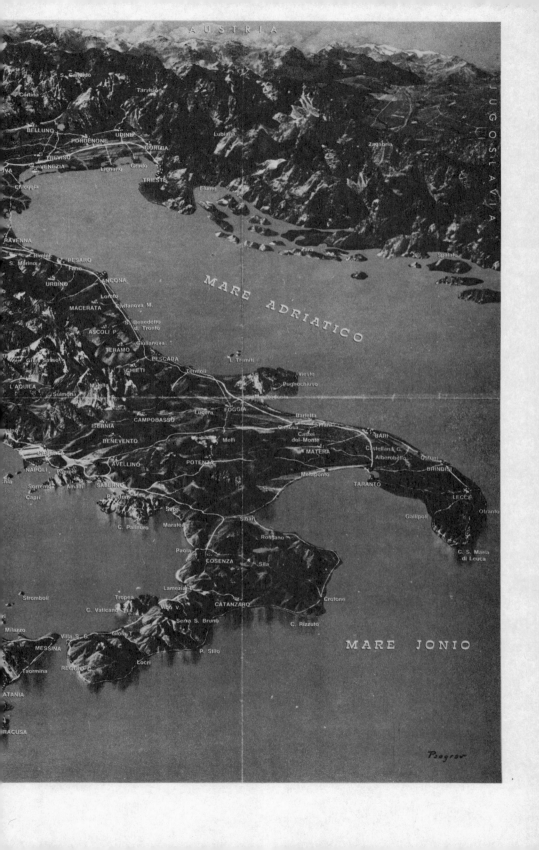

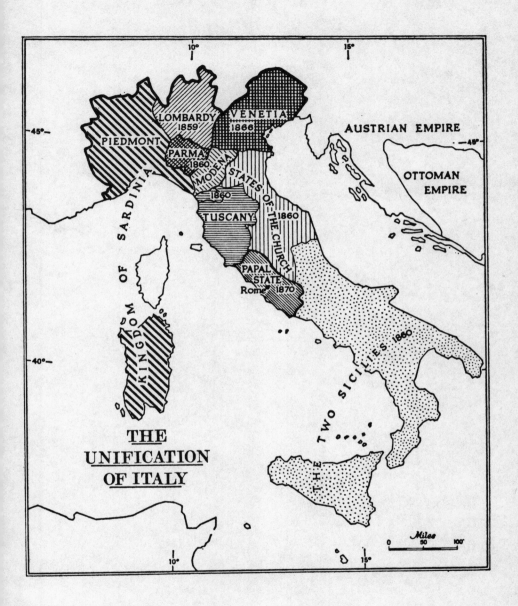

AUSTRIAN EMPIRE

OTTOMAN
EMPIRE

LOMBARDY
1859

VENETIA
1866

PIEDMONT

PARMA
1860

MODENA
1860

STATES OF THE CHURCH

TUSCANY

1860

PAPAL
STATE
Rome   1870

KINGDOM OF SARDINIA

THE TWO SICILIES 1860

THE
UNIFICATION
OF ITALY

Miles
0   50   100

CONTENTS

PREFACE

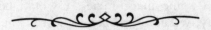

I have had a relationship with Italy for almost half a century. First, as a boy of six just before the war, staying for a year with my family in Alassio. I remember going out to an Italian cruiser in the bay and being hoisted up to sit on a gun on the occasion of an official visit by Crown Prince Umberto. The owner of the hotel we stayed at had known Mussolini, fighting side by side in the army in 1917. He described him, I remember, as "a rough man".

Then, in 1948, I travelled all round an impoverished Italy as an impoverished student, being turned off the Palatine Hill, where we slept, twice by different policemen in the early morning; or spending a night huddled in a crowded cattle truck which served as a railway carriage between Rome and Milan.

Then taking American tourists round the well-known places from Como to Capri in the 1950s. And, finally, I helped to start a school of English (International House) in Rome in 1967 which led to the setting up of fourteen other affiliated schools all over Italy.

It is interesting how valuable schools like this have been for the research this book has entailed. With hundreds of adult students from every walk of life it has been comparatively easy to contact anyone I wanted to, and I would like to thank the directors, teachers and students who have given me so much help.

An Anglo-Saxon writing about Italy will obviously produce a different book from one an Italian would write, and I would like to emphasize here that in criticisms I have made, I am not comparing Italy to Britain or any other English-speaking country. I have written this book as someone who has travelled to many countries as well as Italy and I know that such comparisons, except on a few factual matters, are much too complicated to make. Britain has its own crises and I hope that the old superior attitudes of the travelling Englishman do not exist in this book, although they may sometimes occur in the imagination of the Italian reader. Indeed, I am only too conscious of the wonderful opportunity I have had to explore and research a country as varied and stimulating as Italy.

There are many "facts" in this book and, however hard an author tries, there may be some inaccuracies. I would be most grateful if anyone noticing any, would let me know, just as I am grateful to those who have read the original manuscript and have produced valuable corrections. The question of translating lire into dollars or pounds has been a particular problem with the continual fluctuation of currencies and of the cost of living. Equivalents should therefore be regarded as approximate, giving at least some idea of the sums involved.

I should like particularly to thank my wife, Brita, who shared a lot of my research in Italy; my secretary Jean Peto; Prof Vacciago and Mrs Barsetti of the Italian Cultural Institute in London, for all their help and advice. In addition to those who appear in the text, I should like to thank all the following, without whom this book could never have been written:

Michele Achilli; Sir Harold Acton; Ian Adams; Derek Andrews; Avv. Paola Alfieri; Rolando Argentero; Giovanni Bertolini; Marcella Banchetti; Roy Boardman; Dott. Amedeo Borzello; Dott. Alfonso Bernardi; Claudio Dematte; Betty Cadman; Amedeo Caporaletti; Girolamo Capelli; Paul Cahill; Gen. Capuzzo; Gui Caspani; Dott. Gianni Castellano; John Church; M-Gracia Camineti; Sgr. & Sra Conti; Sgr. & Sgra Corsaro; Lindy Cronin; Robert Culshaw; Dott. Carlo Doglio; Tony Duff; Mme Fargheon; Silvio Favatti; Avv. Alessandro di Ferrari; Avv. Camilo Fré; Martin Dobman; Alison Duigood; Pat Durden; Dott. Fatini; Marco Fiocchi; Antonio Gambino; Prof. Arturo Giuletti; Prof. & Sgra. Gunella; Richard Illingworth; On. Giorgio La Malfa; John Francis Lane; Dott. Andreina Levi; Bill McAllister; Dott. & Sgra Maffioli; Sonia di Marco; Dott. Lucio Messina; Prof. Bruno Menapace; Grace Modolo; Toby Moore; Dott. Morcaldi; Ana Ottaviani; Dott. Padovani; Eduarda & Tim Priesack; Sir Gordon Pirie; Gualberto Ranieri; Maurice Richardson; Lea Roberts; Giancarlo Romano; Sgr. Ruffino; Enrico Sassoon; Philippa and Ken Saunders; Maurizio Schiaretti; Roberto Scrocca; Gaia Servadio; Mario Soldati; Prof. Aurelio Sesso; Italo Somarriello; Anita Riotta; "Happy" Ruggero; Brian Tiffen; Avv. Vincenzo Torricelli; Roberto Trionfera; Prof. Tranfaglia; Villari family; Fabio Zampini; Comm. Ausonio Zappa.

I
BACKGROUND

Some Foreign Views of Italy – A New Country –
Foreign Rule – Divisions – Since 1945

SOME FOREIGN VIEWS OF ITALY

I went to Charing Cross station with a tape recorder to get some general opinions about Italy. "Italians! They're lovely," enthused a girl with fluffy, fair hair. "And all that sun!"

"Italy? It's O.K.," said a tall man in a blue suit and striped shirt. "It's a good place for a holiday. Bit crowded though, if you know what I mean, although they've certainly got a lot of, well, Art!"

"Don't know it!" said a fat, elderly man. "We always go to Spain for our holidays."

From other people, I got more varied comments:

"Barbaric! all that Mafia!"

"They're the most civilized people in the world. They've got a real sense of beauty."

"I don't know. I've never really thought about it! I suppose they're all right. They certainly seem to have a lot of scandals, though."

"They're very good industrially. The North, that is! I mean they really produce some very good things. You find something practical and yet beautiful in the shops and most of the time, it's 'Made in Italy'."

Later, I met a lorry driver who drove every week to and from Italy, and said that Italian Customs were by far the easiest to get through. "Of course you have to give them a few bottles of whisky or the equivalent. Sometimes they may ask for something from your load. But it's worth it in the long run. With British Customs you sometimes have to wait twenty-four hours."

I talked with friends:

"They've given us the best things in our civilization. When you go to Italy you're astounded to realize that so much of our style, even in modern times, comes from them. Not to mention architecture, painting, sculpture. Going right back, even central heating was devised by the Romans."

At an international party in a sunny garden, I listened to people who knew Italy well:

"It's the one European country where nothing is ever what it seems," said an American. "You try to find out how things are organized and you are given a certain version. You then find that in practice it all works differently – but only in the place where you happen to be at the time. Elsewhere, you are given other versions and then find out that in practice this varies too. Everything depends on the locality and the individual. You ought to call your book 'The Labyrinth'."

"Yes," agreed someone who had written an article on Palladian villas for a Sunday newspaper. "It's funny how flimsy the very word 'Italian' is, when you compare it with other nationality words: French, Spanish, German, even Swiss or Swedish – it seems so indefinite. It doesn't really stand for anything, even in the way that Rome or Venice, Naples or Florence do."

"There's this Italian writer, Enzo Biagi, who wrote that Italy does not exist," said a pert Frenchman.

"That's going a bit too far –"

"Of course Italy exists, although it is made up of so many different regions."

"Well," said someone who writes books on general philosophy for schools, "I suppose it depends on what you mean by 'exist'."

A NEW COUNTRY

The "titbit" at the end of the TV news, sometime in the summer of 1983, showed a small, old man celebrating his hundred and eleventh birthday with champagne. In a brief interview, he stated that he was very happy and healthy and that women still meant a lot to him.

Interesting, I thought, motivated by my obsession. Here was someone still cavorting and merry and yet he had been born only two years after the final unification of Italy. While, on the personal level, my grandfather was already twenty-eight when Rome became the capital of a united Italy – largely, though, because he was forty-five when he married a girl of seventeen, and my mother had been the youngest of nine children.

For what they are worth, these calculations do at least bring out the supreme paradox of Italy: how ancient it is culturally and yet how new it is as a nation. What they do not show is how unsuccessful that brief period of nationhood has been, measured so often by the waves of collective enthusiasm which were followed by the deepest disillusionment.

Even before national unity was achieved, the pattern was set. First, by Napoleon, who occupied the whole of present-day Italy except Sicily and then, in 1814, was replaced by the foreign and autocratic regimes which he had previously overthrown: the Austrians in most of Northern Italy, the Bourbons in the South, the Papacy in Rome, whose states stretched up central Italy and the Adriatic coast. Once again, Italy became, in the words of the Austrian Chancellor Metternich, merely a "geographical expression".

The Revolution of 1848, which started in Milan with a strike against the use of tobacco, from which the ruling Austrians derived revenue, was crushed within a year. It did, however, create greater enthusiasm for the idea of a united Italy which led to the defeat of the Austrians in 1859 with Napoleon III's help, the subsequent expulsion of the Bourbons from the South, and plebiscites in favour of unity in the Papal States. This, in 1861, resulted in the centralized rule of most of the peninsula by the King of Piedmont and Sardinia, Victor Emmanuel II, whose name now graces a main street in most Italian towns.

Unification, however, was achieved largely through foreign help. Italians themselves fought on both sides in the struggle. The Austrian navy, based in Venice, was manned partly by Italian subjects, as were many of the regiments in the Austrian army. Venice was acquired in 1866 because Italy allied herself with the Prussians, who defeated the Austrians at the battle of Sadowa. Again, it was the Prussian victory over Napoleon III at Sedan in 1870 which compelled the evacuation of the protective French forces in Rome, and thus allowed the Italians entry. Unification, indeed, was the achievement of Italian diplomacy rather than arms. "If I did for myself what I do for my country, I should be a scoundrel, indeed!" wrote Cavour, the Prime Minister of Piedmont, whose skill was largely responsible.

"The radiant dawn," as a plaque at Bologna town hall describes it, was followed by a dreary period of scandals and political manipulation, which allowed Mussolini to boast when he took power: "I tread on the rotten corpse of liberty!" A report from a local official in Sardinia to the Prime Minister, Crispi, in 1896, reads as follows:

... parties are lively, tenacious, intransigent and aggressive; but they are not political parties nor parties moved by a general or local interest, they are personal parties, cliques (in the strict meaning of the word).... Under the great wings of these large parties ... pullulate microscopic personal parties in the different Communes, all the more spiteful and violent because the reasons for disagreement are closer, and contact necessary every day.... They make themselves dependent on the major parties, from whom they receive in exchange protection and effective aid in little local contests and, above all, personal protection through obtaining favours and through avoiding the consequences of breaking the law, and sometimes even of committing crimes....

If Italians had little cause to feel proud of a government at home where a bill was actually passed simply by giving honours to sixty opposition deputies, they also had sparse reason for pride in their country's achievement abroad.

Whether for good or ill, Italy came in late on the European race for colonies. A politician commented at the time: "Italy has an enormous appetite but rotten teeth." It had the unfortunate distinction of being the first European country to be defeated by an African army, losing four thousand officers and men at the battle of Adowa against the Abyssinians in 1896. Later, in 1912, it did succeed in wresting the Dodecanese islands and Libya from the Turks, but it was not till 1931 that the real pacification of Libya was achieved.

The First World War is known in Italy as the "Italo–Austrian War", and can be considered as a final phase in the movement for Italian liberation from the Austrians, who still occupied parts of Italy in the north and north-east.

The Italians fought gallantly and, in the first two years, pushed the Austrians back, only to be overwhelmed at Caporetto in 1917. Despite the subsequent victory of Vittorio Veneto in the last month of the war, the Treaty of Versailles gave Italy very little consolation for a percentage of casualties to men mobilized that was even higher than Britain's.* Although they extended their frontiers in the north they had no share in the division of German spoils, as did Britain and France.

Mussolini, in fact, was probably unique in giving the masses a sense of pride in being Italian. He forbad the use of local dialects in schools, asserted the apparent strength of central government, maintained order and contained the Mafia. There is little doubt that in 1936, with the conquest of Abyssinia, most Italians felt that they had finally achieved international importance. However, as always, it was not to last. The foundations were absent. As Riboldi Vicende wrote: "You could get

* Italy: 39.1 per cent; British Empire: 35.8 per cent.

away with 98 per cent of public clamour and 2 per cent of solid achievement."

A recent biographer of Mussolini, Enzo Forcella, who was born in 1922, looks back at his youth under Fascism and writes of "the discovery of bonds with *la colletività*, the warmth of the group, what sociologists define as the 'sense of belonging'".

However, he goes on to say that with the coming of the war, everything Mussolini said, his vainglorious objectives, the heroic models he fixed on, "were acceptable so long as they were not confronted by reality and, above all, if that confrontation did not demand too high a price from his subjects".

That price was paid with defeats in Greece, Libya, Sicily and Russia. Forcella describes looking at the photographs of Mussolini and his mistress, Clara Petacci, strung up in the Piazza Loreto in Milan in April 1945. He notes the similarity of Mussolini's swollen and distorted face to that of Popeye, and concludes that, like voyeurism, "after having seen everything one realizes that there is nothing to see."

FOREIGN RULE

The failure of "Italy" as a concept is also linked to the fact that for four hundred years the inhabitants of the peninsula had little reason to identify with any of the foreign governments which ruled them (see map p.ix).

There is an old saying: "The Spanish or the French? It doesn't matter, so long as we eat!" No part of Italy except Piedmont has escaped a long period of alien rule. In Venice it was shortest, as the independent republic lasted until 1797. It was then abolished by Napoleon, Venice was given to the Austrians and became part of Italy only some seventy years later. In Tuscany, the rule of the Medici continued until 1737 when the last childless grand duke, Gian Gastone, who rarely saw his subjects when he was sober, finally expired. Then that region too was governed by an Austrian archduke.

It could be argued that the Papal States were under some kind of "Italian" regime. However, people from that region will often tell you that the reason it is strongly Communist today is due largely to an historical reaction against the laxity, indifference and inefficiency of the cardinals, bishops and priests who once ruled it. Indeed Goethe, travelling through Italy in the eighteenth century, remarked that the Papal States "seem to keep alive only because the earth refuses to swallow them".

However, it is above all the southern part – that long extension of territory which stretches down below Rome and the Abruzzi, which contains provinces with romantic Latin names like Campania and Calabria, Basilicata and Apulia, and ends with the tormented island of Sicily – which has had a succession of foreign dynasties from the break-up of the Roman Empire until 1946. The guide books list them: Arabs, Normans, Germans and Angevins; the Aragonese, the Spanish and the French. Finally, the Piedmontese who, although acclaimed initially, had to send their Carabinieri to fight a bitter revolt between 1861 and 1865.

For a long time, the states of Italy were the bargaining counters of European royal families. In 1737, Tuscany was given to the Duke of Lorraine on condition he surrendered his duchy to Louis XV of France. In 1713, Victor Amadeus II, King of Piedmont, was crowned with great pomp in Palermo Cathedral, only to exchange Sicily for Sardinia five years later. Maria Luisa, daughter of the Emperor of Austria and Napoleon's second wife, was "given" the duchy of Parma and a one-eyed lover, Count Neipperg, to distract her from thoughts of her exiled husband.

Some of these rulers were much loved. Peasants from Apulia and Basilicata marched barefoot to join the Bourbon army in its last resistance to Piedmont and Garibaldi in 1861. Citizens of Parma will tell you even today that memories of Maria Luisa are still fond, despite or perhaps because of her nymphomanic tendencies; although she died 140 years ago, bunches of Parma violets are still sent to Vienna and laid on her tomb on her birthday.

Despite the fact that the Austrians were among the main opponents of the unification of Italy, their rule is remembered for its honesty and administrative efficiency. The survival of its structures and the attitude it created are still regarded as one of the bases for the economic success of Lombardy and the Veneto. A poem in Mantuan dialect about Maria Teresa, Empress of Austria and ruler of a large part of northern Italy from 1740–80, runs as follows:

> Come una bona mama la regnava
> par al bene e'l progres a dla gent
> e tuti i citadini la stimava

(She ruled like a good mother for the welfare and the progress of the people and all the citizens esteemed her.)

Nevertheless, these centuries of alien rule also meant that Italians rarely identified themselves with government. Those who worked in the administration of king, pope or duke during the long centuries represented a foreign power, not the people themselves. The payment of taxes was seen, therefore, not as a duty to the community but as an exaction to be evaded. In an interesting article showing how proverbs reflect Italian attitudes to their rulers, Carlo Lapucci writes: "Italy, particularly, has lived through political changes in the form of a succession of foreign entities with whom, after finding a means of co-existence, it was necessary to break in order to try out new masters, who were even more exigent, greedy and alien.'"* Among other proverbs, he quotes a popular verse:

> Fatta la legge, trovato l'inganno
> Fatta la legge, la malizia é pronta.
> Chi ruba al re non fa peccato.
> Rubare al re
> Peccato non é.

(As soon as a law is made, the loopholes are found and cunning begins. He who robs the king doesn't sin. To rob the king is no sin.)

Recently, I went round a Fiat factory in Turin with a group of Rotarians from Biella, a neighbouring town. We started discussing Italian attitudes to government.

"The government! They're no different from us. They're rogues! Just as we are!" said a sausage manufacturer.

"All we do if we pay taxes is to empty our pockets to fill theirs!" added a man who managed a textile factory.

This is normal talk. Ask any Italian – even one in government. Because Italy is a new country, because of regional differences, because government has never established itself as anything but a group of separate cliques working for themselves, the ancient verses and proverbs are still quoted and still have their modern equivalents.

DIVISIONS

Most Italian towns and cities have a street called Settembre XX because it was on that day in 1870 that the newly formed Italian army breached the walls of Rome. In a humble horse-carriage, the old and disconsolate Pope Pius IX drove away from his palace, the Quirinale, over the river to the Vatican – which still remains a separate State with its own stamps, its Swiss Guard, its diplomatic corps and even its own bank, the IOR, which has recently been involved in two major financial scandals.

* "Le Lingue del Mondo", July–August 1983. Valmartina, Florence.

The choice of Rome as capital has often been criticized. Certainly it has distorted the city. A town of a few hundred thousand, containing unique monuments, which like those of Athens and Jerusalem belong to the whole world, has now become a metropolis of over three millions, teeming with cars and bureaucrats. A broad carriageway laid down by Mussolini covers part of a forum. Temples and baroque churches share walls with government buildings. Shaken by traffic vibrations, ruins become yet more ruinous, are hidden by scaffolding and closed to visitors for the inevitable *restauro*. Over the years, new industry and shanty towns have crept up on the city walls like ancient hordes of Goths, Lombards or Vandals, likewise intent on destruction.

However, the choice of Rome as capital was inevitable. For one thing it disguised the fact that the unification of Italy was essentially a conquest of the South by the North. It borrowed, too, the glory of an empire that in truth has as little to do with modern Italy as the empire of Tsar Dushan has to do with modern Yugoslavia. It also, however, created a division that was to split loyalties still further in this precariously unified State and give the Church the role of the fairy godmother who had not been invited to the feast. In a country which had been the centre of Christendom for fifteen hundred years, anyone who participated in the new national government even as a voter was excommunicated until as late as 1904. The Roman aristocracy boycotted supporters of the "Piedmontese King", and it was not till the Concordat of 1929, almost sixty years after unification, that Church and State were reconciled – at least officially.

A second major division split the country only a few years later. During the last war, on September 8th 1943 at precisely 5.10 p.m., the King, Victor Emmanuel III, left Rome with his Prime Minister, Marshal Badoglio, and a convoy of generals, and made their way to Pescara on the east coast and then down to Brindisi. That night it was announced on the Italian radio that an armistice had been signed with the Anglo-Americans, who had occupied southern Calabria and parts of Apulia and were establishing a bridgehead at Salerno, just south of Naples.

Naturally, the Germans, who already had nine divisions in Italy, reacted to the news and demanded the surrender of units of the Italian army not only in the peninsula but also farther afield in Avignon, Dalmatia and Greece. Perplexed phone calls from local Italian commanders to Rome were answered by a general who stated that he knew nothing because the King's government had left no orders.

Some Italian troops joined the Germans; some the Allies. Others merged with partisan groups which were forming in the north. Those who resisted the Germans with no hope of Allied assistance were massacred. In Cefalonia, south of Corfu, the Italians fought for a week. When they finally surrendered, 4,500 officers and men were shot and their bodies were left in the open. "The Italian rebels do not deserve a burial!" said the German major in command.

As a result, the State broke up into those who still supported Mussolini's new rump republic at Saló on Lake Garda and those who sided with the Allies, with whom the King was now ranged. In addition, an estimated 450,000 men joined the partisans, who fought an irregular war against the Germans and Italian Fascists, owing loyalty to no one except their incipient Communist, Socialist or Catholic parties.

An Italian film, *The Night of St Lawrence*, directed by the Taviani brothers and released in 1981, pictures the chaos and the bitterness when the inhabitants of a Tuscan village steal out at night to join the Allies. Instead, they fight a battle against Fascists of the same village who have pursued them. This takes place in a field of ripe corn, which a few years previously all would have harvested together. Now, they peep above the wind-swept waves of golden wheat under the hot sunlight, take aim, and fire at each other.

Of course, many Italians manoeuvred between both sides. Licio Gelli, the Venerable Master of the Masonic lodge, the P2, which in 1981 was discovered to have percolated even the Secret Service, was a fervent Fascist. He fought in Spain during the Civil War and in Albania. In 1943, when the rift came, he sided with Mussolini. However, a year later he was playing a double game in his native province of Pistoia, working for the Fascists but at the same time releasing Communist partisans who were brought to him for trial. Like many Italians in the same situation, he survived.

War monuments are perhaps the most evocative traces of these divisions. In most Italian towns you come across stone plinths covered with the names of the fallen in the 1915–18 war, crowned with metal angels and the stark statues of soldiery. However, there is rarely a commemoration of those who died in the last war. Only in towns where partisans were strongest do you find framed photographs of those who died, as at Modena behind the cathedral, or at Bologna, opposite the Tower of Re Enzo. However, even this is complicated: in October 1983 a small town, Pedescala, near Vicenza, was given the Gold Medal of the Resistance which even forty years later is still being awarded. The town, however, refused it. Photographs in the newspapers showed the citizens gathered round a war monument pointing at names of brothers, or husbands, or fathers. Because the partisans had fired on the Germans and had then simply fled to the hills, sixty-three villagers had been killed in reprisals.

On September 20th 1945, Italy celebrated the seventy-fifth anniversary of its unification. Yet Italians had no reason to rejoice. "The weight of lost battles," as the Italian historian Sergio Romano calls it, was even heavier. Foreign soldiers were once again on their soil. The grandson of the king who had united them was in exile in Egypt. Mussolini's great railway stations still stood in Milan and Rome but the trains hardly existed, much less ran on time. Factories in the north were in ruins and Turin had lost 37 per cent of its buildings through air bombardment. In a book called *Naples '44* Norman Lewis, a British member of the army of occupation, had written: "And what is the prize eventually to be won? The rebirth of democracy. The glorious prospect of being able one day to choose their rulers from a list of powerful men, most of whose corruptions are already known and accepted with weary resignation."

Europe too was shattered. Other countries, however, did have some historical consolations for their devastation and exhaustion. Britain and France still retained their empires for the time being. Germany could recall astounding victories as well as defeats and a tradition of government which may have spewed up Hitler, but, sixty years previously, had also brought the welfare state. Spain was wretched and threatened but still had a tradition of pride and unity, a memory, in spite of everything, of national success. Russia was triumphant despite its twenty million dead.

Most Italians, recalling the past, could look back with pride only to the time when independent communes, republics and duchies ruled small cities and regions, and produced the artists and architects, the thinkers and saints, the philosophers and scientists, even the generals and admirals, for which the peninsula is renowned. Unity, the State, had brought nothing but sordid cliques. There was no question of breaking it up again, although there was a strong initial movement for independence in Sicily immediately after the war. There was, however, division, despair and a feeling that humiliation could go no further.

SINCE 1945

Since 1945, there has been enormous social and economic progress in Italy – as in so many parts of the globe. As a result of the boom of 1959–62, Italy became the seventh industrial nation in the world, despite the fact that her natural resources are scarce. After the war it was estimated that there were five million illiterates. Today, school attendance is much as it is in any other European country. The contrast emerges clearly from a report made by schoolchildren interviewing old people as part of a project for the 1982 International Year of the Aged. One old lady who has experienced two World Wars and three earthquakes describes life as "a vale of tears". Another talks about the way she went out barefoot and half naked as a girl to collect firewood. One who went with her family to live in Rome says how difficult it was for her to use the buses because she did not know the numbers as she had never been to school.

Now, a survey of 1984 shows that the average income of an Italian head of family is about $7,000 a year after tax. It is difficult to compare figures like these because of fluctuating currency exchanges and cost of living indexes, but this indicates a standard of living similar to, or above that in Britain.

Politically, there has certainly been stability. Indeed Italy is the only Mediterranean country which has never had an army coup d'état – although the wags will tell you this is because Italy has no "état". For thirty years up to 1981, the Prime Minister, or President of the Council as he is called, came exclusively from one political party, the Christian Democrats. The Italian expression *i quattro cantoni*, literally the four corners, describes a game similar to musical chairs where people just change from one corner to another. Italian politics has been rather like this, with politicians like Fanfani, Rumor, Andreotti and, before his death, Moro, popping up in turn to head the government – like figures on a town clock emerging one after another to the sound of the same music, midday after midday.

In many ways, government has not yet adapted itself to the amazing developments of the last thirty years. It is still a little like the eighteenth century in Britain when men like Walpole or Newcastle used bribes, the offer of sinecures and intrigue to get the votes they needed. After all, it took at least a hundred years for this type of government in Britain to adapt itself to the impact of the Industrial Revolution.

In Italy, 1978 was probably the most disillusioning year. On March 16th, the President of the Council, Aldo Moro, was being driven from Mass to his office with a bodyguard of five. Suddenly, a car in front with diplomatic number plates braked and reversed into his car. Gunmen sprang out, killed all five bodyguards and then drove off with Moro, and disappeared.

Fifty-five days later, Moro was found dead in the back of a Renault

Five. For almost three months he had been hidden in Rome itself. Despite road blocks, appeals to the public, detective work and house to house searches, both police and Carabinieri had been powerless.

Moro, one of the founders of the ruling Christian Democrat party, was the first to try to form a national coalition with the Left to deal with Italy's economic and administrative problems. In 1963, he had become President of the Council for the first time, after persuading his party to form a government with the Socialists. Before his capture, he was thought to be trying to end an eight-week political crisis through greater power-sharing with the Communists. This is probably why he was abducted and killed.

In photographs released by the Red Brigade during his captivity, Moro has the dark face and intelligent, soft eyes of the southern Italian. His expression is that of one who has sensed the slaughterhouse. His murder was unique: heads of government have been beheaded, assassinated, blown up, torn to pieces by mobs. Never, though, has a group of terrorists captured a man in Moro's position in broad daylight, held him for three months in the capital city, and then put five bullets round his heart. Never, probably, has a state shown itself so powerless without collapsing. The ultimate insult lay in the place he was found: the Renault Five was parked in a busy street half way between the Christian Democrat and Communist headquarters.

Italy's special characteristic is that she is a new, divided country, stretching down a long peninsula where Milan is closer to London than to Palermo, and where prosperity, vitality and creativity seem to exist in spite of government rather than because of it.

II

THE LAND

~~~~~~~~~~~~~~~~~~~~~~~

DIALECTS AND REGIONALISM

If you compare Italy's shape to that of a man, it seems a monster with an
oblong, oval head, no neck or arms, a small tail, and dwarf's legs. In
relation to other countries on the Mediterranean, it appears to be falling
slightly forward – as if about to kick a football which is Sicily. Another
football, Sardinia, lies further in front.

In Rome you can buy a series of maps called Bella Italia, which
represent the country with an exaggerated high relief of mountains: the
rocky, snow-powdered northern Alps form the hair and the top of the
cranium, those fringing France are the front of the face (see pp. vi-vii).

Below, there is a continuation of the Apennines which form the
backbone and ribs, with a fringe of narrow plain along the coast and
little, flat patches, like those near Rieti, or the Fucino, between the
central bones. Four-fifths of the country is mountains or hills. They go
through the front leg, Calabria, and rise up too in Sicily and Sardinia.
Only in the rear leg, Puglia, do they disappear to be replaced by a
stretch of plain which starts down from above the tail, the Gargano.

Contrary to popular belief, Italy has one of the most varied and
extreme climates of Europe. In winter Venice is colder than London,
and Turin than Copenhagen. Manchester has a milder climate than
Milan, and you can ski in September in several parts of Italy. The
plateau of the Sila in Calabria is on the same latitude as Ankara, Madrid
and New York, and is as cold in winter. In 1980, villagers there were
isolated by snowdrifts twenty feet deep, and had to be rescued by
helicopter; while Etna in Sicily is covered much of the year by snow.

The north is more foggy than London, or southern England. Once,
approaching Turin by air, I noticed a cloud squatting strangely on the

surface of the sunlit plain. It mystified me until we actually entered it and I discovered it was Turin! This was a consequence of industrial pollution, but I remember a friend describing what it was like to live in Modena, one of the most beautiful market towns in Emilia Romagna. "In October," he said, "the fog from the river may well envelop us and stay without pause till spring. If you go out, you can hardly see your hand if you stretch out your arm!'

We drove down the Aosta valley.

At Courmayeur, large, thick slates lay haphazardly on the roofs, and on either side of the valley great escarpments of rock were visible between the shrubs and small bushes.

At the tourist office in Aosta I talked with Dr Boglione, who told me that the town had been built by the Romans as a fort. They then extended it into a town which was half the size of the square mile of the city of Londinium, and called it after Augustus – from which the present name derives. Known as the Rome of the Alps, it still has the massive gate of the Praetorians, the remains of the theatre, and an arch with Corinthian pillars and a sloping tiled roof.

At our first lunch in Italy, a couple at the next table were speaking dialect, as were most people in the restaurant. Some say Aostan originates with the Salassians, the tribe which was here before the Romans. However it seems very close to French, at least in its written form. Most Italian dialects derive in fact from Latin, so, when written, many words are close to Italian or French – or for that matter, Spanish.

It is estimated that only 2 per cent of Italians are unable to speak a dialect. There are regional but no class overtones in speech and the royal family found it more natural to speak Piedmontese than Italian among themselves. During the First World War, and to a certain extent during the Second, operations were impeded because so many in the army could only speak dialect and therefore often could not understand each other. Indeed, there are great differences in the spoken forms: when a Sicilian I know came to London for the first time, someone from Lombardy introduced him to a friend and when they started speaking in northern dialect, the Sicilian thought they were talking English – so alien was their speech! Goldoni wrote in Venetian, and his little-known play *Tasso* was written in Italian only in response to jibes that he was incapable of doing it.

Italian originated as the language of Tuscany. "Tuscans polish the air around them!" is an Italian saying. It was Dante, Petrarch and Boccaccio who made their form of speech more widespread than any other in Italy – although the Florentines are one of the few peoples who speak Italian with a marked difference noticeable even to foreigners: they pronounce "c" like the "ch" in the Scottish word "loch".

It was not only lack of political unity but also the fact that Italy is a long, narrow country, with many dividing mountains and valleys that slowed the development of a national language. Yet even in the flat northern plain of the Po the Lombard dialect is different from Piedmontese, with more German words – presumably because of the Austrian occupation from 1713 to 1861. Venetian, again, is different, with a number of Spanish and Portuguese words probably originating in the fact that all three countries were great seafaring powers at the same time. Indeed, the abbreviation "Ca" in street names emphasizes from all corners of Venice the link with the Spanish word "calle".

When written, though, these dialects can probably be understood by anyone who knows Italian, as can be seen from the following recipe:

In Lombard dialect—"Se preparem di frittadinn (voe unna per personna) che sien bej moresim e suttil e se fan frigg in l'oli."
In Italian—"Prepara tante frittatine (una a persona) che sono morbide e sottili e si fan friggere nel olio."
In English—"Prepare a number of fritters (one per person) which are soft and delicate, and fry them in oil."

South of Rome, the basis of dialect was influenced by Greek as well as Latin. It is often not realized how southern Italy was virtually a part of Greece for hundreds of years before the Roman conquest. It was called Magna Grecia and many Greek legends actually had their setting in Italy. The entrance to Hades through which Orpheus descended to recover Eurydice was supposed to be at Lake Averna, near Naples, whose name itself derives from Neapolis, a Greek word meaning new city. Scylla, who snatched six men from Ulysses's ship, dwelt on the Italian side of the straits of Messina and Charybdis on the Sicilian side. Archimedes, who ran naked through the streets shouting "Eureka" because he had discovered the principle of the displacement of water in his bath, was born and died in Syracuse, in Sicily. Aeschylus, the playwright, was killed in Gela – also in Sicily – by an eagle who tried to break a tortoise's shell by dropping it on his bald head, mistaking it for a rock.

Some of the most splendid remains of Greek temples in the Mediterranean are in southern Italy: at Paestum, near Salerno; at Agrigento, Syracuse and Segesta, in Sicily. Many place names are of Greek origin, including Gallipoli in southern Puglia. In Bova, a village in the Aspromonte mountains behind Reggio Calabria, the inhabitants speak a dialect based directly on ancient Greek. It is probable that during the five hundred years of Roman rule the official language was Latin and the local tongue was Greek. Linguistic reinforcement came after the fall of Rome, as the Greek Empire of Byzantium then ruled over parts of the south for centuries.

Even in the relatively small island of Sardinia there are at least four separate dialects, influenced by the Byzantines, Arabs, and Spanish. The main language, Sardo, seems to have one of the strongest links with Latin, which indicates how some of the inhabitants of that mountainous region managed to keep themselves separate from the influence of invaders, in the same way as the Rumanians, who still speak a Latin tongue. Thus, in Sardo "door" is "yanna", which presumably derives from the Roman god Janus, "ampula" is a jar, and "mesa", from Spanish or Latin, is a table – though where "pizzino", a boy, "tuntono", a mushroom, or "aidare", to speak, come from is another matter.

Refugees have also played a part in forming dialects: in southern Italy, there are twenty-six Albanian villages which originate from Mehemet II's invasion of Albania after he had taken Constantinople in 1453. In Frossimonte in Calabria, we met the owner of a hotel who spoke Albanian with his family. With modern Albanians, though, he found it impossible to communicate as four hundred years of separate development is a long time, and there are different dialects in Albania itself. He also told us with pride that his ancestors had emigrated when their great chieftain Skanderberg had died, after keeping the Turks at bay. In fact, on the label of the *amaro** he made was a face with a horned helmet which represented Skanderberg. One of this chieftain's strategies had been to cut off the heads of cattle, and nail them to palisades round Albanian strongholds. The Turks had presumed the forts were full of soldiers and had retired.

The whole of Italy, then, is still criss-crossed with different dialects, descending from Latin or Greek, and influenced by the languages of various invaders. The fact that until just after the war schooling was not compulsory added to the effect of geographical and historical divisions. Even today you find people, particularly the middle-aged and elderly living in small villages, who speak very little or no Italian: in cosmopolitan Ischia I met a lady who owned a restaurant and spoke only dialect and German – as the latter is the language of most tourists on the island; in Catania, Mario Ferrini, the well-known owner and manager of the television station, Telesud, speaks only Sicilian.

* A digestive liqueur made with herbs.

An interesting example of what escape from the world of dialect can mean was the film *Padre Padrone*, directed by the Taviani brothers. Set in Sardinia, it is based on a near-autobiographical book by Gavino Ledda and is about Ledda's childhood as a shepherd boy some time after the war. Because he is taken away from school at the age of nine by his father, he is unable to read, write, or speak Italian when he is twenty.

He goes into the army, which forbids recruits to use dialects. Gradually, he is taught Italian by a fellow soldier. This opens the outside world to him. The same soldier also teaches him Latin which they practise together as they charge about the countryside in a tank. He has the chance of being a radio mechanic, of going to university. He still expresses his conflicts with his obdurate and narrow-minded father in dialect, but if he wants to prepare himself for anything outside agriculture or the limits of his village, Italian is essential. In the end, he writes his book in the Italian he has learnt – not in Sardo.

In the last thirty years, many Italians have gone through the same sort of experience – if not so extreme – as Ledda. Television is another unifying factor. Inevitably, there is an increase of Italian in the home. The result is that dialect is used in a more limited way.

How long, though, will these linguistic divisions last? My guess is that dialects will disappear as those who are now under twenty grow old. So often you ask young people if they speak dialect and they answer, "A little at home, but my parents speak it well!" Perhaps it will take some fifty years, although this again depends on how Italy as a nation grows politically and economically.

Dialect is, of course, related to one of the most important issues in Italy: that of regionalism. Given the attempt by Piedmont to unify so many diverse areas with a different history and background, a federal structure would probably have been ideal from the start – as it almost certainly was for Germany, also in 1870, for the United States in 1783, and for Switzerland in 1848. However, traditionally the heroes of Europe are those responsible for unification, from Augustus in Roman days, to Russia's Peter the Great, to Napoleon. Unfortunately, the answer to divisions has usually been subjugation, rather than delegation.

Initially, the new government of united Italy did recognize the need for a degree of regional independence. Vittorio Emmanuel's first proclamation, now inscribed on stone in the Museum of the Risorgimento in Turin, at least expresses the intention. But the influence of the French, the great exponents of unification, was too strong, and the first administrative patterns were modelled on theirs. Prefects took the place of dukes and viceroys. Bureaucracy was centralized. This, naturally, was continued by Mussolini and only changed after the war when a Sicilian movement for independence and a turbulent German majority in what was once the South Tyrol made some sort of delegation of authority advisable. Another region, with the long name of Friuli-Venezia-Giulia, was also included in 1963, partly because of the existence of a large minority of Slovenes.

Aosta, on account of its French links, and Sardinia and Sicily, largely because of their separation as islands, were added to those regions which now have considerable control of their internal affairs. Because they are all different and not equally prosperous, the degree of delegation is not identical. Thus Sicily can legislate for its own education, agriculture and industry, while Sardinia cannot. Although rule is by an executive, chosen by the regional assembly, which in turn elects a president, every law passed has to be examined by the Supreme Court to ensure that it conforms to the law and constitution of Italy. In practice, this usually takes months – if not years.

Not till 1970 was a slightly more limited independence agreed for the other fifteen regions. This delay was mainly due to the fear of the Christian Democrats that the Left would dominate in regional parliaments. In the end, full transfer was only completed in 1977. Increased responsibility now includes tourism, encouragement of industry, agriculture and crafts, the building of *case popolari* (the Italian equivalent of council housing), transport outside the towns and the running of the hospital system. However, police and Carabinieri are still responsible to central government and there is a lot of duplication with the Commune, the equivalent of the borough, and with the province, which still has not been abolished – although its main responsibility is limited to roads. It was hoped at the beginning that the establishment of regions would mean fewer bureaucrats in government. In fact it merely duplicated many of them.

Furthermore, government financial control negates true delegation or independence. In 1982, only 6 per cent of regional expenditure came from the regions themselves. In Perugia, a councillor gave me an illustration of this: the government imposed a sum of 27,000 lire as a road tax, and to this the region was permitted to add a mere 2,000.

Government financing is, though, in the interests of the Southern regions who – so a Councillor in Basilicata told me – are terrified that the government may ultimately expect them to depend on their own resources and taxes instead of giving them lavish subsidies. The North, for the same reason, would like to see central government leaving more of the financing to the regions. After all, they have to bear most of the burden of subsidizing the South: they are the richest part of the country, as the following table of expenditure on consumption related to population, in 1982, shows:

North		South	
Piedmont	12.33	Sardinia	8.08
Lombardy	11.88	Apulia	7.73
Tuscany	11.55	Sicily	7.60
Lazio	11.30	Basilicata	6.65
Veneto	10.15	Calabria	6.63

At present, the organization creaks. In order to make it smoother, Spadolini, the Prime Minister from June 1981 till November 1982, had regular meetings in Rome with the presidents of regions, but these were discontinued when his government fell. However, at the other end of the scale, it is an advantage for people to have an authority nearby which they can appeal to. A diplomat who comes from Siena told me that, initially, the Sienese were reluctant to agree to the new regions because Florence, which historically had always been a rival, was chosen as the regional capital. However, this has been compensated by the fact that they now get quicker answers to queries and appeals, whereas previously Rome had always been a remote and silent centre. Also, governments now consist of people they might know locally, rather than distant politicians.

The regions formed after the war were created as a precaution against separatism. Yet in the European election of June 1984 the Sardinian Action Party, whose policy is independence, tripled the number of its votes from 3.3 to 9.5 per cent. This may seem a negligible proportion but there are so many active political parties that even the slightest increase is significant. In this case it illustrates the failure of industrialism in Sardinia in the last twenty years and the sense of neglect and inefficiency on the part of Rome.

In the north-east, in Trentino-Alto-Adige, things are more complicated. The southern province is predominantly Italian, while the northern one is mainly German. In the local administrative elections in November 1983, there was an absolute majority in the northern province of 59.5 per cent for the PPST, the pro-Austrian party – as opposed to 33.7 per cent in the region as a whole. Thus, it is the actual composition of the region which hinders the move to independence.

In fact, the Italian government has done everything it could for Trentino-Alto-Adige, with large subsidies and grants, and it is now one of the wealthiest regions in Italy. One politically minded Italian friend told me that it was about time the British found the same solution for Northern Ireland! However, both Sardinia and Trentino-Alto-Adige are examples of the way links are loosened when the country as a whole begins to falter in its economic and political development.

However, if the old, centralized government still existed, these separatist movements would be even stronger. Regional feeling and force are, after all, in the Italian historical tradition. They still express themselves in surprising ways. John Julius Norwich, chairman of the Save Venice Fund, told me that finance for preserving Venice was held up in the Italian Parliament because many Deputies asked themselves why they should provide money for what, after all, was the capital of just another region. Again, just before the Rome–Liverpool match at the end of May 1984, an article in the Rome newspaper *Il Messaggero* explained to British fans that "Rome is foreign in Italy". The journalist, Fulvio Strinchelli, went on to say: "You shouldn't be surprised, therefore, dear friends who back Liverpool, if in this important match you find your team supported by a majority of Italians." Resentment against other regions and particularly against the capital is often stronger than competition with other countries. When I took Americans on tour round Europe some time ago, we were always greeted in Milan by a local guide, one of whose favourite sayings, delivered to a bus full of foreigners, was: "In Milan we work! In Rome they eat!"

In Italian, *paese* means your local village, or town. Unlike *pays*, the French equivalent, it is rarely used to describe "country" as well.

TURIN AND THE NORTH/SOUTH PROBLEM

We drove down the valley away from Aosta in the sunlight, past towns and castles squatting on rocks which almost blocked the way.

To our west was the Gran Paradiso, 12,000 feet high, centre of a national park, home of 3,500 ibexes and 6,000 chamois – not to mention marmots, blue hares, martens, and the snow vole. Surprisingly, it also shelters birds, including the alpine accentor, the wall creeper, the hazel hen, the alpine chough – as well as that bird with so many exotic, medieval associations: the ptarmigan. The birds are surprising because, normally, in the Italian countryside you wonder what is unusual, and realize suddenly that there is no bird song. Italians go for anything that moves – like cats. In fact, they are such passionate hunters that they – of all people – have killed music in their countryside. Even sparrows only exist in the cities because not even the Italians would have the temerity to shoot them in the streets.

We passed the village of Brand, which Napoleon crept through with his army at night, laying down reeds and sacking in the streets so that the rumble of his gunwheels would not penetrate to the Austrian fortress on the hillside above.

On either side, the escarpments began to lose height. Vineyards lay close to the road. Then, there was "Aosta dice arrivederci" on a sign, and we were at the beginning of the great plain with maize growing everywhere in the sunlight, and Turin and the hill behind it in the distance. Then the beginning of modern apartment blocks and the dirty fronts and stone balconies of older buildings, and, finally, the great tree-lined avenues and stone-block pavements of the city which Montesquieu once described as "the finest village in the world" – the home of the Savoy dynasty, of Cavour who, more than any other, contributed to unification, and made Turin the capital of a new Italy for a brief four years after his death.

Nietzsche finally went mad here and, according to Camilla Cederna, Turin is also supposed to be the city of black magic. With an estimated forty thousand followers, it comes second after the sixty thousand of London, which Cederna calls "the Vatican of Satanism" largely because of Aleister Crowley. Turin's four rivers form, it seems, the ideogram of Tao, and the city lies on the astrological Greenwich parallel of 43°. Also, from the great siege of 1706 and before, it is mined with a maze of tunnels – where secret rites and mystic reunions are said to be celebrated by candlelight. Indeed, for a Catholic country Italy is surprisingly given to astrology: many newspaper advertisements extol fortune tellers, who even indicate their whereabouts by way of illuminated signs in the streets.

Turin, with its eighteenth-century squares, is beautiful if the sun shines. The countryside is nearby, just across the river Po, which runs along the side rather than through the middle of the town. If you go up the great narrow tower of the Mole* by lift, you have a vivid view beyond the river, of trees, and slopes with villas, up the hill of the Magdalena. In no city I know is the division so clear. From the Mole, you can see traces of eighteenth-century planning, where parallel streets predominate. The Via Roma goes straight from the royal palace to the fan glass façade of the railway station. Half way down is the splendid Piazza San Carlo, a stately eighteenth-century square which is

---

* Built between 1863–90. The lift takes you up 275 feet.

marked at one end by two churches which denote the beginning of the section altered under Fascism: there are columns without plinth or abacus, like vertical concrete tubes; unadorned, monotonous façades, where windows seem dark, rectangular, unframed holes.

Arcades are a notable characteristic of Turin. They are even followed by interlinking streets in arches, with plants in pots above. The Via Po, also coming down from the Piazza del Castello, is lined with them, and Rousseau, in a fit of masochistic rapture, actually exposed his arse under one of them. They lead on into Piazza Vittorio Veneto, which with its massive buildings is reminiscent of those series of enormous houses you find in pictures of eighteenth-century Paris. The Piazza is supposed to be the biggest in Italy. Under its arcades are shops and cafés with chairs outside, sheltered from the drizzle. Beyond is the bridge over the river Po, with the pillared church of the Gran Madre at the end of this long vista.

Turin still has some of the trappings of the Savoy dynasty who ruled it from 1045 till 1946. Some shops continue to be "by appointment". If you go to one of the royal castles outside, the old gardener will tell you that ex-king Umberto gave him a thousand lire when he visited the house. Older ladies still remember the ex-king as a handsome young man, and there is a crusty royalist society which meets once a year for dinner.

However, it is Fiat which has really dominated Turin's life in the twentieth century. It was at Fiat that the first attempt at a Communist revolution was organized after the first war. Workers went on strike and took over the factories under the leadership of those who ultimately were to become most prominent in the movement: Gramsci, the philosopher of Italian Communism, and Togliatti, who became the first leader of the party after the second war. Since 1975, the city administration has been Communist and the region Socialist. In the '70s, Turin was prey to the Red Brigade which ordered a whole faculty out of the university and "knee-capped" the teachers. "Turin is a city of workers, employed by the biggest industry in the land," said Giorgio Fattore, the editor of the local, and national, newspaper *La Stampa*u in an interview, "not of the five hundred old ladies who meet to sigh over pastries, or the ten thousand colonels who fought at Vittorio Veneto."

In the last twenty years the city has changed radically, mainly because it doubled in size when half a million workers were imported from the South to work for Fiat. Even mealtimes have changed in conformity with Southern ways: lunch from 12.30 to 1.00 or 1.30, and dinner from 7.30 to between 8 and 9. There are now more pizzerias and

Southern restaurants – although the Piedmontese seem to think, justifiably, that theirs is still one of the best cuisines in Italy.

As an official in Fiat admitted to me, the company itself may well have caused much of the disaffection of the '70s by failing to create the substructure needed for such a massive importation of labour. There were not enough houses, hospitals or schools. Initially, many of the Southerners occupied the more derelict old houses in the centre, and washing hung out on many of the historic streets. Then the richer people, who had moved to villas outside, found it difficult to get into Turin with the increased traffic. Robberies increased. So they returned to the centre, and the Southerners moved to flats which had now been built for them in the outskirts, particularly near the factory of Mirafiori Sud, which is virtually a separate town where people talk about travelling "up to" Turin.

Racism is still rampant, as it is all over the North. Southerners are called *terroni*, which means, literally, "earth people", or peasant – in the sense we use that word in English. Shamelessly blatant jokes express the resentment:

"Someone from the North went to Washington," begins one, "and was invited to a party in honour of a man who had invented a mechanical rat."

"What's the point of this rat? I don't see it," the Northerner said to the inventor.

"Well, you see, it makes a special noise. You put it in the street. And all the rats in Washington come rushing out of the sewers, and the mechanical rat leads them to a lake, jumps in, and they all follow it and are drowned."

"Splendid!" said the Northern Italian. He paused and thought a moment. "I wonder – couldn't you invent a mechanical *terrone*?"

Another refers to Aladdin's lamp which responds to a Northerner's wish and overturns the whole of Southern Italy. Then after four days it does this again. So, all the *terroni* in the North who go back to see what has happened to their relatives get the same treatment!

One of the initial reasons for this resentment was the clash between the outlook of poor agricultural workers and the more sophisticated Northerners. When thousands of illiterate Jews emigrated to London after the pogroms in Russia in the 1880s, middle-class British Jews did everything they could for them because they felt they were the same race. In Italy, however, the South was a separate kingdom from the time of the Romans until its conquest by Piedmont in 1861. Those in the North tend to feel ashamed that Southerners, too, are now Italians: even a tolerant, gentle and broad-minded professor at Urbino university told me that when he went to work in Germany in 1964 he was ashamed of being Italian because the immigrant workers from the South seemed so uncouth – and these were the only Italians the Germans knew.

Northerners, anyway, would like to be thought close to the Europe beyond the Alps, which also is industrial and ordered: to France which has had so much influence in Piedmont, to Germany whose Austrian brethren gave them efficient administration for so long, to Switzerland to which many of those on the borders commute. There is also considerable influence from Britain and, of course, America. The Southerners, they feel, have ruined their dream of being considered as wealthy equals; without them, they would be able to hold their heads high as Italians, no longer associated with Southern casualness, crime and folklore.

Often, you will be told that Cavour never really intended the South to be part of Italy, and it was only that hothead Garibaldi who made it inevitable with his March of the Thousand. Without the South, they say, the North would be the richest country in Europe. This is probably true, although they forget that much of their industry would have collapsed without Southern workers. Now, however, with the increased use of robots and the recession, Northern firms have survived only by reducing their labour force savagely. 90 per cent of the unemployed are Southerners.

Another feeling often expressed is that the South is kept alive only by subsidies. The Cassa per il Mezzogiorno, which until it was given another name in 1984 was Europe's biggest development fund, has since 1950 spent the enormous sum of $17,400 million – much of which should be valued in pre-inflationary prices – on the 40 per cent of Italians who live in the South. In addition, fifteen to seventeen million welfare benefits and pensions, in a population of 56 million, are paid out mainly to Southerners. Then there is the Mafia, which is largely responsible for the distribution of heroin, which has ravaged the big cities of the North rather than the South. A further irritant is the fact that most government administrations and the various police forces are staffed by Southerners who traditionally prefer stable, secure jobs to the adventurous economic enterprise which is at the root of Italy's wealth.

Underlying everything, too, is probably an irritating sense of guilt: the realization that the North is twice as well off, and that it has maladministered and neglected the South since conquering it in 1861. Northerners are proud of working hard and of their success and find it difficult to understand Sicilians, particularly as they seem self-sufficient, at least psychologically, in their island. "In Sicily, everyone has his own truth," wrote Pirandello – who was himself a Sicilian. Southerners don't even seem grateful for what they have received – like the Europeans with Marshall Aid.

Most shocking to a foreigner, for whom racism is probably a dirty word, is the openness and vehemence with which these views are expressed.

In the South, of course, you find balancing attitudes similar in many ways to those of countries which have been colonized. "It is the North which has always exploited us," Southerners will say. "They've used our manpower when they needed it for their industry or their wars. Because we have little here, we invest any savings we may have in their factories. The cost of the Cassa per il Mezzogiorno often goes back to them. Northern firms get subsidies for starting in the South and then go bankrupt and re-export their machinery to the North!"

They will cite the Taranto steel works, where all the overalls used were imported from the North and paid for by subsidies which should have gone to the South. Or the firm which went down to Maratea, bringing its old machinery, and then started a new factory in the North with its government subsidies. They will tell you of the way so many firms have started up just over the line between Rome and Latina where government grants start, and where there is a concentration of industry in the middle of the countryside – although the surrounding region is wealthy enough.

Above all, they criticize the way government money has been used. "We want to start co-operatives," said Dr Eboli of the Cassa per il Mezzogiorno when I visited him in Calabria:

> But it is difficult and centralized plans from Rome are often politically motivated. The result is that aid comes in sudden "showers". Reservoirs are often created without a proper study of agricultural needs. Not enough technical training is organized in schools. In the next five years, we must devolve more to regional councils. It is the people on the spot who know best what they need.

Silvio, a lawyer from Palermo, said:

> We have had so many invaders. They left us to develop ourselves and also to embellish the island. But the worst invaders of all have been the Italians. They have made us lose our separate identity. They have destroyed the structure of our peasant society and left nothing in its place. They could easily have started useful industry here, not these "cathedrals in the desert",

these big refineries and chemical plants which hiccup at the smallest recession. No, we need manufacture linked to agriculture: preserving and canning factories, fertilizers. The autostrada is a great achievement but they have been talking for thirty years of building the bridge over the straits of Messina which could really give us the commercial link we want. After all, we are the natural outlet to Africa and the Middle East. They prefer to give us subsidies to stop us starving rather than the appropriate industries which might compete with those in the North.

Underlying everything is resentment at no longer being an independent nation. It is amazing how unpopular Garibaldi is in both North and South. Neapolitans, particularly, are nostalgic for the eighteenth century when Naples was a capital, the third largest city in Europe after Paris and Vienna. Ever since Italian unification it has declined. The Bourbons are still talked about with interest and affection. After all, their government was not much worse than what Neapolitans have had since. Did the Bourbons not develop the first railway in Italy between Naples and Portici in 1839? Did they not build one of the first steamships in the world? Were they not the first to use gas streetlighting?*

In 1984, the body of their last king, Francis II, was brought to Naples to be buried in the Church of Santa Chiara. "Viva i Borbone!" shouted the crowds gathered in the street to watch the funeral procession – although the Duke of Aosta told me that when he appeared to represent the Savoys, they also shouted in their fickle way, "Viva i Sabaudi!"

Despite the friction, though, this is a problem which really belongs to the past. Since the war, prosperity in the South has increased enormously, principally due to the money that has been pumped in from the Cassa per il Mezzogiorno – however well or badly it may have been distributed. The movement of workers to the North has produced conflict, but it has also meant that Northerners and Southerners have gradually become accustomed to living in one community, not only in Turin but also in Milan and Bologna, Rimini and the small towns of the North. As Fattore, the editor of *La Stampa*, remarked in his interview, Southerners are now being absorbed: "In the primary schools there are only Italian children!"

* In *The Last Bourbons of Naples* Harold Acton gives figures for the financial contributions of different parts of Italy to unification in 1861. The Kingdom of the Two Sicilies contributed much more than the rest of Italy put together – 443.2 millions of gold lire compared to 27 millions from Piedmont, Sardinia and Liguria, 8.1 from Lombardy, and 12.7 from Veneto.

VISUAL ITALY, ALBA, WINE

In Italy, house façades are often similar to those in France, with the iron grilles of non-existent balconies in front of windows flanked by louvred wooden shutters. In the South, there are real balconies with ironwork which is curved because built at a time when ladies wore crinolines. The predominant colour of houses is dark apricot, or rusty red, but there are great buildings of stone, often with a large gateway and a courtyard beyond.

In towns most people live in flats burrowed at all kinds of angles into vast buildings, with creaking, old, black metal lifts which, for moments, seem to have no relation with the shell around them, as they soar between widely separated landings. *Pavimento* is the Italian word for "ground" or "floor", and flats and houses are paved with bright stone or tiles or marble. Washing hangs profusely in unexpected places, under grey plastic coverings in the north to protect it from dirt. Further south, there are banners, or strips of blue and red and green and white, ranged at the windows of the courtyards. In Gubbio, in Umbria, I saw washing hanging frivolously from a window beside a church where velvet drapes were suspended solemnly to celebrate the day of Santa Rita. In Palermo, I was told that washing is often hung to display the quality of one's underwear to neighbours.

Except in medieval cities like Orvieto, streets tend to be broad and straight, part of a vista leading from one piazza to another. Lighting is usually suspended above the middle of the carriageway, so pavements, which often consist of great smooth blocks of stone, are darker. As a result, the streets at night resemble stage-sets, with the lights of shops standing out more brightly, and the streetlighting itself swaying and wavering if the wind blows. As you walk, you notice basements with men, seen through narrow panes of dirty glass, moving around a printing machine or arranging books on shelves in underground warehouses.

At ground level, you find small shallow shops, like those in the ruins of the forum in Rome, or Pompeii. There is a large, white T on a blue background over the doors of a tobacconist, where you can also buy stamps or a razor. The sign of a telephone receiver hangs over bars or restaurants. There are no public lavatories, as any bar has to give access to those in extremities. As so often in Italy, public services and private enterprise are blended. Garages and supermarkets are the only emanations of creeping sameness.

In the south, boxes full of vegetables and fruit block the pavements, and stay "open" till the small hours. Boys step nimbly through the traffic selling newspapers, or teddy bears. Shop spaces range from a cubbyhole where a car is being repaired, bulky in a narrow space, while someone probes or hammers underneath, to a paradise for children, where people sit at tables set on marble floors and eat ice cream – while pastries of every shape and sweetness are ranged, layer above layer, in big glass cases.

The bars all have bright silver-coloured steel counters. I remember suggesting to my Italian partner when we started International House in Rome that we shouldn't spend a million lire on one for our student bar. We could have a cheaper one, built of wood. "Italians won't come if you don't have a steel bar!" he insisted. Particularly in the south, bars have few chairs, and it is unusual to see women there. They are not like pubs but are designed for the man who comes in for a quick drink, or thimbleful of coffee, talks a while with friends, and departs. Scores of bottles stand on shelves behind the counter. Opposite, probably, is a glass case with ornate chocolate boxes in shiny transparent paper. Oranges may be arranged in tasteful pyramids. By a cash desk, lottery tickets are hung for sale. To avoid embezzlement by staff, you have to decide what you want when you enter, and pay the cashier who gives you a little piece of paper in return, which you hand to the barman.

In towns, because Italy is mountainous, you often see the blue shape of hills between buildings, or you look down on steep valleys, or broad plains, from the side of a street or piazza.

I went down by early morning bus from Turin to Alba through flat country, similar to the plain which stretches for 250 miles all the way beyond Venice, to Udine and Gorizia and the Julian Alps. A watery sun shone, and the fields stretched out endlessly on either side, ruffled with great hunks of earth. All over this plain there are rows of young poplars. In autumn their wispy lines of branch and leaf are insubstantial against the sky, as if an engraver had sketched them rapidly and, disturbed for some reason, had left them uncompleted.

Suddenly, there was an abrupt change as we drove over a ridge and down into a different countryside, an almost secret land, of hills and sharp ridges. The road descended steeply, with soft woods on one side and, on the other, straight, black sticks with hard twisted vine roots below.

All over Italy vines are grown in many different ways: in Trento, the grapes hang from triangles of wood set next to each other, like the roofs of terraced houses; in Sardinia, white sticks stand in the fields as if in a war cemetery; in Metaponte on the gulf of Taranto, there are long tunnels with the grapes forming the roof. In northern Sicily, the vines squat like little individuals in the fields, with a bunch of grapes glowing like a purple sporran against the green leaves.

In Alba, I was met by Geoffrey Anscombe, who used to be on the staff of our school in Turin and, two years previously, came to try his fortunes as an English teacher in Alba. He had come over the plain from Turin as I had, and when he breasted the ridge into this broken, varied countryside had fallen in love with it, and decided to stay there.

With Riccardo, a friend of his who worked in a bank, we wandered through the town. It was Saturday, and the main street was almost entirely occupied by a market, with shirts in plastic covers on long tables, and bags full of corks, which are one of the minor products of Alba. It was almost Easter and in the shops were chocolate hens and rabbits. A prize egg was on display in one window. It had been ordered by the choir of a local musical society and the singers were made out of sugar while the maestro beat time with a tiny baton and the organ's black and white keys were clearly delineated. Italians spend the equivalent of eighty million dollars a year on Easter confectionery, and Alba has one of the biggest chocolate factories in Europe, Ferrero.

In fact, the town has a surprising amount of industry despite its rural aspect. Miroglio is a big textile factory which produces seventy-five thousand metres a day; another factory, called endearingly Mondo Rubber, manufactures rubber paving and footballs – not to mention plastic doors. Here is also the firm which prints *Famiglia Cristiana*, the biggest Catholic weekly magazine in Italy. Most of these enterprises are outside the town. As so often in Northern Italy, you arrive at a small historical *paese* and find that, apart from its strong farming tradition, it also employs thousands of people in medium-sized firms which export all over the world.

Like Turin, Alba has doubled in size in the last twenty years, helped by the immigration of ten thousand workers from the South. Unlike Turin, the whole area which stretches down to the Alps to Cuneo is a predominantly conservative region. In Alba, there are fifteen Christian Democrats out of thirty members on the town council. Riccardo told me that there was considerable clerical influence. In the 1970s Alba voted overwhelmingly against divorce and abortion, although in neighbouring Turin the vote had been over 80 per cent in favour of the latter. The authorities had been very skilful with immigration. Instead of lumping the Southerners together, they had distributed them throughout neighbouring villages and a special bus service took them to and from work. As a result, they had been absorbed into small conservative communities. Any rallying of discontent by the Left had thus been made more difficult.

Even before industrialization, Alba was rich. Napoleon, when invited down by the Jacobin mayor in 1796, wrote to the Directory in Paris: "Alba is ours: we are in the best and most fertile region in the world." He imposed a contribution on the town of 123,000 lire, and when two councillors came to complain that it was an enormous sum, he gave a short answer: one of them was shot!

Another irruption occurred during the German occupation towards the end of the Second World War, when Alba declared itself an independent republic for twenty-two days. When we went to meet the mayor, he showed us the Hall of the Resistance in the town hall, with photographs of partisans tramping along dusty roads, and the "government" of this new republic smiling and waving on the balcony outside. The Germans had returned, but resistance had continued nearby in a place called La Morra, a town with a castle on top of a hill, a few kilometres away. From there, it is possible to appreciate the slopes and valleys of this countryside – different from Tuscany because the hills are less rolling, broken by definite lines, with no cypresses and olive trees. The Alps are a snowy fringe in the distance, and this is more a landscape of their foothills, with green grass and woods, while the earth itself is lighter in colour than in central Italy.

In the main street we came across photographs in a shop window. There was one of the black, parallel lines of vine sticks under the snow; another of a landscape of valleys, with the towers of churches and of some of the twenty castles in the region, protruding from swathes of mist; another of Alba itself, nestling in the valley of the river Tanaro, with a few of the remaining medieval towers, of which there were originally a hundred. These the nobles built in many Italian towns, including San Gimignano, Bologna and Viterbo, partly to show their wealth and partly to keep a watch on each other. They also indicated the division of even small communities into the tribal fortresses of the many Montagues and Capulets who must then have existed. Although few towers remain, this tendency still has its traces in the family-centred society of Italy today.

Other photographs showed men in medieval costume, holding up red and white flags during the "Palio", which originated in a celebration of one of the many wars which took place between Alba and the neighbouring town of Asti. In 1250, said Riccardo, the army of Asti, which is about twenty miles away, occupied Alba and were then driven out. Neither town has forgotten it, and when in the 1930s Alba asked if they could take part in Asti's Palio, it was agreed. However, when the people of Alba arrived, they were abruptly forbidden to participate. Now, therefore, Alba have a mocking representation, during their own festa, of the Palio of Asti with mules instead of horses!

It is amazing how the feuds continue, expressing themselves in dramatic and picturesque forms. They occur also in other Mediterranean countries. Pitt Rivers in his *People of the Sierra* gives many examples of the mocking hostility between one village and another near Ronda in southern Spain. In Spain, however, enactments of war are more likely to be between Christian and Moor. Italy in the Middle Ages was divided into innumerable city states, and there is still a lot of nostalgia as well as loyalty to these independent communes. Previous battles with those of another locality will therefore be known in detail by everyone and will be celebrated dramatically on the exact date of the event, or be incorporated into the local saint's day.

Yet another photograph showed a man hurling "an electric ball" in a game which is still played in the streets and in a local arena, and seems to be similar to the Basque *pelota*. Another depicted a man sitting in front of dishes full of what looked like large potatoes, and being handed a medal. He had, explained Riccardo, won a prize at the festa of truffles, held in October. Alba is famous all over Italy for these mysterious fungi, which the early Romans believed were caused by thunder. They are so expensive that they are usually scraped onto food to give it flavouring, or eaten in thin slices. The reason for this is that they are very difficult to find, although they usually grow near oaks and are sometimes indicated by groups of yellow flies. A man will go out with a dog one night, and visit a place where, last year, he found a truffle. He can't actually mark these places because others might discover them. He must remember them. If he is lucky, his dog smells the truffle out, and he starts digging. This is usually done at night when the dog is less likely to be distracted.

Generally, Italians are experts at finding and using a large variety of mushrooms. In towns all over the north, there will be notices pinned to trees or outside town halls, with illustrated lists of mushrooms which are edible and toadstools which are not. This is in strong contrast to Britain, where truffles used to be dug on the South Downs but no longer are. An Italian in Britain told me that in the countryside he found a lot of mushrooms which were used for cooking in Italy but which were left unpicked in England. Particularly well known in Italy are the *porcini* which are used in dishes all over the north.

Alba is also well known for some of the best red wine in Italy: Barolo, Barbera, Dolcetto and Barbaresco. All except Barbera come from the Nebbiolo grape. Barolo is one of the great wines of Italy and needs decanting hours before drinking. There are a number of other excellent wines: from near Venice, Soave, Valpolicella and Bardolino, which was described by an Italian, Zeffiro Bocci, as "wine of friendship and young, sweet, carefree love"; from Emilia Romagna, dry Lambrusco, rather than the sweet fizz which local inhabitants themselves call Lambruscola; from Tuscany, Chianti, Nobile di Montepulciano, and what has often been termed the greatest of all, Brunello di Montalcino; Rosso Piceno from Le Marche; Verdicchio from the Abruzzi, and many others, less known abroad, which come from the South – whether Ischia, Etna or some varieties of Corvo from Sicily.

Local wine, also, is usually excellent. If you ask for it anywhere in restaurants there is usually little to complain of. An Irishman I know who has a small vineyard near Siena produces the most excellent wine, as does an Italian from Naples who has a small vineyard amidst lemons on terraces near Salerno. In Molise, which has only recently produced wine in labelled bottles, there are 34,800 vineyards and 53,000 farms, according to Burt Anderson. In my experience, only sometimes in Rome do you get served with vinegary mediocre wine, as an expression perhaps of weariness induced by so many tourists.

All told, Italy is the biggest wine producer with, in 1982, more than seventy million hectolitres – about one fifth of the world's total. It also produces more types: Burt Anderson, in his classic *Vino*, refers to a list made by Gianni Bonacina of 3,811 individual wines. As a basis, Italy produced no less than twelve million tons of grapes in 1982, of which about 85 per cent was used to make wine. Apulia is the biggest producer, followed by Sicily. Much of this is exported either as table grapes, or simply to fortify French and German wines.

What is interesting, though, is that individual Italian wines are little known abroad, compared to French. In London, I asked the owner of a wine shop why he stocked so little Italian wine, and he said that ten years ago it was so bad that he stopped ordering much, and had never resumed. For most English people, Italian wine is Chianti, although the straw round the bottles which used to make it distinctive is often now replaced by plastic. For the Americans, it is also Lambrusco. However, the small bottles of wine you get on airlines or at self-service restaurants are still almost invariably French.

One obvious reason is the English habit of drinking claret and burgundy, formed over centuries, dating back perhaps to the Hundred

Years' War and the English occupation of Bordeaux and Aquitaine, which lasted 299 years. Another is the very real difficulty of pronouncing the names of many Italian wines. There is, for instance, a good, light, red wine called Cacc'e Mitte di Lucera from Puglia. Cyril Ray in his *The New Book of Italian Wines* says that this means "taking out and putting in" in dialect, referring to the way the wine is made. Imagine going to the local liquor store and asking for it, or seeing it in a Safeway advertisement!

Another reason used to be that given by Amerine and Singleton in *Wine: an Introduction for Americans*, published in 1965:

> Thus, in summary, the wines of Italy are made from small vineyard holdings in mountainous areas on promiscuous culture, and the many untrained winemakers use rather primitive techniques. The wines do not enjoy sufficient distribution among critical consumers either inside or outside italy to force an improvement of the quality. The average Italian consumer is not critical of the quality of his wines.

In Alba, we visited Gigi Rosso in a one-storey, modern winery with leaded windows and vast bottling rooms inside. To him, the comparison between Italian and French wines is invalid. Of course, there are various French grapes which have been imported into Italy: the Cabernet grape, which is used in Bordeaux wine as well as in north-east Italy, or Merlot, the grape which provides the basis of excellent wine in the same region, yet which originated in France and gives softness and delicacy to clarets such as St Emilion and Pomerol. However, the land and climatic conditions are quite different in the two countries. Anyway, you can't compare a Barolo to a Burgundy, said Rosso, "they are different personalities".

The real reason why the great Italian wines seem relatively unknown, according to Rosso, goes back to *mezzadria*, or share-cropping. Under this system, which gave 50 per cent of the crop to the tenants, and 50 per cent to the owners, vineyards tended to belong to town dwellers, and not to those who worked them. Thus, a lawyer might save money and decide that he would like to buy a place in the country. So, he would call on the priest who, more than anyone, knew people in the locality and who would recommend a "reliable person". The lawyer would then buy some land, and make an agreement with his new tenant. Every year on November 11th, St Martin's Day, they would share out the crops.

The lawyer, probably, would not be very interested in his property, regarding it as a side issue; while the tenant, given that he was going to lose half his crop, would not be greatly involved either. There would be clashes of ownership between them. The laywer would want to come down at weekends with his family. Rosso had even seen *mezzadria* contracts which stipulated that the tenants' children were not allowed to play football in the courtyard on Sundays because this would disturb the landlord's siesta!

The result was that no one was motivated, or able, to go out and sell their wine abroad. Most parts of Italy had their own wine, anyway. It was therefore enough to produce what could be consumed locally.

In the last few years, however, everything has changed. *Mezzadria* has been abolished and the government has given credit to tenants to buy their land at an interest of only 3 per cent. There are new technical inventions and improvements, although complete mechanization is difficult because bad wine is produced if leaves and branches are also sucked into harvesters. Nevertheless, the local production of grapes has increased by five times in twenty years. Before the last war, Rosso's firm employed one man for two hectares, whereas he can now look after ten hectares. Everyone now takes wine-making more seriously. In Alba, there is a special college where students are taught the wine trade, professionally.

Another development is the drawing up of categories for good wines, similar to the Appellation Controlée in France. In Italy, it is called Denominazione di Origine Controllata, or DOC – usually pronounced simply "dock". Above this, there is a category of "super wines": DOCG, the added G representing "Garantita".

DOC was first granted in May 1966, and by 1981 it included 201 wines, which represented between 12 and 15 per cent of the known total of major vintages. The first DOCGs have already been granted, but they become official only in 1985. They include Barolo and Barbaresco, Nobile di Montepulciano and Brunello di Montalcino. Requirements for both are complicated: the wine must come from a definite zone and be made from grapes which have been grown in that region for at least ten years; minimum alcohol levels are set, as is a limit on the total production of each area; with blended wines, the proportion of the different grapes used is also laid down.

Cyril Ray in *The New Book of Italian Wines* comments on the bureaucracy involved where the grower must keep a record of each step in wine production, and the relevant documents must accompany the wine at every stage. He also asks how judges can assess whether the wine's description is exact when it is described with words like "delicate", "harmonious and of good body" which, by their nature, are subjective terms. He also complains that the categories exclude many good wines like Sassicaia, which at a wine-tasting organized by the magazine *Decanter* in 1978 was held unanimously to be the best out of a group of thirty Cabernet Sauvignon wines. The reason for exclusion is that this grape is not recognized in Tuscany as DOC, although it is in other regions. The same applies to another good Tuscan wine, Tignanello, which Cyril Ray describes as a "fine wine, worth ageing in a bottle". Further south, in Sicily, the well-known Corvo wines are ineligible because the grapes are from all over the island rather than from one area.

Nevertheless, the introduction of these categories has meant that Italian wine now has guarantees for the customer. It has also stimulated the growth of what are called Consorzios. In Florence, I talked to the manager of the Consorzio of Chianti Classico, which has a black cock as its symbol. This goes back to competition in the Middle Ages between Florence and Siena, when it was agreed that a horseman from each city should ride out at dawn, and the border between them would be fixed where they met. The cunning Florentines starved a black cock so that it would crow and wake their horseman at the first glimmer of dawn. As a result, they obtained more territory.

The Consorzio of Chianti Classico was one of the first, starting in 1923. It is a voluntary organization which covers about a third of the wine-making in the region and controls the quality of 1,000 associates' wine. Grapes are bought from small vineyards, and profits paid back in proportion, while the EEC helps pay for distillation. The great advantage, too, is that the Consorzio can disseminate know-how and organize exports on a scale that owners of small vineyards cannot undertake.

One afternoon we drove out to one of these associates, Sergio Manetti, who lives nearer to Siena than to Florence, in a house on top of a hill incorporating a tower dating from 1000 AD and an Etruscan arch. The slopes of the hill are covered with vines, and near the house is the vinery, where new, red wine was gurgling up and down tubes connected to a large vat.

In 1982, Manetti and his German partner won a Consorzio's gold medal for their red Monte Vertine wine. They also produce a white wine, another red, and Grappa – a highly intoxicating, almost transparent, spirit which is more popular in Italy than brandy.

Manetti bought the vineyard in 1963, just at a time when emigration from the land to the industrial North was reaching a peak, which meant that vineyards were absurdly cheap. He himself was part of a reverse process, as he escaped from a job in industry in an attempt to find a less frenzied life style.

He told me he had never regretted his decision, although the amount of work needed was phenomenal at all times of the year. The Consorzio itself was a great help. "I've just sent off some bottles to a wine tasting in London," he said. "This I would never have done if I was on my own. The Consorzio is organizing it and paying for everything – except for a contribution of 50,000 lire [about $20] payable by each participant."

And what of the future? "Good," he said, "at least for Chianti, although there is an immense surplus of wine in Europe. I was reading only the other day that the Italians themselves are drinking less wine. Believe it or not, beer drinking, here, increased by 14 per cent last year!"

Back in Alba, Gigi Rosso also talked about the future. His firm was a bigger enterprise than Manetti's, with thirty men working for him in addition to help from his wife and sons. He, too, worked incredibly hard, including Saturdays and Sundays. "We're all such individualists," he said, "and if we've built up something, we never like to let it slide. Even the variety of names in the wine trade is part of this individualism. Look at the situation here: the Marchioness of Barolo has her own wine, which is made from Nebbiolo grapes. So is Professor Cavazza's on the other side of Alba, but he calls it Barbaresco. Another owner names the same kind of wine Nebbiolo di Alba. And another, with the same grape again, calls it Roero. Now, though, the younger people who haven't had to fight so hard are less competitive, and are beginning to form co-operatives. My sons are much more in favour of this than I am. Young people don't want to work so hard these days; they like to enjoy themselves more!"

Certainly, the general effect of hard work and of changes in organization has been to improve Italian wine and make it more marketable. Burt Anderson, speaking at the Italian Wine Centre in London in January 1983, said that Italian wine production had gone "from the verge of disgrace to world-wide respectability" in the previous fifteen years. He also said that Italy now has twice as many oenologists (wine technicians) as any other nation, including France. He summed it up by stating: "I would not hesitate to describe the rapid revolution in technique, concept and legislation as the most extensive overhaul of any nation's wine industry in history." No less than 60 per cent of American wine imports is now Italian, while wine exports represent almost a third of Italian production.

We said goodbye to Rosso and went off to lunch in the Castle

Grinzane, which once belonged to Cavour and has now been bought by the regional council as a local show place for wine and cuisine.

We started with Albese, a special local dish, consisting of raw meat, flaked paper thin, with vinegar and small slices of cheese on top. With it were tiny bread rolls, with meat inside and a kind of fondu round them. Then we had tagliatelle, which is a form of flatter spaghetti. Then choices of meat with mushrooms or with wine, or asparagus with a fried egg.

With our meal we drank various wines: Barolo, Dolcetto and Barbera, brought to us in appropriate glasses. With our Barolo, we were told to hold the glass at the base so as not to heat the wine. With Barbera, though, we were given what resembles a brandy glass and held it under the cup to warm it with the hand.

We finished with Tume, a creamy goat-milk cheese which, if kept a long time, turns into a kind of strong Gorgonzola. Then, a variety of sweetmeats and a tiny black coffee.

As with most things in Italy, it is in the *paese* and the family that pride and the search for perfection lie.

NORTHERN TOWNS, COOKING, AGRICULTURE

If you fly high up over the great plain in the evening, it is peppered with the lights of small towns and villages, so you feel there must be very little countryside left.

There are three lines of major towns, with Milan in the centre of everything, which perhaps explains why its original settlement was made there, as it has no river, no hill to crouch on.

To the north, you have the towns fringing the Alps: Varese, one of the richest in Italy, and a morning's walk from Lago Maggiore; Como at the southern end of its lake where, surrounded on either side by high, steep hills, sunrise is much later and sunset much earlier; Bergamo, with a lower and an upper level: a modern one on the plain and an older one in the foothills above, with palaces decorated with the Lion of St Mark – it belonged to Venice for 350 years.

Then, Brescia, the heart of the private steel and small-arms industry; Verona, with the remains of an amphitheatre which was one of the largest in the Roman world and was admired by Goethe. Close by, to the north-west, is another lake, Garda, which cuts deeply into the Alps. It, too, has high, fringing hills, particularly on the western side. As a result, from Riva at the top of the lake, an old, illuminated Venetian fort seems a space machine suspended in the night, and the headlights of cars are like moving stars as they turn and twist along invisible mountain roads.

Then, beyond Verona, is Vicenza, birth place of Palladio, the sixteenth-century architect, whose domes and columns embellish the city. Further on, you are in the Veneto, with towns like Feltre and Belluno, up in the foothills of the Alps.

From this fringe of lakes and mountains, rivers flow down across the plain into the river Po, which is 420 miles long if all its windings are included. From Lago Maggiore flows the Ticino; from Como, the Adde; from Lake Garda, the Mincio.

The line of towns along the Po includes Piacenza, with its famous equestrian statues of two rulers, the Farnese, posed in front of the thirteenth-century town hall. Then Cremona, a beautiful, clean, almost Austrian town. Here, Stradivarius worked at the turn of the eighteenth century, and there are still sixty workshops where seven hundred violins are made a year. However, Stradivarius's house and the church of Santa Domenica where he died were destroyed in 1935, and no one knows where his bones are.

Further, on the same latitude, is Mantua, Virgil's dreamy city, surrounded on three sides by a lake formed by the river Mincio. From the other side of the causeway you see it almost as an island, with its towers and the mass of the Palazzo Ducale, which has 450 rooms and fifteen courtyards. It seems extraordinary that such a small city could have a palace as large and as splendid as Fontainebleau until you realize that this is one of the richest plains in the world with several harvests a year.

War swept this whole area from just after the French Revolution. First, Napoleon's battles: Lodi, the bridge at Arcoli, Marengo where he was almost vanquished by an Austrian general of eighty-four. Then, the clashes of the Risorgimento: Novara and Custoza where the Piedmontese were defeated; Magenta and Solferino where, with the French on their side, they were victorious. Then, further east, the endless advances and retreats of the First World War on the river Isonzo just beyond Venice. And, finally, the German occupation which lasted right to the end of the war in Italy on April 25th 1945.

South, there is the Apenpine range with great forests of chestnut, oak and beech and good pasture on the upper slopes. Skirting them is the third line of notable towns: Parma, one of the most peaceable in Italy which the Red Brigade left untouched, and which *Le Monde* recently denoted as first in Italy in prosperity and quality of life. Indeed, all along this line, each town lays claim to being one of the richest in Italy.

Reggio Emilia is the first city of Italy for ballet, where, according to Camilla Cederna, "dance schools grow up like mushrooms". Yet 10 per cent of all the pigs in Italy are produced here, with 1,500 sows giving birth to 20,000 piglets a year. The methane from their excrement produces enough electricity to illuminate a whole quarter of the city.

Modena and Bologna are also part of pig country, which has had a great influence on the cooking, supposed to be among the best in Italy and including the famous sweet *prosciutto* of Parma and San Daniele, *zampone* (pigs' trotters) and *culatello*, from the softest part of the pig's posterior. Bologna itself is said to be the capital of gastronomy: Bologna *la grassa* it is called.

I remember asking a Senator what Italians like to spend their money on. He thought for a moment and then said, "Food." They spend as much as 38.8 per cent of income on food, of which only about 4 per cent goes on restaurant meals. Italians are therefore not only considerable consumers, but also practising cooks – both men and women.

Can it be said, though, that there is a national style of cooking? Yes – but mainly because different local styles have overflowed into neighbouring provinces. There is, in common, the tendency to use the herbs of the region and often to spice food – although this rarely goes to extremes.

There is also the use of pasta from one end of the peninsula to the other. In factories in Naples, three hundred different types are created. There is not only *spaghetti* but also *tagliatelle* which is flatter, *rigatone* which in cross-section is rectangular instead of round, and even a shape like little ears, *orecchiette*. Then there are variations of *lasagne* – pasta cooked in slices. There is the "container" type of pasta, where meat is enclosed, in *ravioli* in little cushions, or in *cannelloni* in tubes. Then there are different colours: white is natural for the hard durum wheat used, but pasta can also be green if spinach is added and reddish when tomato is included.

There is also the flavouring: *spaghetti* with mushrooms or shellfish; *carbonara* which, it is said, American troops invented during the war by adding their rations of bacon and dried egg. Then the sauces: *bolognese*, which is tomato, garlic and some minced beef; *pesto*, which originates from the Ligurian coast near Genoa and consists of chopped basil, olive oil, garlic and parmesan cheese; *napoletano*, which is tomato, garlic and olives; and, most spicy, *all'arrabbiata*, literally "furious", which consists of tomato, garlic and as many chillies as are thought advisable.

When you actually multiply the three hundred forms of pasta with the available colours and different sauces, you probably have more than three thousand possible variations. So, although pasta may be a national dish, it can certainly be eaten in a diverse way all over Italy, and many of the forms are regional.

Another national similarity is the staging of the meal: first, antipasto, which may be a kind of hors d'oeuvre, probably consisting mainly of cold meat and, on the coast, including cold fish but with anything native to the region added on. Then pasta. Then fish or meat, and what are called *contorno* (vegetables), usually served on a separate plate but not as invariably as in France. Then a dessert which may be fruit or some of that delicious cake (which seems in the North to be an inheritance of Austrian rule) or some form of ice cream, which was brought to Sicily by the Arabs and refined by using the snow on Mount Etna. Cheese may or may not be included, although it tends to be regarded more as something to be used in cooking.

This is often followed by coffee, and a liqueur, which may be an *amaro*, a digestive made of local herbs. To a foreigner tasting it for the first time it resembles cough mixture, although he usually gets to appreciate it in the end. Or the liqueur may be *sambuca*, which is the Italian equivalent of *ouzo*, or *rake*, or *anis* – one of those versions of aniseed which every Mediterranean country seems to have.

Nowadays lunch in towns is not as heavy as this, although even in cities working people are rarely prevented from returning for a family meal. It is surprising how well adjusted such meals are. The only "heavy" element is the pasta and that seems comfortably digestible within the hour.

As far as meat is concerned, it is surprising how many well-known dishes are made from veal, as cattle farming is not widespread in Italy, except in the North. Among these is veal dipped in egg and breadcrumbs. Or, also from Milan, *osso buco*, which consists of veal shanks, sliced with the bone marrow in the middle and stewed with vegetables, garlic, oregano and lemon juice. Or, again *saltimbocca alla Romana* which is literally "jump into the mouth". This is veal cutlet with ham, fried in butter and oil and then cooked in white wine.

One explanation I heard for the popularity of veal is that Italians now want to eat the whitest and tenderest meat they can. Those who remember the days up to twenty-five years ago, when they ate meat only once a week, wanted to compensate. So the custom began.

At the agricultural department of the University of Perugia they told me how wasteful the eating habits of Italians are in this respect: they want only the whitest and leanest meat and the rest is wasted.

With lamb it is different. Some Italians say they don't like the smell.

But it is eaten particularly in Rome and in the Abruzzi, the mountainous region to the east, and also in Sardinia where most of the cultivation of sheep takes place. The favourite time is Easter when lamb has garlic, rosemary, and ham inserted and is then soaked in lemon and white wine, and roasted as a traditional dish. The sale of very young lambs helps the dealers. In 1984, they got 5,500 lire per kilo for a forty-day-old lamb, and 3,500 lire for one of a hundred days. When the extra care and the possibility of illness and early death are included, it is worth selling the lamb very early even though there are fewer kilos on it.

I often find, particularly when eating at home with Italians, that you get some new, delicious dish which you have never tasted before. Sometimes you even feel that it has just been invented as a result of the kind of experimenting which Italians love. I remember a friend whose father, a hotel owner, died suddenly. He knew nothing of cooking, so he asked an old man who had cooked at the hotel years before to come and teach him. Among other things he learnt were twenty-seven ways of serving rice, which included mixing mushrooms, truffles, chestnuts – not to mention various kinds of shellfish.

When you add the variety of cooking along the extensive coasts of Italy you get a further dimension: prawns and shellfish, a wide variety of fish, many of them, such as the John Dory, virtually unknown in Britain; and, in Sicily, swordfish and tunny. The further south you go, the more fresh vegetables there are, particularly tomatoes, which are extensively used for Neapolitan pizzas. Fruit is phenomenal. When confronted with large juicy peaches, melons, apricots, cherries and grapes, you begin to realize what a stoical fruit the apple is. I remember in Sicily, in September, a stall by the side of the street, with hundreds of water melons, piled one on top of the other, looking like children's old beach balls, with broad swathes of faded light and dark on the rinds.

Cheeses, too, are varied and, like so much in Italy, some go back hundreds of years. Thus, Pecorino Romano is first mentioned in a work, *De Rustica*, of the first century BC, while the Grana cheeses, such as Parmigiano Reggiano and Grana Padana, are first mentioned in the twelfth century AD. Gorgonzola is said to have originated in the year 1000 when a wandering shepherd, leaving a container of milk, went to dally with his girl-friend and, on his return some time later, found the container full of a blue-veined cheese.

In the South, the best-known cheeses are Mozzarella, a sweet, rubbery cheese made originally from buffalo's milk, and Ragusano, from Sicily, whose rind is grooved because of the mark of strings when the cheeses are hung during the ripening process.

Broadly, cheeses fall into a number of categories: the flaky, hard Grana from near Parma; the creamy, fatty Fontina, originally from Aosta; and the smooth firmer cheeses like Gorgonzola, Taleggio and Provolone. However, like wine, it is possible to find a local cheese, originating often from sheep or goat milk, in most parts of Italy.

Italian cuisine is based on the healthy principle of using fresh foodstuffs: processed or tinned food is not popular. And there are the ancient traditions, coming from years of scarcity, of using whatever the countryside can offer, from herbs to mushrooms.

Underlying Italian eating and cooking habits is the pattern of agriculture.

Massimo is a teacher of mathematics at an elementary school. His home, a small farm in Umbria, is on two floors and has fifty acres, much of it forest land. On the ground floor, grapes are pressed and the juice passed into barrels to produce 600 litres of wine. There is also an oven made of iron which, when heated, remains hot for twenty hours, so you can bake bread at leisure. A dovecote, set in one of the outside walls, means that the person whose bedroom is behind wakes to the sound of cooing. Massimo also breeds pheasants and geese, chickens and turkeys, and a bantam cock which looks like an old lady scurrying along with her handbag.

The view from the terrace is over a broad valley with fields divided not by hedges but by the type of crop. Great jets of water spread over them, like plumes of smoke when the wind blows. On the slope behind there is a village with houses of rough stone and red tiled roofs. Behind, high hills with oak woods are broken by fields on which olive trees grow in ordered rows. On some fields, there are white sticks supporting vines. Much of the neighbouring land is owned by a property developer from Catania who allows it to decay. The part down the valley belongs to someone who prefers to live in a modern flat in a neighbouring town. He has a good bailiff from the village, though, who tends the crops efficiently.

Massimo has two straggles of vine in a large field. He has put his other fields down to clover because the previous owner grew wheat for nine years and the soil is exhausted. He sells the grass and clover to a neighbour who comes and mows it several times during the summer. By law, even the trees are cut in rotation, so they are all renewed over twelve years. From them Massimo gets enough logs to heat the house throughout the winter, to bake bread and to cook. He is helped and advised by an old man whose family tease him because he is teaching a *professore*!

Massimo's farm was designed to make the family which once owned it self-sufficient. Now, it is typical of those farms, particularly in the hills, whose owner is part-time. The developer from Catania is typical, in another way, of the owner who keeps his land in the hope that it will increase in value, even though he neglects it; the owner in the valley, on the other hand, is typical of those who regard land purely as a commercial investment; while the former owners of Massimo's farm sold it because they were getting old, and none of their sons wanted to take it on. They were part of the old world of peasants, scratching out a living under the *mezzadria* system (see p. 33), or as small, independent farmers.

Since the war, Italian agriculture has changed radically. Whereas in 1950 40.8 per cent of the population worked on the land, only 12.8 per cent do so today. In the South, the big estates were broken up and small farms were given to peasants, with all the modern equipment they needed. However, psychologically this didn't work – as with so much of the help then given to the South. The *contadini* were accustomed to living in big villages, even though this meant spending three hours a day "commuting" to work. They were not used to solitude, and having to make their own decisions. No sooner were these reforms under way than emigration to the booming industrial north of Europe, particularly to Germany, began. Foreign firms sent missions to South Italy to recruit workers. Even in England the brick companies in Bedford emptied two villages in South Italy, and 10 per cent of the town is now Italian. By 1983, it was calculated that there were no fewer than five million emigrants living abroad with Italian passports. Many of them left derelict land behind them.

Today, Italy is still the major producer in Europe of wine and olive oil, of hemp and oranges, of pears and peaches, sugar and tobacco. It is second to France in wheat and maize. Unfortunately, though, there has not been enough consistent planning. Thus, there was an excess production of sugar in the late 1970s. The crop was therefore reduced so much that it is now necessary to import it. Ministers of agriculture, so a director of the Banca Agricola told me, have been neither sufficiently expert nor sufficiently involved. The drain of labour from the land has continued because salaries still do not compare with those in other professions. Farming is rejected by younger people because it seems a return to the poverty and sweat of the past; while those who come back from abroad are experts in some industrial skill and prefer to use their talents there. Also, inflation has been the highest in Europe, with retail prices increasing to 513.7 in 1982 on a base of 100 in 1970, and this has affected exports.

The North, as might be expected, has benefited most from the last twenty years. The plains of Emilia Romagna and Lombardy have seen a development of agriculture similar to the wheatlands of America. Trees have been cut down, and co-operatives share modern machinery on vast areas of land. As a result, the production of corn has tripled in twenty years, with yields as high as eight or nine tons per hectare. Irrigation is more effective through the use of hoses rather than ditches.

Before the war, life in the fringing mountain areas was hard, with only a few vines and vegetables on small plots and charcoal burning as the main occupation. Now, big firms have taken this over and have turned the land into pasture, while the fruit yield has increased in the Imola hills. Also, between 1970 and 1982 the number of pigs increased by 130 per cent in Lombardy and 54.9 per cent in Emilia.

In Orvieto, in Umbria, I talked to the ex-mayor who, like most elected officials in Umbria and Tuscany, is Communist. He criticized the government for never putting in enough money, except in the South. In central Italy, large firms have taken over. There were two foreign ones down the road. No one knew anything about them. After the emigration of the '60s and '70s, people came back and returned to the land, but as workers. There were no local *padroni* any more and too much competition from those with modern machinery. Of course, the export of wine was going well, but there used to be a lot of fruit-growing, which no longer took place because the "juice-war" was too intense. Now, even tomatoes were imported.

In Rome, I heard further tales of woe. The problem is really lack of confidence and, consequently, of investment. People with money prefer to invest in government bonds which give tax-free interest above the rate of inflation. Olive oil is in crisis because the cost of labour is too high and olives are difficult to collect. The Common Market favours the North because, in the interests of Holland and Germany, it prefers to subsidize milk, meat production and wheat, rather than the fruit and vegetables produced in the South. Here, there is also mounting competition with Israel and Spain in citrus fruits. As a result, tons of lemons have to be ground over by tractors, in order to keep up prices. Soon, California too will be a competitor.

In Depresa, in Apulia, we stayed at a castle, with bougainvillea round the courtyard, belong to Barone Riccardo Winspeare. His family came to Tuscany from England in 1702, and his great-great-grandfather was the Ambassador of the Kingdom of the Two Sicilies to the Court of Turin, just before the war of 1861. He said that his family only live by selling off pieces of land as the income from them does not increase. The

EEC is reluctant to subsidize because Italy has tried too often to defraud them. However, Apulia as a whole is richer now because aqueducts have been built. Before, only olives and wine had been grown. Now, there are artichokes and flowers; carnations are being sent to England.

On our way back to Bari, we stopped beside a field which fringed the sea. Two men were using a little machine like a lawn mower. It ploughed up the land, while a bar behind created a furrow. Another man was sowing, spraying the seed from a bag he held on his arm. Like most farmers, they complained. You could only get 30,000 lire for 100 kilos of wheat. It hardly covered the expenses of labour, petrol, or the maintenance of the tractor. If it didn't rain in March or April, the crops were ruined. They didn't get any subsidies. Money went to those who had it already – not to those who didn't!

In Bari we were told by the director of tourism, who came from Tuscany, that Apulia could be like California. Its red wine could become as famous as Chianti. The trouble was that few people had the experience or expertise to export. At the Festa of the Artichoke at the town of San Fernando di Apulia, in 1983, the Under-Secretary of Agriculture, Signor Zurio, bitterly attacked the associations who received subsidies and then wasted them, did nothing, or made too many mistakes. "We need," he said, "to develop a continuing process of training and education."

In Naples, I met Dottore Roberto Pasca, who said that much agricultural planning had been distorted by interference from the political parties. Obviously, more votes could be obtained if loans and credit guarantees were made to small farmers with large families. Also, it looked better to help poorer groups although they were not as efficient. On a large scale, money spent this way brought in more political support than a long-term project like a dam. Although they had spent a lot on agriculture it had been a great mistake of government to put more money into industry which, in the South, had not been particularly successful. Now, the Italian agricultural deficit was equivalent to four billion dollars in 1982, while the industrial surplus only just balanced this at five billion.

If agricultural production were increased, he continued, this would provide more income to stimulate industry, diminish unemployment, and help the balance of payments. Although there were surpluses in wine, wheat and dairy products, there was still scope for expansion in market gardening. Meat was more difficult, as the cost of forage made it uncompetitive.

The crucial need is water. In the Metaponte, on the Gulf of Taranto, more than a hundred thousand acres have been reclaimed, and now grow oranges, grapes and market produce. In Cosenza, in Calabria, I was told that there had been a real agricultural revolution in the last twenty years. In 1954, it had been necessary to buy water at the chemists'. Because Calabria and Basilicata are mountainous, the water supply has now been harnessed.

Even now, though, a third of the water is wasted in transit and 12 per cent used for cleaning cars. Because drinking water is used for agriculture and industry, Cosenza is short in summer for some of the day. There were bad droughts all over the South in 1981 and 1982. Demand is now overtaking supply again.

Sicily has plenty of water, a few feet below the surface in the centre of the island. However, much of it is controlled and limited by vested interests, particularly the Mafia. In Erice, west of Palermo, I remember seeing, in 1983, a well-dressed man with a smart car loading up cans of water from the village pump.

In 1982, ISTAT, the government statistics office, published figures on changes in the agricultural situation since 1970. These were disappointing. Worst was the fact that cultivated land in Italy had diminished by 9.7 per cent. Much of it has been abandoned, or devoured by growing cities, new roads and factories, or by building speculators. As worrying is the fact that the average size of farms has remained almost static. This means that, although there have been more big farms in the Centre and the North, the majority are still small, without the technical resources to modernize. In comparison with the rest of the EEC, Italy still has the smallest average size: 7.5 hectares per farm, compared to 26.9 hectares in France and 64.9 in Britain.

The agricultural situation in Italy is, therefore, complicated. Wine, it has been noted, has made great strides – largely due to modernization and government control through the DOC system. However, most of the successful wine is in the Centre and North where co-operatives are numerous and the systems efficient. In the North, agriculture is almost a model, with plentiful yields of rice, wheat, fruit, pigs and cattle. In the ISTAT survey, the number of pigs has gone up by as much as 48 per cent in twelve years. As so often, the South has been left behind. Yet it is precisely in market gardening that expansion there is possible.

Italy, though, has more or less maintained her position since 1970. Yet it is because economic expansion was so rapid during the previous twenty years, from 1950, that Italians are so critical and disappointed. Now, though, they are no longer surging out from south of Eboli, beyond which, in Carlo Levi's novel of 1935, Christ didn't travel.

Fortunately, there are no longer extremes of poverty, even in Southern villages.

Italy is now a complex modern State, involved with the EEC. There is a need to balance industry and agriculture, North and South, the tension between political patronage and efficiency – without losing the impulsiveness and energy which, hitherto, have taken its people such a long way in such a short time.

FESTAS

We came to Gubbio, a medieval town of hard, grey stone, clustered within its walls, at the bottom of a high hill with the church of its patron saint, San Ubaldo, at the top. Here, Saint Francis of Assisi made friends with a ferocious wolf, and San Ubaldo became renowned because he persuaded Frederick Barbarossa to spare the town in the twelfth century.

Gubbio is in Umbria. It is just over the stretch of Apennines which divides the long, flat northern plain from the rest of Italy. To the east is the perched, independent Republic of San Marino, where whisky is £2 a bottle, and where different streets seem to specialize in either German or British visitors. As a compromise, I saw a notice there advertising a "Schwimming Pool"!

Beyond San Marino is the low strip of land running along the Adriatic coast from the holiday town of Rimini, down to Ancona and Pescara and the beginnings of the long plain of Apulia. To the south is the Abruzzi with a national park spreading over tall mountains. To the west there is a unique grouping of ancient towns: Assisi, Perugia, Spoleto and Orvieto in Umbria; and, in Tuscany: Florence, Siena, Lucca and Pisa. This is the heartland of Italy, where small towns lie on their hills, or amidst their vines and olive trees, self-sufficient in their beauty, aware that their past is their present, and that they have so many treasures that there is no reason to change or replace anything. The outside appearance of most buildings remains as it has been for hundreds of years. Inside, though, new wealth has meant alcoves becoming shower rooms, old kitchens being modernized, ancient windows equipped with double glazing, and central heating appearing along the walls. The social structure is different, also, with palaces and convents now divided skilfully into flats or art galleries.

We arrived in Gubbio, called the City of Silence, on May 15th, the day of San Ubaldo. Everything was in tumult, and the whole town seemed to be gathered together in the large Piazza della Signoria.

Although the crowd was thick, we managed to squeeze our way through. Italians don't resent you pushing gently. After all, everyone has to progress, and there is always a small space somewhere that you can fit into.

The piazza is built on arches with a forty-foot drop down to the lower town, giving a view over the countryside. On one side is the Palace of the Consuls, with its crenellated tower and tall windows. On the stone platform in front trumpeters stood in fifteenth-century dress with dignitaries and guests behind. Above, the bell tolled, moved round with regular kicks by a boy who somehow clung to the superstructure. Below, a procession consisting of the Communist mayor and town officials began to make its way through the crowd. They approached the balcony and presented the key of the town to the elected captain of the festa, as a sign that for one day authority over the town was his. Next, a cross advanced through the masses, and the bishop, accompanied by priests in white, also went up to the balcony, and blessed the key.

The trumpets blew again. Slowly, the doors of the palace opened. A great cheer went up, as the nose of the first of the Ceri appeared. These are long structures, sixteen feet long and weighing half a ton, shaped like a rocket in two stages, with a small image of the saint they represent at the top. Rapidly, the first Cero was carried through the crowd by a team of ten men. Two others followed. With them, the teams also carried wooden supporting structures which were laid on their side, in the middle of the multitude, while the Ceri were nailed to them. This done, the captain of each team threw water onto the connection, and then hurled the jug into the crowd, where it shattered. Around it, everyone scrabbled for a piece, which brings luck.

The Ceri were then pulled into a vertical position and stood, tall and sinister, like long, hard-shelled insects which had somehow infiltrated themselves into this vast, excited crowd of soft bodies. After a pause, each was lifted to the shoulders of their ten bearers, who set off at speed. Everyone gave way without panic, pulling small children to one side, as these great rocket-like objects bore down on us. Three times, the Ceri went round, and then left a furrow as they made their way out of the piazza to tour the town.

The morning's events were over, and we went to look around Gubbio. Crowds were everywhere. Medieval flags fluttered from balconies, and the bars and ceramic shops were open. Every town in Italy seems to have its own speciality, whether leather or truffles, cars or asparagus. Since medieval times, Gubbio has been well-known for *ceramica*, and one artisan, Maestro Giorgio, produced a famous iridescent red lustre, the secret of which was never discovered by neighbouring towns.

After lunch, we went to see a family which owned a butcher's shop – friends of friends. We sat round a table in their small flat and drank coffee and grappa. Some of them had come over for the festa from Tome and Perugia, where they worked. All of them preferred Gubbio to anywhere else: "But what can you do? There's not enough work!" Some of them belonged to the clan of San Giorgio and others to that of San Antonio. The Cero of San Ubaldo always wins the race in the afternoon: "But of course! After all, he is the Saint of Gubbio!" Then comes San Giorgio and then San Antonio. "But the Pope has abolished St George!" I said inadvisedly. "He has no right! We shall abolish *him*!" came the reply.

We talked about the way the festa is important to the people of Gubbio. There are records of the ceremony dating back 825 years, but a French historian, Herbert Boyer, has said it probably represented the development of a sylvan rite going back thousands of years. Cero means candle and there is another theory that it came from the custom of taking votive candles up to the church of San Ubaldo. Indeed, until the sixteenth century the shape of the Ceri was that of a candle. Of course, others say that it was a phallic rite of spring, and there is some substance in this when you consider the shape and the water spilt on the newly erected Ceri in the piazza. However, the important thing is that, rooted as it is in the history of Gubbio, it is a rally which allows everyone to express the loyalty they feel for their home town. Emigrants from Gubbio in the United States celebrate it there, and even in Somalia before the war a group of workers organized their own festa of San Ubaldo, with a Cero formed of two empty barrels which had once contained smoked herring, one on top of the other.

When I asked how religious the festa really was, Antonio, the young man working in Perugia, said that religion was undoubtedly part of it. The various clans were represented by saints and, as we would see that afternoon, the day ended in the church of San Ubaldo. However, that didn't mean that those who took part were necessarily believers. In Italy, it is difficult to make such distinctions. Gubbio, like other Umbrian and Tuscan towns, is ruled by a Communist municipality and region. But Communists celebrate as enthusiastically as anyone else. After all, he, Antonio, voted Communist, and was a devoted member of the clan of San Giorgio. It was only natural that the bishop and the Communist mayor should both take part. In fact, they got on very well together.

We went out again into the crowded streets, with people moving in all directions, greeting friends, shouting up at those in the windows of the surrounding houses. Suddenly, the Ceri were upon us once more, long, dark obelisks, moving rapidly through the crowds, like the spikey fins of fish swimming strongly below the sea of people. Three times, recently, the Ceri have fallen: San Ubaldo in 1969, San Antonio in 1971 and San Giorgio in 1982 – fortunately with little damage except to the asphalt.

We started running. The object now was to get to the church of San Ubaldo on the top of Monte Ingino, which looks down on Gubbio, 2,690 feet above sea level, before the Ceri arrived. Once away from the procession, we strode up through paved alleyways, past the massive stone sides of churches and palaces, through a gate in the walls, and started the mile-long climb to the top of the mountain. A broad dust path went straight up through the trees, and doubled back several times. At the end of each stretch were stalls where drinks and sandwiches were sold. As we climbed, the panorama of the plain, with the surrounding hills and the stone mass of Gubbio below, became more evident. Crowds wandered casually upwards, with little groups resting by the side of the path, or beginning to form fringes of spectators.

At the top, there was a café hanging over the mountain side, and steps led to the closed doors of San Ubaldo's monastery and church. In the sky, a hang glider swooped and rose, advertising cement, of all things, on its wings. Boys climbed trees which soon seemed full of chattering, as in the jungle. Below, the crowd got thicker until everyone seemed suspended only by the pressure of bodies, and a small girl was raised up, kicking petulantly.

Suddenly, the small yellow image of San Ubaldo on the top of his Cero appeared from further down the path, moving fast up to the church. Everyone cheered frenziedly, or sang. "San Ubaldo!" they shouted. Apparently, it had taken only eight minutes to get all the way up the hill, and the bearers' faces were shiny with sweat. The Cero was lowered to a horizontal position. The doors of the monastery were opened and, slowly and carefully, the Cero was borne into the courtyard beyond. At intervals of a few minutes the other Ceri arrived, first, San Giorgio and then San Antonio in the prescribed order. If either of them were too far behind, the doors could be shut by the bearers of the previous Cero, which represented defeat. As it was, they too arrived in time and were taken into the church to be fitted onto specially made stands, near the altar, where the unputrefied body of San Ubaldo lay in his glass coffin.

In the church and courtyard the spectators cheered and sang. Standing there, too, were the Ceri for the younger people. Those for the adolescents weigh 400 lbs, and the ones for the children seem like toys, weighing only a hundred pounds. These would be carried in similar processions, one the following week, and one at the beginning of June. In this way the young people of Gubbio get accustomed to the ritual, and participate in the processions at an early age.

We went out on the terrace overlooking the plain. Above us, the hang glider swooped suddenly down, diminishing against the green of the fields below, giving a final flutter as it landed. The sky began to get dark.

Below, the piazza was almost empty. Over at one side, a bare-chested fire-eater entertained a small crowd, belching out flame into the night. Coca Cola tins crunched metallically underfoot, or were kicked, clanking, down streets.

The festa was over. However, it was only the first. Next week, there would be the processions of the younger people. On the last Sunday in May and the first in September, there was to be a cross-bow contest, dating from 1461, with the team from the neighbouring town of Borgo San Sepolcro. On August 15th, there would be another contest, this time between different quarters of the town – a competition in tossing flags. Already at Easter there had been a procession of images: Christ taken from the Cross, and the Virgin Mary, accompanied by penitents in white Ku Klux Klan robes, singing thirteenth-century mourning hymns. At Christmas, lights are arranged over the whole of the façade of Monte Ingino to form a large, illuminated fir tree with a star at the top of the mountain. As has happened for hundreds of years, the quiet of medieval streets alternates with the frenzy of preparations and festas.

As we had discussed, the motivation is not purely religious. Nor is it just touristic, although money is made. Nor is it merely a competition, as in the Palio of Siena where ten horses representing ten parishes compete in a race round the splendid Piazza del Campo, and everything, from hitting a neighbouring rider to bribery, is allowed. Perhaps it is all summarized in the words of that day's newspaper, the *Corriere dell' Umbria*: "The Ceri are part of ... a tradition in which merge sacred and profane elements, which themselves constitute the indestructible roots and essence of a people."

In contrast, there are few national festivities. On September 20th 1984, the significance of the celebrations for the entrance into Rome of the Italian armies in 1870 was diluted because it was also Sophia Loren's fiftieth birthday. Indeed, the only heartfelt national celebration recently was when Italy won the World Cup in 1982: "Italian flags were hanging everywhere!" commented a friend. "We'd never seen so many and wondered where they'd all come from. Had some entrepreneurs manufactured them overnight?"

Yet every city, town and village has its festa or saint's day – even Milan and Turin. Some involve the carrying around of obelisks. In Nola, near Naples, eight of them are borne about the streets. In Viterbo, there is one ninety feet high, called the Macchina di Sant Rosa. Its design is changed every few years and it is illuminated with tiny oil lamps. In May 1984, when the Pope visited the town, it was brought out suddenly and unexpectedly: it was startling and moving to glimpse the illuminated image of Santa Rosa appearing suddenly above the roof tops, against the cloudy, night sky, just near the piazza where the Pope was talking to a massive crowd.

Many festas, like that at Gubbio, have evident pagan elements. At Cocullo, a little village in the Abruzzi mountains, there is a procession of the local saint, Dominic Abate, during which everyone carries a serpent they have collected in the neighbouring countryside. Even the statue of the saint is festooned with them. This apparently originates with the offering of serpents to the pagan goddess, Angizia. Now, though, the Church has a strong part to play. Priests bless the symbols, as they do the Ceri in Gubbio, and the tooth of St Dominic is also carried in the procession as a balance to the serpents. Some festas originate in religious stories, like the cruel one in Madonna del Arco in Campania where, in the fourteenth century, a boy flung a ball against the fresco of a madonna which started bleeding, and the boy was executed.

Local patriotism and tradition join to keep these festas alive, while the Church sanctifies them and often gives them their drama. Thus in Bari, on May 8th, pilgrims come to the town from all the neighbouring villages. Saint Nicholas is then taken out in a special boat into the sea, followed by scores of others bearing people who worship and buy a coloured reproduction of the saint.

Many festas, naturally, are associated with Easter or the day of the Magi. On the island of Procida, near Ischia, convicts from the local prison take part in a procession in which four floats, depicting some of the miracles of Christ, are borne through the streets. In Enna, in Sicily, the style is more Spanish, with penitents in hoods following floats. While in Piana degli Albanesi, near Palermo, the Easter Mass is Greek Orthodox, and boiled eggs, stained red, are distributed to children.

Some festas seem to have little religious element, and are mainly fairs. One evening in September we drove up to Arola, a little village in the hills above Sorrento. The streets and piazza were decorated with illuminated peacocks, shooting stars and sprays of flowers. In the piazza, a Neapolitan traditional dance group performed fandangos in peasant costume on a specially erected stage. Afterwards, we went to a friend's house and watched one of the most magnificent firework displays I have ever seen. Great sprays of colour came out of the sky; umbrellas of fire stood for a moment and then collapsed into kaleidoscopic rain. "It's very good this year!" said Mario, our host, "It depends on how much money the Commune has in the kitty!" It turned out that one of the biggest firework factories in Italy is in Naples. Probably some benevolent, rich man in Arola had shares.

Local pride also expresses itself in artistic festivals, particularly in Central Italy, where the very towns themselves seem to demand artistic expression. In summer, with the gentle, clear evenings and the sound of crickets coming from nearby vineyards and olive groves, they provide a perfect setting for opera and concerts. In 1984, Florence had its forty-eighth *Maggio Musicale*, or "Musical May" – to translate literally – directed by the Italian composer Berio. The range of concerts and operas is vast and they take place in superb settings: the courtyard of the Palazzo Pitti, or the Church of Santa Croce. In 1936, Alessis's opera *Savonarola* was staged in the Piazza della Signoria – the very place where the fanatical monk was burnt in 1498.

Even small towns have their artistic festas, like Montepulciano, which has only 15,000 inhabitants yet which has had international artistic workshops since 1976. In 1984 these consisted partly of courses: in mime, directed by Marcel Marceau, with others in modern dance, oboe and cello. Spectacles included Finnish dancing, performances of Giraudoux's *La Guerre de Troie n'aura pas lieu*, and a concert in which the major piece was Britten's *War Requiem*. One of the declared objects of this festival is to bring culture to the local inhabitants. None of the participants is paid, but fares and expenses are covered, and they are put up free by local families. Funds for this and for sets and direction are provided not only by local government, but also by radio and television companies who broadcast performances.

Italians seem to make none of the distinctions between poetry, theatre, music and everyday living that we do in Britain or America. "Culture" is not regarded as something pretentious or "sissy", an attitude which probably starts at school when an artificial division is often established between the "intellectual" and the games player. I was amazed to find in *Stop*, one of the popular Italian weekly magazines, which was full of articles about a Roman prince, John Travolta, astrology and television stars, that there was also a piece about Leopardi, the nineteenth-century poet, and one of his poems was printed. It was illustrated with sad portraits by Vespignani, a contemporary painter.

In Italy, foreign culture is welcomed, perhaps with excessive deference. Often, at these festas, you miss the native contribution. Italians themselves will tell you that in a small town a play by someone from another Italian region or city is as alien as the work of a Frenchman or an Englishman. Verdi, after all, comes not so much from Italy as from Parma, Rossini from Pesaro, and Puccini from Lucca.

Perhaps because Italian culture has influenced Europe from Roman days, the people of Italy feel little chauvinism about it. "Culturally, we are all Italy's children," as Peter Nichols wrote. They are, more than the people of any other country, at the root of much of our music, painting, architecture and theatre. Often they must feel they are receiving a version of what they have already sent out.

The link to Europe rather than to Italy is a real one. Apart from giving so much, they have been ruled by other Europeans for so long, and have sent millions of their citizens out all over the world. Indeed, it is interesting how often you are told in Sicily that the island should really be linked, in its own right, to the EEC rather than to Rome. Among the town treasures of Gubbio, there is nothing which can be called "Italian" rather than local. However, a Council of Europe flag, with a representation of the Palace of the Consuls, surrounded by twelve stars on a blue background, was presented to the mayor, in December 1982, by an official representative of German nationality. It has been prized ever since.

Carnival is another manifestation of local custom. The most famous are those of Viareggio, of Arcireale, near Catania in Sicily, and of Oristano, in Sardinia, which is also renowned for its extraordinary equestrian feats.

At the beginning of March 1984, we visited the Carnival of Venice, which was resurrected only five years ago. It was a superb festa. On the afternoon of our arrival we went to the Piazza San Marco where there was a ball. At one end, a band was playing on a big stage. People were already dancing, among them some disguised in masks and many different forms of fancy dress. A dragon charged at St George who was complete with flag, hao and visored helmet. A family of black imps gambolled between those disguised simply by pale white masks; a man stood dressed in a white cape, over which was stretched a fishing net, while on his head was a fully rigged sailing boat. By Florian's café, a strange figure with witch's hat and different coloured ribbons hanging below black wings, squirmed and moved round a pillar, as if making love to it. False nuns walked along with reddened lips, and from the balcony of the Doge's palace a "Pope" with white hair, skull cap and surplice, resembling John Paul II, blessed the crowd.

We watched a Punch and Judy show at one end of the Piazza. A little girl went up to it and lifted the concealing drapery, revealing a young man holding a puppet on each hand. He stopped. "You shouldn't have done that," he said cheerfully.

We talked to three soldiers in the doublets, ruffs and hose of the sixteenth century. They came from Milan, they told us. They came every year. The whole family helped them make their fancy dress. Next year, they would wear something else. They kept all their discarded disguises in a cupboard. What motivated them? They looked a little bewildered. Why not? It was what you did at carnivals. Why were we not in fancy dress ourselves?

Next day, the weather broke, and it actually snowed. The Piazza San Marco was two feet deep in water, and scores of thin-shoed visitors found themselves in a small shop, clamouring for gum boots, which were smuggled through in boxes by four assistants.

Fortunately, that afternoon the snow stopped and the water seeped away. Apart from the crowds in the piazza and the streets, there was a whole programme of activities. There were no tickets for Strauss's *Die Fledermaus* at the Fenice opera house. It was necessary to have booked months before. There was a great ball at the house of Prince Orlofsky with the orchestra of the Fenice and the Bella Musica ensemble from Vienna. The programme invited "all the lovers of the Carnival and the theatre to live Venice, Vienna and waltzing". However, tickets were fifty dollars each. There were, however, street balls in many piazzas, an exhibition of masks throughout the ages at the Palazzo Grassi, Argentine tangos in the Teatro Malibran, and a masked ball with an Andaluz folklore group in the Teatro Tenda Ca' Savio – to mention only a few of the innumerable activities from all over the world which took place every day.

One afternoon we went to see *The Intrigues of Harlequin* at the tiny Teatro a L'Avogaria with wooden seats for about forty people. The theatre is both a workshop for young actors and, as part of this, has a permanent company of those who are training and being prepared. On stage, there was an impressive performance of Commedia dell' Arte, based on a seventeenth-century script, with its masked Harlequin,

Pantalone, Colombina, Pulcinella, Scaramuccia and company, all indulging in the series of simple intrigues, drubbings, servant cheating master, master worrying about his money, which have always characterized this ancient and influential theatrical tradition.

The Carnival, though, really expressed itself spontaneously in the streets. There was a market of masks in the Campo dei Santi Apostoli with blue ones, golden ones and many deathly pale, like those of clowns. In the Piazza San Luca, a group from Southern Italy suddenly started dancing a tarantella. Several youths drummed in time. A trumpeter, passing by, joined in, impassive with his white mask over his instrument.

There was no brawling, no disorder. At one stage, we went along to the police to find if there had been any trouble, but there hadn't been. The great thing in Italy is that drink is simply something which goes with meals, and Italians are used to enjoying themselves without it. In fact, at the police station we found only a disconsolate Englishman who had come from Bologna with masks he had made, and had had them confiscated when he tried to sell them. He had not got a licence, explained the policeman. It was not fair to allow strangers to come from outside to compete with Venetians during their Carnival.

By the canals, it was cold and damp. But the whole city was on fire, crackling, warming, without sudden outbursts of destructive flame. As so often in Italy, much of it was a family affair. Apart from imps, you would suddenly come across an entire eighteenth-century family, with a father, mother and two children in tricorn hats and powdered wigs, as if the Doge were still in his palace.

On the walls, though, some posters reminded one of "reality". One from a Communist organization complained what a scandal it was to spend so much money on festivities when there were 3,000 people without lodging in Venice, while a Catholic organization emphasized that the carnival spirit might exist but that, underneath, the state of man's soul was the important question – not this triviality and exuberance.

Carnival, after all, has always been the last fling before the expiation of Ash Wednesday and the rigours of Lent.

CATASTROPHES

We took a hydrofoil from one end of the volcanic zone to the other. One afternoon we left Naples, which is flanked on one side by Vesuvius which last erupted in 1944, and on the other by Pozzuoli, a town subject to bradyism, which means it can go up or down as much as five or six centimetres a year. Then we surged over the sunny sea, through the straits between Capri and Sorrento, and on to the Eolian isles, where, according to the Greeks, a god keeps the winds imprisoned in a vast cavern. From these islands on clear days you can see the Sicilian coast, with Etna a tall smudge behind.

On the door of the hydrofoil's bridge was a notice which forbad entry. However, as we approached Stromboli, everyone crowded in to catch the view ahead. Girls chatted in the big chairs either side of the pilot. People behind craned over their shoulders as we approached a Gothic, volcanic rock, with sharp peaks and a white lighthouse, which lay close to Stromboli. As so often in Italy, this easygoing tolerance delighted me. Why not? It gave people pleasure, including the crew, and did not disturb.

The Eolian islands are so beautiful that the inhabitants say you should really have four eyes to see them. We went to Panarea, which has no cars, no street lighting and, until last year, no telephones. It was emptied by emigration after the last war, and people still don't know who some of the land belongs to, as owners vanished long ago to Australia or Canada. Behind the fishing port clusters a small, white village, and above it there is a spinal hill, covered with brown scrub and thousands of cactuses with prickly oblong paddles, shaped like those of turtles, or like light-green ping-pong bats.

At the port, masted sailing boats come in on pleasure cruises from Sicily or Naples. Once, we saw a large motor launch captained by an elderly self-important man who was accompanied by six stern bodyguards. At night, one of them sat on a chair in the stern, guarding the boat which seemed part of a Mafia holiday.

One afternoon, we set off in a small fishing boat with twelve Italians to visit Stromboli, three hours away. We went right round the island. Every few minutes, a blob of smoke came from the top of the volcano. One slope was black and smooth with newly ejected lava. As each small eruption occurred, magma was thrown down and burnt with a puff of smoke above the waterline of black sand. The town was on the other side, with white houses against dark rock, and between the streets, small vineyards which produce the sweet, local Malvasia wine. After visiting it, we returned to the boat and ate a delicious meal on the small deck. Then, as it was getting dark, we set off back to Panarea.

A full moon had risen and above us was Stromboli, emitting little spurts of lava which now were incandescent. As we got out of the lee of the island, the wind blew stronger, probably out of the gods' cavern, and the sea got rougher. The boat with its small engine churned on, swaying alarmingly from side to side, with water coming over the gunwales. It was impossible to sit or stand so everyone lay on deck. Two girls lay together in the bows, and one of them leaned over the side and was sick.

The scene was like one of those early romantic paintings, with bodies slumped in the dark boat, the full moon silvering the tempestuous waves, the volcano spurting fire in the background.

Tormented, we arrived safely. Everyone was suddenly cheerful in the moonlight. There were none of those petulant accusations that the captain had been "irresponsible" for setting out. One of the pleasantest characteristics of Italians is that they rarely blame individuals – particularly afterwards. Too much goes wrong anyway, and they are used to it. In any case, as Dr Pasca said to me, sitting in a hotel between earthquake-shattered Naples and the oscillating city of Pozzuoli, "Danger is our daily bread."

Living in calm, northern pastures, it is difficult to imagine the effect of innumerable earthquakes, eruptions and floods on another nation's outlook. Some major disaster seems to happen in Italy every year. The 1980s started with the earthquake at Irpinia in the mountains east of Naples, on November 23rd 1980.

Suddenly, at 7.35 in the evening, Italy twitched slightly towards Yugoslavia and over an area the size of Belgium whole villages crumbled, and tall buildings in the cities collapsed. It was 6.2 on the Richter scale and included the major towns of Naples, Avellino and Potenza. Over five thousand people were killed and eight thousand injured, and more than 250,000 people were made homeless at a time of year when snow was on the higher hills.

The Neapolitan newspaper *Il Mattino* during those terrible days is full of personal stories of tragedy. Two lovers, Lucio and Antonietta, were sitting in a car when an entire cathedral fell on top of them. A woman lost her family of ten. In the little village of San Angelo dei Lombardi, a thousand people died or were injured. Whole streets suddenly turned to rubble, burying everyone underneath. A bell which had been suspended in a church tower for seven hundred years, and which had survived previous earthquakes, plummeted down and crushed the refectory in which a priest was talking to his family, who had come to see him: grandparents, parents, brothers and sister. All but one were killed. In many places the lights went out and there was no water. In Naples, a yellow liquid came out of the taps.

Chaos reigned for forty-eight hours. Over ruined houses, desolate people stumbled, looking for relatives. Below tons of masonry, others lay in the paralysing cold for a whole night, and perhaps for days, until they died or were rescued. The army arrived, but they were mostly teenage conscripts with no experience of this kind of relief work. President Pertini toured the devastation and was greeted with abuse, as if everything were the government's doing. One woman cursed him with her dead child in her arms. When he returned to Rome, he broadcast on television and asked why no precautions had been taken, when provisions had been voted in Parliament. He recalled the village of Belice in Sicily which had been completely destroyed in 1968. Although the government had granted quantities of money it still hadn't been completely rebuilt. Who had stolen the money? Why did nobody care? Some politicians, particularly those from Salerno and Avellino, protested, and the Christian Democrats described the speech as "a stab in the back".

The earthquake was the climax of those which had occurred in the previous ten years: Friuli, in the north-east, in 1976, when a thousand people were killed; Tuscania, north of Rome, which was destroyed in 1971. In the Naples area the damage will probably never be put right. Eighty streets were still closed in 1983. Many of these were like narrow alleys, full of branchless trees, with crossed girders to keep the two sides from falling in on each other. There were still 100,000 homeless, many of whom had abandoned empty, shattered villages, which now were nothing but prefabricated settlements, or caravan encampments, or armies of tents.

Nearer the epicentre in Potenza, a hundred miles away in Basilicata, the main street on the ridge was a mass of girders above the heads of passers-by, through which thin slices of sky could be seen. Wooden walls still prevented bits falling off the roofs, although the five-storey, modern buildings on the slopes had survived virtually untouched.

"The trouble is that the government only granted money for reconstruction six months after the earthquake," an official in the regional government told me. "Also, it's a question of how many skilled specialists are available. It is, above all, the medieval buildings that have collapsed – although that is perhaps our fault for loading them with extra storeys. Left alone, they might have survived."

"Isn't it possible to build anti-seismic structures?" I asked.

"Of course. There's a village called Melito Irpino which was destroyed in the earthquake of 1962. It was rebuilt with the advice of experts, with no houses more than three storeys high or ten metres tall. Now this earthquake has hardly affected it. However, where do you find enough specialists? Anyway, do we want to forget our heritage and construct soulless towns? It's mainly the historic centres that have been destroyed."

The shortage of expert manpower was emphasized again in Naples, particularly with the restoration of works of art. "The trouble is that Naples was never maintained after the earthquake of 1930," I was told at the office of the Beni Culturali, a ministry roughly equivalent to the Historic Buildings Council in Britain. "We need help in the restoration of frescoes, stucco work, churches. We haven't got enough specialists ourselves. So we employ Romans and Florentines. But in Rome they're doing a lot of work on the Forum, so they haven't many people to spare. There's a marble arch which collapsed in the Castel Nuovo and needs special work, but we can't find anyone to do it. In general, the Neapolitan extremes of heat and humidity don't help, either."

Since 1980, there have been other disasters, mainly in the north which is also prone to earthquakes, as shown by those in Friuli and Tuscania. In October 1982, earth tremors shook a large area in Umbria, round Perugia, and made thousands homeless. Then, in December, a massive landslide destroyed hundreds of houses in Ancona, and the earth split open along a railway line. This was followed in 1983 by an earthquake extending from Parma to Turin, although as building is more solid there, little damage was done. Then in May 1984 there was an earthquake in a remote village of the Abruzzi which extended to Gubbio and Assisi. However, in the case of Assisi, press reports exceeded reality. I was there shortly afterwards, and everyone said they had suffered no damage but, because of television reports, eighteen groups of tourists had cancelled their bookings. The town was pleasantly calm and uncrowded!

Geographically, Italy is afflicted by the movement of "plates" on the Earth's crust. The African plate pushes north and goes under the one moving east from Iberia, forming molten rock which pushes upwards through the volcanos of Etna, the Eolian isles and Vesuvius. The Apennines have been crunched up by pressure between the Apulian and the Iberian plates, which meet down the middle of Italy. Because these three plates, all moving against each other, clash in, and under, the peninsula, eruptions and tremors are frequent.

Etna normally erupts ten to twenty times a century. It is pocked with over two hundred small craters, as lava can break out anywhere on the mountain. In 1979, a sudden eruption killed nine tourists. Another occurred on March 17th 1981, from a chain of vents above the little town of Randazzo. Normally, the lava moves slowly, but this time it covered two kilometres in twenty minutes. It blocked a railway line and buried farms. The townspeople formed a procession, carrying a picture of St Joseph, their patron saint, in front of the magma. Next day, the lava stopped, a miracle was proclaimed and a local sculptor, Gaetano Arrigo, fulfilled a vow and carved a statue of St Joseph out of volcanic rock, and put it up in Randazzo.

In April 1983, a further eruption occurred which lasted seven weeks. A flow of lava descended towards Catania, the second city in Sicily, which it had last reached in 1669, when it filled the harbour, and destroyed a new Benedictine monastery. This time, about twenty-five houses, the funicular – the most modern in Europe – and a restaurant, La Quercia, were overwhelmed. In the magazine *Oggi*, there was a description by local hunters of how animals were affected: birds with nests on the ground were overwhelmed. Others flew crazily around and, tired, alighted on burning lava and were immediately frazzled. Rabbits and foxes both found refuge in their burrows and were baked alive. Only the hares escaped.

On this occasion, there was an attempt to divert the lava away from towns and villages, under the supervision of a Swede, Lennart Abersten. Over a hundred men dug an alternative canal, and forty charges were then exploded in the cooled wall of the channel down which the lava was running. The experiment was only partially successful. The risk was high: charges had to be placed in the wall which still was very hot. In the end, the wall was only partly breached but, by good fortune, a rock was hurled into the middle of the lava channel, thus diverting it in part. Soon afterwards, in any case, the eruption ceased.

However, the worst of recent afflictions have again been in the Naples area at Pozzuoli, ten miles west of the city, where Sophia Loren was born. For thousands of years Pozzuoli has been afflicted by bradyism, and here, on October 4th 1983, there was another earthquake of 4.4 on the Richter scale. Fortunately, only one person died, and that of fright. But most people fled, or were evacuated.

When I went there, a month later, it was almost a ghost city. Eight hundred rooms had been found in hotels along the coast, villas and apartments had been requisitioned, and 350,000 lire were given to anyone who could make their own arrangements. We entered one of the few shops open, to buy our lunch, and met the owners who had lived in America for a long time. Although their house behind was unsafe, they came in every day to sell food to those who remained.

The evening of the earthquake had been particularly terrifying, they said, partly because everyone presumed it was a repetition of two years earlier. If there were no further tremors before January, they would be allowed to come back again and repair their house. However, Pozzuoli seems ruined. The fishing port no longer functions, partly because the quays have risen, and the sea is so shallow that few boats can come in. Now the town goes down in summer and rises again in winter, partly because the sea evaporates when it is hot, and weighs down more heavily when there is more water in winter – as if Pozzuoli were on a kind of lever, with the sea accentuating or reducing the pressure on one end.

Even without an earthquake, the buildings crack as they rise or subside. Between them and the molten lava, there is a crust of rock two or three kilometres deep, which is also pushed up and down, according to the movement below. Of course, if you live in Pozzuoli, you get used to it. After all, it has gone on for thousands of years. You only have to walk round the corner to see the Temple of Serapis, which in Roman times had been in a busy square, but which now is flooded. There are marks of marine molluscs on the marble columns almost six metres high, showing that, at one time, it was virtually submerged.

If we wanted to get a sense of the danger and instability, we ought to go to Solfatara nearby, said the shopkeeper. We did. It is the animated crater of the volcano, close to which Pozzuoli lies. Within it, you walk on hot ground, between parts marked off with rope. These bubble gently, emitting clouds of smoke or steam which smell of sulphur and shroud you as, cautiously, you advance. If you throw a piece of paper on the ground, it ignites suddenly, and you wonder if at any moment you may sink into the molten lava beneath, or be hurled into the air, a cinder in a sudden eruption. Once across the crater, you come across a little stone cabin. From behind it, a lady emerges surrounded by fumes, like one of the witches in *Macbeth*, and tries to sell you a little plastic bag full of pieces of volcanic rock of different colours.

What is the likelihood of an eruption, similar to that 17,000 years ago, which provided the ash layer on which Naples is built? If it occurred, it would probably finish the whole area off. Giuseppe Longo, an Italian seismologist, calculates that there is a cubic kilometre of lava below Pozzuoli, compared to the 2.5 cubic kilometres which destroyed Pompeii and Herculaneum in 79 AD. The present rise in level indicates that magma is building up. The same thing happened in 1538 when an eruption created Monte Nuovo, a four-hundred-foot hill, in just two days. Certainly, British seismologists seem worried: in September 1984, two hundred British troops attached to NATO were evacuated because it was felt that the whole area was unsafe.

Similar worries have been felt about Venice ever since November 1966 when the Adriatic breached the great defensive walls, completed in 1782, only fifteen years before the end of the Doges' Republic. These walls are fourteen feet thick at their base and twenty feet high, made of gleaming, six-foot marble blocks, fronted by an enormous breakwater of heaped up boulders. At the high tide on November 4th, the sea breached them in ten places.

Floods occur in Venice when the barometric pressure on the sea is low, so that the surface rises, and when a sirocco blows north and pushes water tumultuously up the Adriatic for long enough to keep successive high waters enclosed in the lagoon. In this case, the sirocco blew force 8 and the barometer was down to 744 mm, and the flood lasted for twenty hours, so that three tides were contained. As a result, the water in Venice rose to six and a half feet above sea level, which was a record.

There have always been floods in Venice, at least since the first chronicles in 1240. However, the situation is different now, as John Julius Norwich, chairman of the British Venice in Peril Fund, explained to me. For one thing, the big industrial complex at Marghera, on the mainland north of Venice, has encroached on the lagoon, making it smaller and capable of taking less water. The piles on which Venice is built, made mainly of petrified larch, are still sound, even after a thousand years. However, below them there is a crust of earth, some forty to fifty feet thick, and below that a further reservoir of water, from which the Venetians originally drew their drinking supplies. Now, however, the demands of modern industry for water are phenomenal. At one stage, the factories at Marghera were drawing off hundreds of gallons a minute. An aqueduct has recently been built and this danger has ceased; but a lot of damage has been done and there is still a fear that Venice could subside through this crust. Already, it has been sinking year by year, which partly explains why there were over forty major floods in the fifty years before 1966, compared to only seven between 1867 and 1914.

Also, the combination of sulphur from the industrial complex and the salty atmosphere of the sea has meant that the outer surfaces of marble and stone become like sugar. The rain then gets into the pores and expands when it freezes. The whole process then begins again until columns and facings are destroyed.

After the 1966 flood, over £200 million was raised as an international loan. However, since then nothing has been done, apart from limiting the harm caused by the industrial complex at Marghera. Various projects were discussed and a contract was won in 1982 by a consortium. Their plan was to create flood barriers which would stay on the bottom until needed, when they would be raised – similar to those across the Thames. However, in September 1983 this contract was cancelled because the National Auditing Tribunal in Rome stated that the firm had not gone through the proper channels, and that different tenders had not been proffered. Now, however, approval has been given. Over the years, the barriers will presumably be constructed – if it is not too late; there are now over two hundred floods a year in Venice. Many of them are slight but each takes its toll.

Italians are accustomed to precariousness. Perhaps it is this which gives them flexibility and their ability to improvise. After all, the very creation of Naples or Venice was a hazardous venture. It needs a special temperament to accept disaster and re-build. Perhaps the legend of Sisyphus, rolling his rock up the mountain and having it crash down again whenever he reached the top, originated in Greek Neapolis. Perhaps, too, the Italian attachment to their *paese* or city enters in. After the earthquake near Naples, it was proposed to build another city, fifty miles away. However, few were interested in moving.

Italians have not expected "security" for thousands of years. It may not have kept them all alive, but the sense of continual danger has probably given them alertness and stimulated their ability to absorb themselves in the moment, and enjoy it.

III
INSTITUTIONS

∽⟞⟞⟞⟞⟞⟞⟞⟞∾

Parliament – President or Monarch? – Mussolini's Heirs –
Party Politics – The Communists – Bureaucracy

PARLIAMENT

From the Piazza Venezia, where Mussolini made his speeches, you
plunge into Renaissance Rome. You tread through a sombre-grey city
of palaces and government offices, of straight streets leading to
monumental piazzas. Between them, alleyways wind alongside
baroque churches and convents which have been turned into schools, or
skirt little shops encrusted in massive walls. Remains of Imperial Rome
appear unexpectedly round a corner: the Pantheon whose dome was
used as a model by Brunelleschi when he built the Cathedral at Florence
and which, therefore, is the ancestor of all the domes in the world; or
Piazza Navona which was once the Emperor Domitian's race-course.

About three hundred yards up the Via del Corso from Piazza Venezia
is the nucleus of Italian government: the Chamber of Deputies with,
beside it, the Palazzo Chigi, which houses the offices of the President of
the Council, or Prime Minister. The Senate also is nearby – a five-
minute walk to Piazza Madama. Not far, either, are the headquarters of
the Communist Party in Via Botteghe Oscure, and that of the Christian
Democrats in Piazza del Gesù.

The Chamber of Deputies is in the Palazzo Montecitorio, built by
Bernini. It was once a private palace and then the Papal Hall of Justice.
Now, men in dark suits walk self-consciously in front of it as if they
were famous, or were likely to meet someone who is. The Italian flag
hangs above the doorway and two soldiers in battle dress stand either
side, tirelessly saluting everyone who goes in. Mussolini called it a
"bivouac of manoeuvring". In fact, it is one of the most dramatic
theatres in Italy.

Before it in the piazza is an obelisk, dating from the sixth century

BC, brought from Egypt by Augustus. Here, as so often in Italy, time is united in one place: the obelisk constructed when Rome was a struggling Republic, brought over by the founder of its Empire; then the view of Renaissance buildings beyond the piazza from a palazzo built in the seventeenth century, which was an official centre when the Popes were rulers of Rome; now the complex of a parliament and the parked cars, the modern bar opposite, the soldiers in khaki.

Inside, the Deputies' seats are ranged in a horseshoe with desks equipped with microphone, inkwell and voting button. The President sits on a dais above a long table which has seats for Ministers and their Under-Secretaries. It is interesting that the Deputies speak facing the Ministers rather than each other. Psychologically, it must make a difference: a Deputy is not attacking serried ranks opposite; he is communicating principally with the Cabinet. Also, the division between Government and Opposition is blurred.

Above the Chamber is a stained-glass roof and an Art Nouveau frieze where naked figures of both sexes stand, lie, sit on lions, or droop over each other. "It's by a Sicilian, Massili," said an usher, whose work on a crossword I interrupted. "It is supposed to represent the Virtues of Italy: Labour, Hope, Generosity." Even at the turn of the century, there was little visual prudishness in Italy. As in the times of the Romans and Greeks and in the Renaissance, the naked body had allegorical significance, quite apart from sexual attitudes. Perhaps the frieze was a gesture of defiance to the Pope, who had recently been supplanted. After all, Sixtus IV insisted on loincloths for Michelangelo's nudes in his "Last Judgement" in the Sistine chapel, and was depicted in Hell as a revenge. In Britain, the equivalent decoration in public places in the late Victorian era consisted of Romantic knights in armour with smooth schoolboy faces, or Rossetti maidens with pure but yearning expressions.

Six hundred and thirty deputies use the Chamber, including thirty Ministers and fifty-nine Under-Secretaries. Over at the Senate, they have a smaller, more comfortable Chamber for three hundred and fifteen, yet their powers are very similar. The Senate is the "graver" house, with six representatives from each Region and various life Senators, appointed for their achievements, including ex-Presidents of the Republic.

Compared to the British or American systems, there are a number of differences. For one thing, everyone over eighteen is supposed to vote by law. "A vote is personal and equal, free and secret," says article 48 of the Constitution. "The exercising of the same is a civic duty."

Officially, failure to vote is marked on the citizen's criminal record, and it might affect getting a job.

Today, this is not adhered to so rigidly, but after the war voting was a sign of support for the very idea of democracy, which after all was won from Fascism, rather than inherited over hundreds of years. Professor Negri, head of the parliamentary administration, summed this up when he told me that when his children said they hadn't voted, he lost his temper, "I spent two months in a Gestapo prison for your liberty!" he snapped, "and now you're wasting it!" At the election of June 1983, there were fears of blank votes as a protest, and yet 82.6 per cent went to the polls, a slight decrease on 1979 when 85.8 per cent voted. Italians even travel back from abroad or plan their holidays with the election in mind. Yet they are not voting for a government as in Britain or the United States, but for a party, and there are no fewer than ten of these. After the election, the President of the Republic chooses a possible Prime Minister, who then sees what coalition can be formed. Since 1981, two of these premiers have been heads of minority parties: Spadolini from the Republicans with only sixteen seats, and Craxi from the Socialists, with seventy-three.

After listening to the views of Liberal and Social Democrat Party supporters in Britain, it is interesting how many people you meet in Italy who would prefer the British or American systems because they feel they would produce more decisive government. There has also been hot debate on the idea of making everything more manageable by excluding any party which has less then 5 per cent of the overall vote – although so many parties would be affected that vested interests are unlikely to be overcome.

The voting system itself is complex, based on a form of proportional representation devised by a Belgian sage. Other differences include an obligation on all parliamentarians to declare their private income. In 1984, the Christian Democrat Guido Carli, former director of the Bank of Italy, was the richest with 435 million lire ($230,000) and one of the poorest was the late Communist leader, Berlinguer, with 23 million ($10,000). Members of Parliament receive a salary of about 24 million lire ($10,500) a year but their board in Rome is paid and they can eat cheaply. They are also allowed to follow their professions.

As far as actual legislation is concerned, one difference is that Deputies can vote secretly. This means that a Prime Minister cannot be sure of support even from his own party, and that the system of party whips is hardly practical. Thus, when Craxi, the Prime Minister, tried to pass an amnesty on illegal building in September 1983, he failed to get it through, despite the fact that all the parties in his coalition were officially in favour. A group of thirty anonymous "freelances", as they are called, defeated the motion.

In this case, the measure had already been made official in the form of a "decree law". This means that a decree becomes law immediately, but Parliament must confirm it within sixty days. The result in this case was embarrassing as some people had already paid the fines that were laid down as the price of an amnesty. It also meant that as they had "confessed" they were liable to prosecution under the old laws, which were now still valid.

Laws can also be passed in committee as long as no more than 10 per cent of members do not vote against. This use of committees means that members of minority parties can take part in legislation, even if, like the Communists, they are in opposition.

A further way for public opinion to express itself outside the limits of government initiative is through a referendum. This takes place if anyone organizes a petition with over 700,000 signatures. In the 1970s it had great influence because it was thus that both the divorce and abortion laws were passed against the will of the Church and the Christian Democrats, who dominated the government. Because it was a referendum, it was also a national debate. Arguments even went to the extreme of the MSI – the neo-Fascists who also were against abortion – parading with placards which asked what people would feel if their favourite football player had been aborted! Psychologically, the verdict of a whole nation was a crushing blow to Catholics, and to the elected government.

Other external factors which limit the power of the government are extensive regional government (see p. 18) and the need for all legislation to be within the written Constitution, which describes Italy as "a Republic founded on work". Many clauses are principles framed in 1947 to counter any possibility of a return to Fascism. Thus, the Constitution guarantees the rights of man, ethnic minorities, public meetings without arms, and religious freedom. It forbids censorship, supports free trade unions and the rights of the family as the basic unit of society. It represents the ideals of a democracy which believes in the welfare state and a mixed economy: State education should be without charge, and free medical treatment to the needy is guaranteed. Private enterprise is also encouraged, as long as it does not run counter to the well-being of society, or constitute a danger to security.

It is an admirable document but, inevitably, some of its clauses are only aspirations. Thus, it emphasizes women's rights but these were not really established till thirty years later. It also states that everyone should share in the expenses of the State according to their "contributory capacity", which vague phrase has not been fulfilled, as tax evasion is still widespread. Often, it is difficult to interpret, and a Constitutional Court was set up in 1955 to give decisions on whether laws were constitutional or not. This has proved an additional complication in a slow-moving and excessively intricate machine.

The existence of a Constitution also implies rigidity, and produces results which seem alien to the Italian temperament. Thus when ex-king Umberto was dying in 1983, there was a widespread feeling that he should be asked back to Italy, and buried in the old Savoy capital of Turin. However, the Constitution states that no "pretender" or direct descendant of Vittorio Emmanuele III (who co-operated with Mussolini) should be allowed into Italy. This humane gesture had therefore to be abandoned as it was too difficult to amend the Constitution. So the exile died in Switzerland and was buried in the Abbey of Hautecombe in Savoy, now French, but once the original fief of the family. Many Italians were shamed and indignant, although it was accepted that any alternative was impossible.

Because the modern State of Italy is a cerebral rather than an organic creation, conceived at a time when strong government connoted Fascism, its weakness is that decisive action is difficult. But then perhaps ever since the French Revolution, since Marx, we have exaggerated the importance and influence of government, per se, without considering that it is the collective energy and will of a country which is the most important factor. This, though, is difficult to assess. It is much easier to judge the British by Thatcher, the Russians by the Comintern, the Chileans by Pinochet, and the Italians by the fact that they change governments on average every eight and a half months, and that rule seems corrupt and chaotic.

PRESIDENT OR MONARCH?

We waited in the sunlight outside the palace of the Quirinale until all the directors attending our International House conference had assembled. The Quirinale was built in the sixteenth century by a Pope, Sixtus V, who had been born a shepherd boy; it was perhaps the shepherd in him which had caused him to enclose such a large part of the Quirinale hill for this immense, long palace, the colour of faded oranges.

We were waiting to see the sixth President of the Italian Republic,

Sandro Pertini.* The director general of our Italian organization had written requesting an interview, and the answer was positive.

President Pertini was born in 1896. He fought in the First World War, and recounts how his regiment's machine guns grew so hot they had to be cooled with urine. Later he became a Socialist, which he still is, and after taking a degree in law fled to France in 1926 where he worked as a mason and washer-down of taxis. Returning to Italy in 1930, he was arrested and spent thirteen years in a Fascist prison until released by the Allies, when he became a partisan. He was on the committee which sentenced Mussolini to death and that same morning in Milan passed the Duce on the stairs of the palace of Cardinal Schuster who was trying to bring about an armistice between Germans and Allies.

Nevertheless, Pertini was disgusted by the way Mussolini and his mistress, Clara Petacci, were strung up in Piazza Loreto in Milan, and sent a lorry to take their bodies away. His impartiality and humanity are shown by the fact that he admired Clara Petacci, who could easily have escaped to Spain with her family but chose instead to stay with her lover. "She was a brave and loyal woman," he said.

The President has more power in Italy than nominal presidents like those of Switzerland and Germany, but less than those of France and the USA. Pertini is head of the armed forces, can dissolve Parliament, and is responsible for choosing the Prime Minister. He has his own political staff, can make political moves on his own initiative, and requires the Prime Minister to work closely with him. He is chosen by members of both the Chamber of Deputies and the Senate, along with three delegates from the Councils of the Regions, and is elected for seven years. In the election in 1978 Pertini obtained a larger majority (86 per cent) than any of his predecessors. Since then he has been widely admired for his spontaneity and willingness to speak his mind, and also for his absolute integrity. During the Naples earthquake, he denounced those who had appropriated government money and those responsible for the slow reaction to the tragedy (see p. 59).

His New Year address to the nation in 1984 attacked the way Italian troops in the Lebanon were being used for American purposes: "... let's speak clearly," he said, "the Americans are not there to defend the peace but only to defend Israel." He announced this at a press conference on December 22nd and in spite of reactions from America and Israel, and the fact that only the Communists supported him

*In June 1985, President Pertini was succeeded by Francesco Cossiga, a former Christian Democrat Prime Minister.

publicly in Italy, he refused to change a word.

President Pertini also expresses his emotions openly in public. He has been known to weep publicly at funerals for those killed by the Mafia. In 1981, a six-year-old boy, Alfredo Rampi, fell down a narrow well shaft, and for two days the whole nation sat in front of their television sets to watch the rescue attempts. In the end, these failed and the boy slid further down the shaft and was suffocated. Italians saw their feelings expressed when the President sobbed uncontrolledly. Pertini, indeed, shows all the warmth and personal concern which characterize so many Italians. The country as a whole is his parish, and the normally divisive loyalty to family or work-place, *paese* or political party, does not distract him – it gives him strength. He is essentially a Socialist with a Christian heart.

Outside the Quirinale, a Carabiniere beckoned and we followed him into a large waiting room with a lapis lazuli table and big, open doors, which revealed a view of the first courtyard. A distant car was parked by a colonnade in the emptiness. Then the Carabiniere beckoned again, and pointed up a straight stone alley. No one led us as we walked along, but officials appeared suddenly from doorways and pointed again, like human signposts. We walked past a vast garden in the hot sun, with sculpted bushes and palm trees, until we came to the official residence, a pavilion set in the far corner of the building.

Here we were led up a curving staircase to the second floor, past open doors which revealed officials working on Louis XVI tables in a gilded room. Then into a larger *sala* with a parquet floor and elegant chandeliers. "The President is seeing an Ambassador," said an aide, "he won't be long."

We ranged ourselves round the walls. Then, "The President is coming." A small man with white hair and tinted glasses came through the door. I read my speech and in the middle thought it too long for a man of eighty-seven, standing listening, and quickened my pace. However, I needn't have worried. When it was over, Pertini sprang immediately to shake hands with everyone, while I introduced them and told him which country they were working in.

"Ah, Spain!" he exclaimed, as he greeted a Spanish director. "A great country with long traditions! I remember last summer sitting next to Juan Carlos, watching Italy win the World Cup. It's ridiculous that Mitterand opposed her entry into the Common Market!" he added indiscreetly. "Just for a few vineyards! After all, we have our vineyards too. Spain will also compete with us, but that's not a reason for barring her!"

He looked around. "Aren't the refreshments coming?" he asked one of his aides, and little glasses of fruit juice were brought in on trays. My wife, Brita, presented him with a pipe we had brought as a present.

"Grazie tante!" he said, "Grazie. That will be exactly my nine hundredth!"

He talked about Britain and how he had fought beside English troops as a partisan. Last year he had met Mrs Thatcher. Although she had an iron will, her soul was gentle.

"Don't you agree?" he turned to me provocatively.

"I don't know," I burbled, "I haven't met her."

"What do you think of Michael Foot?"* he was asked by someone. Probably the pronunciation of the name was unfamiliar, because he looked blank. "Are you sure you're translating properly?" he said, flirtatiously, to Susan Denton, whom we had brought along, also from one of the Rome schools, as a bilingual interpreter.

"I'm not official!" she responded, and he laughed.

He told us he had first gone abroad when he was eighteen. "I would give anything, the Quirinale itself, to be eighteen again!" he said. "I'm still a free man, though," he joked, "except when these secretaries tell me what to do!" He waved towards his aides.

He turned to go. "Love Italy!" he called, as he went through the door.

Later I visited the leading member on Italian soil of the royal family of Savoy. The Duke of Aosta is in his early forties and lives at his farm, Il Borro, in the village of Loro Ciuffenna, in Tuscany. He is the son of the admiral who devised the human torpedoes which sank so many British warships in the harbour in Alexandria during the last war. His uncle was in the army and was Commander-in-Chief of the Italian forces which were defeated by the British in Ethiopia and Somaliland, in 1941. He himself attended the Naval College in Venice, but hadn't been able to take up his commission because of his royal blood. The Liberal party asked him to become a candidate in the elections of 1983, but this started an enquiry into the fact that he had actually voted in nine elections, although the Constitution forbids "members and descendants of the House of Savoy" from voting or holding public office.

We sat in his low, comfortable farmhouse, with a green lawn and gardeners cutting the bushes outside. The drawing room seemed very English with a profusion of carpets, low beams, and models of warships his father had commanded. Portraits of his eighteenth-century

* This was just before the 1983 British and Italian general elections.

ancestors, kings of Savoy and Sardinia, looking like unclipped sheep in their powdered wigs, gazed from the walls.

He told us how he had been at Our Lady of the Cross preparatory school in England after the war. The English boys had mocked him for his uncle's defeat, and called him a Wop, which, he said, came from a classification in American immigration offices, and stood for "without official papers"*. However, when he felt persecuted he could always take refuge with the French, who were there in great numbers as the school was an international centre for "aristos".

He had always had close links with Britain, and particularly admired the Queen as the ideal monarch and, at the same time, a very warm person. He also felt close to King Juan Carlos of Spain. His family had ancestral associations with that country: the Aostas were direct descendants of Amadeus who had been invited to become King of Spain after the revolution of 1868, but had given up after a few years in despair.

Juan Carlos gave hope to all royal families who had lost their thrones, said the Duke, because he had so recently recovered his father's crown. Italians were monarchists at heart, too, and were discontented with the present system, but this didn't really show itself. Certainly, it was unfortunate that Victor Emmanuel III had linked himself so closely to Mussolini, but he had, after all, dismissed Mussolini in 1943. If there hadn't been a king, there would have been no way of getting rid of the dictatorship, as in Hitler's Germany.

The great advantage of kings, or queens, continued the Duke, is that they are trained for their task from childhood, and one should always remember that there are more monarchies in Europe than republics. All the "royals" know each other, and this makes relations between countries smoother and more personal.

"And what are the chances of a monarchy in Italy now?" I asked.

"Well, who knows? It's impossible to be certain about anything these days. My guess is that it may come during the life of my son, but not in mine."

I asked him about the present "pretender", Victor Emmanuel, who lives in Switzerland and, like another exile, Bonnie Prince Charlie, speaks his native language with a foreign accent. He has the reputation of being a playboy and once shot a German tourist, Dirk Hammer, who was sleeping in a neighbouring boat in Corsica. Hammer died after a

---

* Charles Feltmann, in his *Wine in the Ancient World*, says it comes from the Latin word for insipid vinegar, "vappa", which survives in the Neapolitan dialect as "voppo" and found its way into American English by way of Southern immigrants.

hundred and eleven days of agony.

"There hasn't yet been a trial or a verdict," protested the Duke. "It's not certain either whether Hammer died because of bad medical treatment, anyway."

"Maybe, but it's hardly good public relations."

"No – that's the trouble."

We got up to go. A dachshund barked. Outside, in the hall, people with appointments rose to their feet as the Duke showed us out. He was very impressive, I thought: still young, confident, eloquent, lively. Informal, too – he was wearing jeans with an open shirt, and dark glasses because he had burnt his eyebrows with a lighter.

However, he was not the heir, and his cousin, Victor Emmanuel, was too impulsive and discredited, always in the papers because of some upset. The most recent was that his Minister of the Household (with the diabolical name of Marquis of Lucifer) had just resigned. So had two executors of ex-King Umberto's will. Victor Emmanuel had even been rash enough to describe Gelli, the head of the masonic lodge P2, as "a pleasant person, a good man with whom it was possible to do business".

In Rome, I visited an exhibition at the headquarters of the Monarchical Union, a palazzo rented from a Socialist senator in Via Rasella. There was no mention of Victor Emmanuel, or the Duke of Aosta, but mainly evocations of the past: a photograph of Queen Elena distributing food to the poor; family trees; a newspaper cutting about the murder of King Umberto I in Milan in 1900, describing the assassin as a well-dressed and handsome man. Also, a poster distributed round Rome in 1983 when Umberto III died. Under a large photograph of the sad, wrinkled ex-King, it stated: "He always spoke only of brotherhood, of justice and of peace and for this reason he was condemned to exile."

I approached a small group and, excusing myself, asked them why they were monarchists.

"Because the monarchy made Italy! Everything is a shambles now under the Republic!" said a thin, greying man, with small, intense eyes. "A king gives dignity, which is what Italy needs above everything."

The others nodded. "Italy is a divided country. It needs a symbol to unite it."

"But isn't President Pertini a symbol?" I asked.

"He's a Socialist! And God knows who will come next!"

As we talked, I began to feel that it was the pomp, the past, their own role in an aristocracy clustered about the monarch, that interested them. President Pertini seemed to have many of the virtues they extolled in a king. Now, the Monarchists have no political party. Once, in 1948, they had forty deputies led by the dynamic shipbuilder, Achille Lauro, who recently died bankrupt.

Rome is the home of faded monarchical hopes. Francis II lived here, sadly, for nine years after his expulsion from Naples. Napoleon's formidable mother died here. Bonnie Prince Charlie drank himself to death in Rome, and his elder brother, Henry, abandoned hope of worldly success and became a cardinal, now, their tombs are in St Peter's.

MUSSOLINI'S HEIRS

Bologna's buildings are tomato-red. You can walk right through the city under arcades, which fringe both sides of the medieval streets. They protect you, either from a heat which reaches 40° in summer, or from frequent snow in winter. Because of these tall arcades the streets are narrow and dark.

On the outskirts there is a market with tents and stalls which sell shoes, ranged out on the ground, ceramics, pots and pans, new clothes hanging from bars, with little canvas changing rooms behind. A knife grinder has his machine mounted on a motor-cycle with scraps of rag at the side to test the sharpness of the knives. At one side, a small plaque shows a smiling man with a round cap and underneath his name: ORESTE BIAVATI. "Who was he?" I asked a stallholder.

"Beh' – he got this piazza for us. He fought against the *signori* for the workers, arranged that we should all pay rent to the Commune, allotted stands."

Bologna has always had a strong radical strain. Since 1945 it has had a Communist majority on its council, and it is now one of the wealthiest towns in Italy, often held up by the Left as a model of order and honest administration, with an efficient school system and sensible schemes for rehousing the poor and for the restoration of the historic centre. It has also given subsidies to industry which have induced factories to move out of town and settle along the Via Emilia.

I was surprised, therefore, to see posters all round town advertising "Mussolini e la Cultura", a meeting to be held in the enormous Palazzo dei Congressi as part of the centenary celebrations of Mussolini's birth in the neighbouring village of Predappio on July 29th 1883. In Italy nowadays one is continually confounded in one's "logical" Anglo-Saxon expectations: Fascist rallies in Communist towns; Communists kissing bishops' hands; Socialists forming governments with Christian

Democrats, and even much talk, in 1977–78, of a Communist-Christian Democrat coalition. Is it expediency, or lack of fanaticism? Probably something of both. Also, perhaps, the feeling that life goes on anyway, with or without political parties, and that one joins them mainly because everyone in this complex life needs a "tribe" to give protection, social identity, and help in need.

Indeed, Bologna itself was the scene of a reconciliation between the Communist mayor and the archbishop, Lercaro. In 1956, the archbishop rang funeral bells all over Bologna when Hungary was invaded. He constructed a great seminary on the hill overlooking Bologna, where building is frowned on, but there were not enough seminarists and it had to be sold to a firm which makes crutches. The mayor was particularly annoyed by what are called *frati volanti*, priestly hecklers, who appeared regularly at political meetings. Finally, however, mayor and archbishop got used to one another, began to like each other, and when the archbishop returned from the Papal Council in 1963, the mayor actually welcomed him officially at the station, wearing his tricolour sash!

At the Palazzo dei Congressi there were only a few Carabinieri. Couples in their Sunday best smiled at us conspiratorially as if we too were Fascists attending a meeting of our brotherhood. Inside, by the book exhibition, I talked to a councillor from a neighbouring Commune where there was a Communist majority. He was the only MSI* representative.

"Do you have rows?" I asked.

He shrugged his shoulders. "We disagree, but 'correctness' is necessary."

Six years ago there was a lot of friction, he said. However, a Professor De Felice, from Rome university, had begun publishing a four-part biography of the Duce, which examined him impartially. As De Felice was a Socialist, he had credibility. Now people were beginning to get over their prejudices and realize that Mussolini had done a lot for Italy. It had been very much "Fascismo all' Italiana", not really a tyranny because the people were behind him, particularly at the time of the victory over Abyssinia in 1936. There were more political prisoners in jail now than there had ever been under Fascism. Of course there used to be manipulation of press and radio. Now, though, it was just more subtle. He himself was a Fascist partly because his father had been. "That sort of thing runs in families," he said.

I spoke to another party member about present policy. "Of course,

* Movimento Sociale Italiano: the official name of the neo-Fascist party.

times have changed," he said. "We no longer believe in dictatorship.
Our real object is to ensure the Communists do not get into power. We
want to remedy some of the disorder in Italy. After all, only Mussolini
ever conquered the Mafia. It was the Allies who brought them back.
Now, we support the Atlantic Alliance and the Common Market –
although we do feel we should be stronger there."

"And the trade unions?"

"Of course we're in favour – although we feel they should be
controlled more strictly."

We went into the meeting in the splendid hall with comfortable, red
upholstered seats which swept down towards the stage. There was
room for a thousand and about half the space was filled – mainly I
noticed by the middle-aged.

Vittorio Mussolini, the Duce's youngest son, presided. With masses
of white hair and a beard, he looked more like Peter Ustinov than his
father. He began by reading out a list of representatives of Fascist
groups all over the North. The leaders each came up to the dais, were
kissed on both cheeks, and given a certificate, to strong applause.

Then the lectures on "Mussolini and Culture" started. A rhetorical
professor stated that there had always been an assumption that
Mussolini was not cultured. This was nonsense. "Fascists are the
opposite, as far as seriousness and integrity are concerned, to the
Socialists and Liberals, with their confused thoughts, their endless
gossip and their uncertainty!" – more rapt applause.

As I looked round, I wondered what these people had experienced of
Fascism. You had to be almost sixty now to have fought in the war.
Perhaps some of the older ones had been in those appalling campaigns in
Russia, or had surrendered in Tunisia, or had belonged to the Young
Fascists fighting the partisans in northern Italy. I wondered how much
enthusiasm there had really been. The Italians surrendered so easily not
because they were cowards, as many older people in England seemed to
think. They did, after all, fight fiercely enough in the First World War
against their hereditary enemy, Austria, to reclaim what they regarded
as their territory.

In the Second War, though, they had nothing to fight for, dragged as
they were to Greece, Albania, North Africa to struggle with outdated
equipment against those with whom they had no immediate quarrel.
The Italians are essentially a realistic people. Because they have always
been rooted in their regions, they don't sympathize with dreams of
empire, glory, national prestige. That is why they were so suspicious of
Britain when we fought for the Falklands. "Tell us! What is there in the

Falkland Islands?" they kept on asking a diplomat I know who was in Rome at the time. "Is it oil under the Atlantic? Mineral deposits beneath the South Pole? There must be something!"

I looked at my neighbour, a man in his late fifties, who was listening with rapt attention. I imagined him as a member of the Young Fascists in his black uniform, roused by speeches from a balcony, marching away afterwards with the band playing, spouting dramatic slogans about things of which he probably knew nothing. Even here, in this hall, it was probably the sense of occasion, of being with so many of his companions, the rhetoric from the platform which entranced him. "The Italians are like the Welsh," said Richard Burton, "very good actors. It is the bad ones who become professionals."

We got up to go and, outside, paused to look at the book exhibition: *The Problem with Democracy*, *The American Sickness*. On the walls behind there were posters: one of the Falange in Lebanon with Arabic letters; another of a ferocious Viking, standing against a red, Valhalla glow, threatening with his battle-axe. "Is he supposed to be good, or bad?" Brita asked a young attendant, provocatively.

"Good, of course!" came the terse reply.

Another poster showed a youth with SS signs above him, with a gun over his shoulder and a knife in his hand, as he sprang out like a panther.

As I confirmed when talking later to a MSI Deputy, there is little on the surface that moderate Right-wing politicians in any country would disagree with. As always, however, it is the sentiments and attitudes underlying policy which are most important, and it was this emphasis on violence, on élitism, on machismo, this scorn for others' "decadence", which obtruded here, along with innocuous lectures on the Duce's cultural prowess.

Historians will discuss Mussolini for centuries and may ultimately conclude that he was abler than we think, that he had been misunderstood, his image deformed by propaganda. However, the fact remains that his heritage is also one of personal violence, of compulsive force, of heavy-handed intolerance.

In the last fifteen years, the only plots against the government have come from the Right: Prince Valerio Borghese's farcical conspiracy in 1971; a plot to capture Rumor, the Prime Minister, with his Cabinet in 1974; Gelli's "conspiracy" of the P2 (see p. 216) most of whose members were Right-wing, while Gelli himself was an ex-Fascist.

Much of the violent provocation has also come from this direction:

there were Black Brigades as well as Red. However, whereas the Red Brigades were firmly rejected by the Left-wing parties, Black Brigades seem to have had some sort of link with the Fascists and also with the army and the secret service. The object of both groups seems to have been the same: to create such confusion that government would disintegrate. But, whereas the Red Brigades were anarchist rather than Left-wing, the Blacks were almost certainly thinking in terms of a Fascist takeover. In the tangle of the Italian political underworld, it is difficult to be sure of anything. However, it does seem that Right-wing groups were responsible for the twelve people killed by a bomb on the Italicus, the Florence-Bologna express, in 1974, the horrifying massacre caused by an explosion in the waiting-room at Bologna station, where over eighty people were killed in 1980, and the bomb on the Naples-Milan train which killed twelve people in December 1984.

More than two and a half million people voted for the MSI in the election of June 1983, and it is the fourth party in Italy after the Christian Democrats, the Communists and the Socialists. In percentage terms its votes jumped a point and a half to 6.8 per cent – roughly the equivalent of the electoral support Mussolini had in 1922 when he took power. However, the vote for the MSI has fluctuated round this figure for the last twenty years. In fact, in the long run it has actually gone down. At the regional elections of 1971, the MSI vote jumped for a time to 13.9 per cent. Part of their backing is a reaction to disorder, or the threat of it; part, also, a transference by the Right wing of the Christian Democrats when they fear their party is going too far to the Left.

However, the neo-Fascists are still in the wilderness, certainly internationally. Theirs is the only political party which is not invited to the Queen's birthday party at the British Embassy in Rome, and is one of the few entities held in equal disgust by both Americans and Russians. In Italy itself, the MSI has never formed part of a national governing coalition, and the riots in Genoa and other parts of Italy in 1960, when Tambroni's government relied on neo-Fascist votes in Parliament to stay in power, has served as a warning which is still heeded. Indeed the Christian Democrat tendency, ever since those days, has been to form Centre-Left governments.

Thus, despite the fact that one in fifteen Italian voters support it, MSI influence is minimal. It appears very little in the press. It has a persuasive and eloquent leader, Almirante, who was a volunteer in the Ethiopian War, and joined Mussolini after he formed his German-dominated Republic of Saló in northern Italy in 1943. However, Almirante is now seventy and no charismatic successor seems on the horizon. Although he has shed many of his former extreme views, and stated when the bomb went off on the Italicus that he had nothing to do with it, it is difficult to see how the party can ever be drawn into national government in the near future. Its heritage is too daunting, even if its period of power before and during the war is being examined more dispassionately.

PARTY POLITICS

A trade union leader in Palermo gave me a vivid description of how politics function, particularly in Southern Italy.

A politician sits in his office and is rung up by someone who wants a favour. So he remembers a person who might help, and rings him up. This man replies that of course he will do everything he can. But he himself is in difficulties and he wonders if the politician can do something in return. The politician agrees and rings up yet another person to see what he can do. This contact proves fruitful, so he calls back to give the good news to the second man, who therefore agrees to do what he can for the first man, whom the politician then rings up, proudly, to tell him that what he wanted is possible.

This process can be elaborated endlessly. It goes on most of the time, so a politician cannot really get any work done. However, he is at least achieving one thing: everyone will remember how he has helped them. Not only they but also their sons, daughters, uncles, aunts, parents and grandparents – not to mention innumerable cousins and close friends who will now, almost certainly, vote for him in the next election.

Gathering votes like this is more productive, said the trade union leader, than doing something for a thousand people whom you don't know and who will not be grateful in the same way. It means that everything is kept on a personal basis and communities are much closer. But in the process, politicians are elected who are not implementing policy but spending all their time helping individuals.

Given that institutions don't work well, this is the only way of organizing society – which means that institutions work even less effectively and become sources of favours: jobs to people who may not be good administrators but are friends of friends; funds for projects which may not be needed but please influential people; contracts to those who are powerful, or will generate money for the party.

In Italy, almost everyone seems to have a political party. The newspapers they carry are almost badges: *Il Popolo* for the Christian Democrats, *L'Unità* for the Communists, *Avanti!* for the Socialists. Their Their influence percolates everywhere. In June 1984, there was a row about the party composition of the board of RAI, the national television network; and in an interview with the British magazine *Nature* (May 12 1983) Professor Leonardi talked about La Scala: "The members of the board are all representatives of the political parties, to the point that when they enrol the musicians they ask what political party they belong to – yes, the players!" Even the governors of the newly founded Italian Association of Sociology are divided into 30 per cent Christian Democrat, 30–40 per cent from the Left, and the remainder from what are known as "lay parties".* Proportions reflect roughly the percentages won during the elections, whether national, regional or communal. Bargaining goes on, also taking time: "You can have more representatives on the Biennale if we can have a few more on the Festival Committee." More "jobs for the boys", contracts for printing and design to friends and relatives.

It seems incredibly complicated to an outsider but in its way it works. It has gone on so long that patterns have been established. Also, it is a form of wider family co-operation, which Italians are used to. As the trade union leader remarked, it is personal. How can one stand alone in a cold world?

At grass-roots level, relations between parties can be vitriolic. I remember a poster on the wall of a Communist union of co-operatives in Rome which ironically advised people to vote Christian Democrat. There was a picture of Cain, and underneath: "Vote DC because we are all brothers." Then Herod and the Massacre of the Innocents: "Vote DC because we know how to get on with the Young!" Then, a picture of an atomic explosion and below: "Vote DC and you will be secure!"

At the top level, though, there seems to be more understanding, at least until recently. Arrigo Levi, the well-known Italian author and political commentator, told me that the party system in Italy was like a pyramid, with people very far away from one another at the base, but close together at the top. At this level, political conflict is often like Barzini's description of the way battles were conducted in the Middle Ages, when armies with knights in resplendent armour, riding splendidly caparisoned horses, wheeled and feinted like flocks of bright

* Called *Laici* in Italian, they include all the parties who are neither Christian Democrat nor on the Left: Republicans, Liberals, MSI, Radicals and Social Democrats.

birds. At the end of the day, they would retire with not a man killed, to negotiate an agreement which usually resolved their differences.

Levi puts this down to the need for consensus. There has been so much polarization: regions; North and South; agricultural interests; industrial influence; the Church. Then the threat of a Fascist revival, of possible revolution from the Left, of the Red Brigades, the Mafia. If these divisions had been allowed to express themselves in bitter party conflict between an established majority Government and a real Opposition, the country might well have broken up. As it is, through its present system Italy has had the most stable government in Europe since the war, with great continuity, whatever the crises. There may have been forty-four different governments since 1945, but most of them have consisted of the same people and parties, with the result that there has not been that see-saw typical of Britain, as one government undoes the previous one's achievement at regular intervals.* The Italian government's apparent ineffectiveness may have been its strength, ensuring reform through compromise.

Even the many parties have a certain continuity, going back historically to well before the war. The Republicans are the heirs of Garibaldi and Mazzini, of those who wanted a United Italy but without a monarchy. Now they are practical, down to earth, "good housekeepers", resembling one of those "solid" parties in Holland or Scandinavia. They are in favour, as one of their leaders, Giorgio La Malfa, told me, of a balanced budget, of a definite framework for treating with trade unions, of tax reform so that everyone pays. At the same time, government expenditure should be limited. As might be expected, they are strongest in the North, and Spadolini, their leader, won a triumph over the Socialists in Milan at the European elections of June 1984.

The Liberals represent those who ruled from 1871 to 1922. They represent the haute bourgeoisie, and are more to the Right than one would expect from their name: "All Gucci handbags and alligator shoes", as one person remarked. One of their leaders, Aldo Bozzi, heads a committee for the reform of the Constitution, which may or may not come off.

Another party, the Social Democrats, split off from the Socialists in the 1950s and is now further to the Right, although it is even more

---

* Gore Vidal puts it well when he writes: "for most Italians, a political party is never a specific programme, it is a flag, a liturgy, the sound of a trombone practising in the night." (*The New York Review of Books*, October 25, 1979.)

difficult to define Left and Right in Italy than elsewhere. As has been seen, parties are really tribes. Their object is to survive and exercise influence. Their underlying belief is that politics is the pursuit of power, whatever may be done with it. When Goria, the Christian Democrat Minister of the Treasury, complained that his job didn't allow him to keep up friendships and that he neglected his family, a popular journalist retorted that he should be put in a straitjacket. He must be mad to make such remarks when he had all that control and the delight of signing cheques for billions of lire!

The Radicals are the jokers in the pack. Only Italy's system of proportional representation would allow such an eccentric party to exist. Founded by an eloquent showman, Pannella, they are what might metaphorically be called a torch to illuminate areas of political activity which have not been examined before. The party is highly dramatic. To protest against what he considered restrictions on his freedom of speech, Pannella spent a whole twenty-minute slot on television, gagged, with his hands bound. His party campaigns for idealistic good causes: for the prohibition of hunting, for giving billions of lire to developing countries, for prison reform. In the latter cause it has welcomed people like Toni Negri and Enzo Tortora, who were in prison for a long time without trial, as Radical Deputies (see p. 237). Despite disagreement from ex-addicts, Pannella has recently been campaigning to give out heroin free as a means of eliminating Mafia profits.

The Christian Democrats, known usually as the DC, is the party that has dominated Italian politics and government since 1945. It originates in the Catholic opposition to government, which was a *sine qua non* of Italian unification when the papacy was deprived of its secular possessions. Called the Popolari, it became a party after the First World War, founded by a Sicilian priest, Don Sturzo. Backed by the Allies after the Second World War as a balance to Communism, it had the advantage of being able to ensure Marshall Aid – a poster in 1948 showed a loaf of bread with a knife cutting away half of it, if the Communists won. Priests all over Italy told their congregations to vote Christian Democrat and those who worked actively for the Left were excommunicated. As the government in power, they have also had the resources to offer rewards and jobs to their followers.

"Please! We are not Conservatives!" emphasized a Christian Democrat. In fact they do represent every shade of opinion, as only Italian parties can. They include workers – they have their own trade union, the CISL – bishops, socialist-minded supporters and others who are almost Fascist. However, very few people who are against the Church vote for them.

The DC's contribution to modern Italy has been immense. Arrigo Levi sums it up in his *The DC in an Italy which is Changing*:

> The DC has been Italy for more than thirty years. The DC has meant the "choice of civilization" that is Western European, transatlantic; the DC was the "economic miracle" and the great State industries; the DC was the Welfare State *all'italiana*, spendthrift, generous, badly administered. The DC was also Italy of the scandals, and of "the palace", attacked for its arrogance, its dark labyrinths of power in a country become sceptical and diffident. The DC was the "comfortable" Italy of corporate favours and the abyss of the budget deficit, of galloping inflation and, finally, of economic crisis. The DC was also Aldo Moro, the main target of terrorism, and also the principal barrier to it.

To me, the DC gives an impression of dusty benevolence. As one of its members said to me, they have been impresarios, masters of compromise with other parties for so long that they have lost their edge. You go to their headquarters in Piazza del Gesù, in a big, old palazzo, and wait endlessly for an interview in a broad corridor with great gilded mirrors on the wall, with sun and wistaria coming through the big window. You note an air of genteel shabbiness, of neglect, while fat, prosperous-looking men also sit waiting. One Christian Democrat told me that because they are Catholic, life after death is more important to them, and they find it difficult to be hard, materialistic, efficient. As they stem from the Church, they have an intricate, secretive organization, a lack of real policy apart from the vague sense that humanity is there to be helped, and ultimately saved. Because they are Italian, they are not clerical puritans but also bon viveurs, tolerant of corruption, sinners at Confession, but always with hopes of redemption.

Their Secretary, Ciriaco De Mita, is an intellectual from Avellino in the South. He has a sad, white face with dark eyes and a sloping bald head, and always looks worried and distraught, like Humpty Dumpty about to fall off the wall. Since he was elected in 1982, he has tried to introduce a new policy of "rigore", the same kind of hard, realistic approach as the Republicans recommend.

In the elections of June 1983, not only he but almost everyone in Italy had a shock. The party which ever since 1948 had gained about 40 per cent of the vote suddenly plunged by 5.4 per cent to 32.9 per cent, losing one in seven of their voters, with only three points above the

Communists. In a country with a different system, this would not have been so significant, but in Italy an era seemed to have ended. The DCs, as one of them said, were no longer a government. They had become a minority party.

What had happened? Roberto Formigoni, leader of a dynamic Catholic group, the Movimento Popolare, said that it was partly because there had been little real electoral organization and also that the DC was no longer closely associated with Catholicism. Since the defeats over divorce and abortion, Party and Church had drifted apart. De Mita's policy was now no different from that of the lay parties. "People don't vote only for political reasons," Formigoni said to Arrigo Levi, "but for culture, for ideals." Others disagreed: religious feeling was changing in Italy; to many people the DCs were still too much of a Church party, and not "modern" enough.

Of the reports from provincial secretaries, thirty out of sixty-eight felt a principal cause was "attribution to the DC of responsibility for the economic crisis and for misgovernment". Another twenty-eight thought that there was "insufficient emphasis on anti-communism". Certainly, the spectre of the Communist alternative has always been a potent electoral asset for the DCs, but it has diminished over the years. In June 1983, a poll showed that only 21.3 per cent felt that the Italian Communists were similar to those beyond the Iron Curtain. "Italians don't like Moscow," ran the heading of this report in *La Repubblica*, "but they're no longer afraid of the Communist Party."

The recession has meant fewer resources for *clientelismo*, or political patronage, which has always been a principal creator of votes for the DCs. Also, since the death of the Dalla Chiesas in Palermo (see p. 180), the belief that the DC is linked with criminal elements has become more widespread among the people, who have become increasingly horrified at the whole Mafia phenomenon. In fact, this suspicion found some confirmation in the arrest in 1984 of Victor Ciancimino, who was DC mayor of Palermo in 1970 and is charged with links with the Mafia.

The great DC fear in 1983, though, was that this was only a beginning, and that in successive elections the party would shrink and shrink. Fortunately for them, this did not happen at the European elections of 1984, although the Communists actually overtook them by half a point – perhaps partly on account of the sympathy evoked when their leader, Berlinguer, collapsed and died when speaking at a meeting in Verona, and was given a moving farewell ceremony in Rome attended by over a million people. Indeed, by the local elections of May, 1985, the DC seemed to have recovered their votes.

However, the worst effect of the 1983 election for the DCs, was that the Socialist leader, Craxi, insisted on being Prime Minister of the new government as a condition of his party joining the coalition. Without his 73 seats in the Chamber of Deputies and 38 in the Senate, the DCs were not strong enough to create a majority, and had to give in.

For the last few years Craxi has been the strong man of Italian politics. A play on his Christian name, Bettino, with Benito is often made. He shares with De Gaulle the distinction of being the protagonist of the old joke about deciding on a suitable burial place. "What about Jerusalem?" someone asks. "Oh, no – the Israelis will charge me too much and I shall only be there for three days!"

Piccoli, the president of the DC, talked to me about their dilemma. "This is one of the most difficult periods for us since the war," he said. The danger was that Craxi would gain votes at the European elections. He had already achieved a lot, splitting the unions and tackling the whole question of reducing the inflation-linked wage increase ("Scala Mobile") head on. On TV he gave the impression of being a strong man. "Italians like a chief," said Piccoli, "and if they admire him, they wear his uniform." The DCs couldn't get rid of Craxi. "People ask 'Where is the DC?' We are just at the window watching!" In the report of their recent Congress the Socialists gave only ten lines to their collaboration with the DC. But at least they hadn't hissed at them as they had at Communist leaders.

In fact, Craxi's vote at the European elections in 1984 went up by only 1.9 per cent to the small percentage of 11.9. It may seem strange that a Socialist Prime Minister should attack the salaries of the workers and disrupt the unions. However, Craxi calls his policy *decisionismo*. He is, like so many, pragmatic rather than dominated by inherited ideas. In a cartoon about the choice of a Prime Minister, De Mita was shown saying: "Well, rather than give the post to a Socialist, let's give it to Craxi."

Indeed, Socialism like so many creeds in Italy is difficult to be precise about. In Arezzo, I asked the Socialist mayor to give me a definition, and he said they always encouraged "active" economic activity, which benefited and involved the community, rather than "passive". As an example, he talked about the setting up of a factory. Land was needed but its owner would obviously try to sell it at the maximum price, which would have to be recouped by increasing the cost of goods which the factory would ultimately produce. The DCs would accept this. The Socialists, however, would expropriate the land, pay little compensation and give it cheaply to the factory so that costs and therefore the price of goods produced would be lower. In other words, they would reduce the price of industrial production at the expense of the landowner. They would, nevertheless, be getting one form of free enterprise to subsidize another.

The previous Socialist leader, Francesco de Martino, said in 1984 that nothing remained of the party he knew except its defects and, as Campbell Page reported in the *Guardian*, "Socialists see his [Craxi's] leadership as nothing but a triumph of style, and fear that Italian Socialism has become nothing more than Mr Craxi's tenure of power."

Nevertheless, at the Congress in May 1984 Craxi was acclaimed by his followers, and there was no opposition. Despite the insignificant increase in his vote in the subsequent European elections, it is possible that the Socialists will still be the beneficiaries of DC confusion. The Communist Party, too, is in a period of change and it looks as though the traditional, organic approach which has achieved so much, but left many problems unsolved in the last forty years, may be at an end.

THE COMMUNISTS

The Communist Party in Italy used to be known as "The other Church", with its "Holy See" and "Pope" in Moscow, with its part in a world organization, and its belief, reinforced by the "Holy Writ" of Marx, that it could not fail. Abroad, it was regarded as similar to any other Communist Party, except that it was the biggest in Europe. Over the years, its possible assumption of power seemed a nightmare for NATO and the Western Alliance: Italy would enter the Russian sphere of influence, with disastrous effects on the independence of neighbouring Yugoslavia and the balance of power in the Mediterranean. It would also mean the end of Italian democracy, Italy's adhesion to the Warsaw pact, and, probably, the eclipse of the Papacy.

In fact, as with so many things in Italy, the word "Communism" now means something very different. Italians have voted for it for years not because they all subscribe to Soviet Communism but because, since the war, it has been the only powerful party of protest. I remember an Italian secretary of mine who typified this. She was gentle and traditional, but was disgusted with the inefficiency and corruption of Italy in the 1950s. I used to call her teasingly, "the Conservative Communist".

In 1921, Bordiga, a leading Socialist, split the party conference at Leghorn and absconded with a minority of followers to form the Communist Party. From the beginning it was an intellectual as well as a workers' movement, partly because it was inspired by Gramsci, a remarkable political philosopher who seems to be less well-known outside Italy than perhaps he should be.

Gramsci was born in a small town in Sardinia in 1891. When he was four, he fell down some steep stairs and injured his back. A girl working in the house used him as an excuse to go and see a doctor with whom she was in love, travelling over bumpy roads in an ox-cart, which did him no good. As a result, Gramsci grew up a hunchback, and was so sickly that a coffin was kept ready for him in the house until he was fourteen.

Sardinia seems to have been the breeding place of Communist leaders: Togliatti, who led the party after the war, came from Sassari in the north, and Berlinguer, who was General Secretary from 1972 to 1984, was a Sardinian. Perhaps this was because the island was one of the most oppressed and backward areas of Italy. Feudalism was only abolished between 1836 and 1840 and many of the lords were still Spanish – a heritage of the time before 1720 when it was part of the Spanish Empire.

Even as late as 1950 1.8 per cent of proprietors owned 44 per cent of the land, and in 1961 a whole village was put up for sale by the inhabitants because they could no longer support themselves.

Gramsci tried to escape the misery around him, what he later called "the sewer of my past", by study. He went to high school in Cagliari, and starved himself in order to stay there. As he wrote later: "I began by not having coffee in the morning, then put off having lunch until later and later, so that I could do without having supper."

From the *liceo*, Gramsci won a scholarship to the university of Turin awarded by the King to celebrate the fiftieth anniversary of the Unification of Italy. Much of Gramsci's philosophy came from these beginnings. Thus he had no idealistic view of the "people" as such, common to middle-class radicals from Robespierre to Tony Benn. His motivation sprang from the miseries he had seen around him, and a desire to create systems which could relieve them. As Garuglieri wrote in his *Memories of Gramsci*: "to be mocked at because of his deformity developed in him a great love for all those who suffer unjustly, and the need to succour them drove him to sacrifice himself generously for their cause."

At the same time, his extensive studies in Turin convinced him that "every revolution has been preceded by hard critical thinking, the diffusion of culture". To him, a revolutionary was a teacher. As an outstanding Marxist scholar he knew enough to make comparisons with other philosophies and his historical sense led him away from generally accepted beliefs about Marxism. Thus, economic laws are not immutable but laws of tendency, which depend also on the environment and the historical development of different countries. This implied that Italy could evolve in a different way from Russia and much of the dogma of Marxism he regarded as inappropriate.

Later, Gramsci was arrested and imprisoned by the Fascists. During this time, ill with consumption, he wrote the *Prison Notebooks*, which expressed his thoughts about everything from politics to "Notes for the Study of Grammar". Gramsci died in the prison hospital in 1937, a few days before he was due to be released. His notebooks were published between 1948 and 1951 and, as Jonathan Steinberg wrote in *The London Review of Books*, "he gave posthumously a lustre to the PCI [Partito Comunista Italiano] which no other Communist Party in the world had been able to equal". This was continued by Togliatti, the first post-war Secretary General of the party, called "The Professor" by Stalin, who said of him: "He is a good theoretician. He writes good political articles." For twenty years after the war the Italian Communists had almost a monopoly of the "intellectuals" – whether writers, theatre or film directors – and it is still difficult to find one now who is neither Socialist nor Communist. Typical of their cultural commitment is *Rinascita*, as serious an intellectual magazine as any in the West. After Berlinguer's death in 1984, Alessandro Natta, an ex-schoolmaster who has himself edited *Rinascita* and can make a speech in excellent Latin, was appointed Secretary General.

Since 1945, when a small cadre of 5,000 grew to a popular political party of over two million members, policy has rarely been one of confrontation. They were part of the government until 1947, which meant compromising initially with the monarchy and, throughout, with the Church. Since then, they have been in opposition. However, unlike Communist parties in countries nearer Russia they have never tried to stage a coup. In 1948, Togliatti was wounded in an assassination attempt, and workers throughout the country declared a strike within a few hours. However, as he was wheeled to the operating theatre, Togliatti told his companions: "Keep calm and don't lose your heads!" The mass movement was contained.

In Parliament, also, the Communists have only occasionally been obstructive. One occasion was in 1953 when the so-called "Legge Truffa" (fraudulent law) distorted democracy by proposing that a party with a majority should automatically get more seats. In Parliament, any deputy can speak for forty-five minutes, with the result that it is easy to block everything for weeks if not months with the two hundred odd deputies which the Communists have. The other obstruction was more recent: in 1984, when they challenged Craxi's move to limit the inflation-linked wage increases (Scala Mobile).

This they did because they felt the measure had been imposed rather than discussed with them. For several years the Communists have become used to sharing in government decisions although they are in opposition, largely through the way laws can be passed in committee. Dr Chiodi, the Parliamentary Secretary of Virginio Rognoni, leader of the DCs in the House of Deputies, put it very well when he told me: "At one table, the Communists are in opposition. But at another they are part of a team." During the worst crisis of the 1970s, Berlinguer, who was then Secretary General of the party, supported the government closely. When Moro was kidnapped, the Communists were firm in refusing to compromise and in rejecting Red Brigade demands. In 1977, they were almost brought into the government which would have meant an extreme of "consensus", with Lamb and Lion* lying down together – inconceivable in any other democratic country in peacetime.

Now, they have gradually broken their links with the Soviet Union. They accepted the invasion of Hungary in 1956 but demurred at that of Czechoslovakia in 1968. The invasion of Afghanistan and, particularly, the moves against Solidarity in Poland brought the ultimate disillusionment. In 1981, Berlinguer, the Secretary General, had already suggested that the Soviet Revolution of 1917 had outlived its validity as a model for Eastern and Western Europe. In the Congress of 1983, he attacked the imposition of martial law in Poland which he said "struck at the essential principles of the Communist and Socialist concept of things". The *strappo* as it is called, or wrench away from the Soviet Union, was now complete, and it looks as though it will last. An amendment at the Congress: "We believe the conditions exist to inject vigour into the thrust which flowed out of the October Revolution" got the support of only 5 per cent of delegates.

The party statutes have now been re-written to include the following heterodoxy: "It [the PCI] is aware that the Christian conscience of the contemporary world can become the stimulus for a struggle for the socialist transformation of society." Berlinguer's widow is a fervent Catholic, as is Natta's wife, and in 1983 Berlinguer on a visit to the Church of St Francis in Assisi was invited to lunch with the friars and was photographed standing at grace. In Arezzo, the bishop told me that

* Who is Lamb and who is Lion is difficult to determine.

the Church now got on better with the Communists.

Berlinguer and, after him, Natta have committed themselves to what they call *la terza via* (the third way). This is essentially pragmatic. In an interview Berlinguer stated he was in favour of the rich paying for their medical prescriptions. This is an example of the "rationality" with which the Communists regard every area. It is important to get away from personal interests and graft, and decide on things which work efficiently for the whole community. As examples of what has previously been done, he talked of "pharaonic" motorways used by few cars, of hospitals built without considering population needs, because only individuals or small groups benefited.

A Communist councillor I went to see in Perugia said that now the party is opening its doors to any group of anti-capitalistic protesters: feminists, socialists, even Catholics. So many concepts are changing. Workers now are not just those in factories or on the land. There is a big growth in technicians in modern Italy. White or blue-collar workers must be considered, and the party has to adapt to this. People are also much better off. It is difficult now to talk of "the proletariat". In foreign relations, Communists are now in favour of the EEC and NATO but, in the case of the latter, they are also working to make it out of date.

In Rome, I went to the inconspicuous building near the Chamber of Deputies, off the narrow Via Uffizi del Vicario, where most of the political parties have their offices cheek by jowl, often sharing a floor. I went to see Napoletano, one of the leading Communists who has often been proposed as party leader, but whose "liberalism" has been a disadvantage. As his name suggests, Napoletano comes from Naples, and he has close links with England: when I met him, he had just returned from a conference in Cambridge.

He has long been in favour of softening the party line and of forming an alliance of the Left through co-operation with the Socialists. "There should be no barriers!" he said. He was also against the lines of demarcation between Communists and Socialists. "It's necessary for everyone on the Left to rally to progressive causes in a new United Europe," he said. "Old ideologies should be dispensed with. Flexibility is essential."

Planning too, he maintained, had to be more professional: the managerial situation as well as the workers' needs should be considered. He accepted that private initiative could produce a surplus which benefited the workers. However, greater control was essential in the challenges of today such as reducing unemployment and the development of advanced technology.

It was also important to defend the achievements of the past, such as the Welfare State. Priority must be given to ensuring that there was no de-industrialization, and the transition to the new computerized society must be watched carefully. Many reforms were needed. Thus, on pensions it was ridiculous to subsidize bogus invalids in order to sustain the poorer communities of the South. Much better to use the money to ensure that all workers got 80 per cent of their salaries when they retired.

While many of his ideas naturally assume a dominant role for the State, Napolitano's view is essentially pragmatic, up-to-date, and seems reconcilable with any modern Socialist party. Few of his recommendations are rooted in atavistic Socialist ideas from the past.

"Are people afraid of the Communists, in Italy?" I asked.

"Some –"

"Why?"

"They're afraid we're not really democratic."

"And are you?"

"Of course. Look at Florence or Naples. We've lost our majority there. But we haven't hung on to power. In a Communist-dominated city like Bologna we're more tolerant of opposition than in a city where the DC have a majority, like Palermo. One barrier is that people are afraid we're still linked to Russia. Italians know nothing of the Russians. They've had nothing to do with them since the Crimean War, except for the veterans who were there in the last war, fighting on the side of the Germans. They only want to go there for hunting or to smuggle diamonds. Yet everyone would like to go to America!"

On the question of democracy, I later talked to Signor Tucci, Communist President of the Regione in Emilia. "People say you're wolves in sheep's clothing," I said, "and that if you get power you'll be just like any other Communist party in Rumania or Czechoslovakia."

"Well they're wrong! Haven't we been part of the democratic government for the last forty years? We don't bribe our way to power like the DCs!"

"Aren't you likely to lose votes as people get richer? Bologna is supposed to be the richest city in Italy."

"Yes it is. But, most factory owners or shop-keepers here are workers who have made good – or the sons of one! My father was a peasant who became Communist because he worked as a *mezzadro* [see p. 33]. I was brought up on his patch of land. Politics runs in families, too. And now the people here are grateful to us for what we've achieved for them since we came to power in 1945!"

In Naples, the situation was different. The local elections of November 1983 had reduced the Communist majority from 31.5 per cent to 27 per cent with a loss of five seats. There was no mayor. The government in Rome had sent down a commissioner to take over as there was deadlock between the parties and therefore no way of forming a coalition.

I talked to the ex-mayor, Valenzi, who is also a well-known painter. Born in Tunisia in 1911, he had flown to Naples in 1944 disguised in the stolen uniform of an English officer, for at that time the French were doing all they could to prevent Communists from coming to Italy. When he arrived in a Naples which in his own words was "a city of great cultural traditions, but full of ruins, lacerated with gaping wounds, so dirty that it was agonizing", he found everyone going round like clowns with white, powdered faces because the Americans had sprayed DDT everywhere. This was the city he adopted. In 1975, when he was sixty-four, he became mayor.

He seemed depressed. Once he had had a splendid office in the town hall. Now he sat huddled in the Communist headquarters, wrapped in a mackintosh. People treated him with tenderness. Downstairs, they had spoken to him with gentle concern. His one secretary, who shared the office, gave him a kiss on the cheek as she left.

We talked about State industry. How far did he and his party believe in nationalization? "In Italy, State industry doesn't work. It's just a vassalage of the State. Here only small industries are successful!" What of Naples? How far had he applied a Communist policy? "Our policy is to clear up problems as efficiently as possible. Yet there are countless difficulties: pollution, defiance of building permits, traffic, the way sewage goes into the sea. I wanted to build a garage for 27,000 cars outside the city, but that was sabotaged. The purification equipment will soon be ready but it is already out of date. There are too many personal economic interests behind it. As there were in building houses after the earthquake in areas in the middle of the city which once were green and open."

It was difficult being mayor of Naples. One could make plans but carrying them out was another matter. I heard from other sources that there had been a scandal with the transport system, where false invoices for repairs had cheated the Commune out of millions of lire. "You can be an honest Communist," had said my informant, "but that doesn't mean that your administration is clean!" The Communists had been the largest party in the Commune when Valenzi became mayor but with only 41 per cent of the total votes.

"Don't you think, though, that Communists have lost their identity? Now their policy is not very different from that of any Socialist Democratic party. Yet they still have to suffer from all the negative associations of the word 'Communism'."

"Perhaps."

"Do you think they should change their name?"

"That would be difficult. We'd lose the votes of those who have worked for our Communist Party for years."

Both the giants who kept the peace for so long seem, then, to be weakening at the knees. In the European elections of 1984 the Communists may have become the largest party by half a per cent. However, since their peak of 34.4 per cent in 1976, they have lost almost 5 per cent – just as the DCs did in 1983. The *strappo* with Russia may have made the fall in support less dramatic but at the same time it has obscured the true nature of the party, just as the loosening of the bonds with the Church has blurred the image of the DC. At the same time, they have the slurs of the past and their own conditioned reflexes to contend with. In the Communist fight against missiles, they still talk openly of the West disarming. I remember in Bologna two street banners, one from the Communists attacking Cruise missiles, and another from the DCs attacking SS 20s. When they talk of "imperialism" Communists still mean the West, despite their condemnation of Afghanistan and General Jaruzelski.

Now, the Communists have as little chance of entering government as before. A cartoon, previous to the 1983 election, shows Berlinguer leaning against a wall and saying: "Vote for the PCI. I can assure you we will not win!" Napolitano's call for a union of the Left is unlikely to come about so long as Craxi heads the Socialists, because it is inconceivable that the Communists, unlike the DC, would allow him to be prime minister of their coalition. What has changed is that the PCI is no longer consulted as before, no longer regarded as a party whose agreement should be sought. As a result, they are more aggressive, as their blocking the vote on limiting inflation-linked wages shows.

This is a pity in many ways, as Communists seem to be the most honest and dedicated of Italian politicians – excepting perhaps the Republicans. In 1979 they could go to the country in the elections with the slogan "We have clean hands". They have never been involved in any of the major scandals: the P2, Sindona, Calvi. They have always been uncompromisingly against the Mafia and terrorism, and it was a Communist Deputy, La Torre, who proposed the law which now permits the investigation and confiscation of Mafia funds.

Meanwhile, it is the little parties in the middle, which are not ideological, that are making progress. It will probably take time for them to make significant headway, as parties in Italy are communities, and the floating voter is a new phenomenon. However, as both parties of consensus lose strength under a prime minister who is ambitious and belongs to neither group, battles are beginning to be waged, not just with feints and manoeuvres, but with real fighting.

An example of this is the way Andreotti, the Grand Old Man of Italian politics, a leading figure for forty years, was accused of corruption in Parliament in November 1984, largely through Communist instigation. This contrasts vividly with Andreotti forming a government in July 1976 only because the Communists refrained from vetoing him in a vote of confidence.

According to Arrigo Levi, now that the "years of lead" are over, the Red Brigade defeated, the Mafia more exposed, the emigrants to the North better absorbed, there is less polarization and therefore less need for consensus, more likelihood of conflict.

Of course, given the weakness of the governmental system and the appalling inadequacy of the bureaucracy which is responsible for putting decisions into practice, how much does this matter anyway? Government in Italy is like the clash of waves on the surface of the sea, its movement caused not so much by its own momentum as by deep currents and the buffeting of the wind.

BUREAUCRACY

"We are an adrenal race," said Enzo Marrotta, who has a job in a bank in Aquila. "Life in Italy is so exhausting. Every situation has to be negotiated. It's like living in a sagging tent without a pole in a gale: you have to hold it up yourself, or it collapses."

I tried to get to London from Turin by air for Easter. There was a queue for all destinations which never moved because the people in front were handing in the luggage and tickets of some dozen friends. From behind, a small blonde lady managed to squeeze herself in front of me. "Excuse me, signora," I protested, "I was before you." She shook her head and ignored me disdainfully.

The last call for London was announced. I shouted down to the registration clerk that five of us were going to London and it looked as if we would miss our flight. So he gave us priority. The blonde lady insisted, though, that she was first, although she was going on a later plane to Milan.

We were given boarding cards and rushed frenziedly past the people waiting for passport inspection, only to be told by an angry policeman to get to the end of the queue. Yet when we explained that we would miss our plane and that it wasn't our fault, the people in the queue smiled, and waved us to the front.

As a result, we arrived just in time. When, however, I got to my numbered seat, I discovered that it was occupied by a large, red-haired man. I asked him to move, which he did, turning someone else out of his seat, who disrupted a couple who in turn went off to find their seats, so that half the passengers on the plane had subsequently to move – which made me feel ridiculous.

One problem in Italy is that no one trusts organization. Because of this, the people in front of our queue had helped their friends. The same applied to the little blonde lady's initiative. The queue for passport inspection on the other hand had helped us because they were not in a hurry, and they knew what it was like to be obstructed by an official. Finally, it had been a very English mistake of mine to insist on my numbered seat. I had presumed that it would be an advantage to stick to the system. The Italians, however, presumed there was no system and that, if there were, it would not work.

In Italy, the idea that any official organization is there to serve the citizen is not only unfamiliar – it is laughable. That civil servants should ever be called "civil" or "servants" and actually sign letters "Your obedient servant" – as they did in Britain some twenty years ago – is additionally perplexing. For one thing, bureaucracy in Italy was for long centuries the instrument of foreign autocracies and, for twenty recent years, it was a means of enforcing Mussolini's dictatorship.

For another, people join the bureaucracy not to do a good job but mainly because they want stable employment where little hard work is expected, and where you can therefore earn your living in other ways. After all, in government offices in Rome they only work from 8 a.m. till 2 p.m. Status is also part of the job because you can withhold favours if you are not treated with respect – while the bureaucracy is so dense and tangled that any complaints will usually be lost in the undergrowth.

Government employees think in terms of rights not obligations: a friend of mine who was attached to the Italian army at the end of the war told me that he had never eaten such good food as in the officers' mess. However, when he visited the NCOs and the privates, he realized why: their food was atrocious. When he mentioned this to his fellow officers, they looked surprised at his objections. "But why else should we be officers?" said one. This may be some time ago but the same attitudes apply.

In his *From Caesar to the Mafia*, Luigi Barzini comments that too many books on Italy, particularly those by foreigners, pay no attention to bureaucracy, which he regards as one of the principal keys to understanding the country. Because of the innate conservatism of bureaucrats, Italy, he believes, has been given stability and protected from extremism from the Left, particularly in 1919 and 1945. As far as efficiency is concerned, he compares them to a vast menu promising everything from *antipasto* to *zabaglione* in a restaurant without cooks or kitchen.

He puts much of the blame on traditions of administration handed down from the Church, as does Paul Hofmann in his *Rome*: "The leisurely bumbling of the Roman Civil Service is in part a legacy from the age-old work habits of the Papal Curia, which itself is heir to the majestic slowness and legal quibbling that characterized the administrative machinery of the Byzantine and Roman Emperors."

Hofmann gives an example of a girl, Norma, employed in the Industry Ministry who in fact uses her office and time to study for her degree in medicine. Because her mother is lonely at home, she brings her in to sit in a corner of the office, where she knits. No one else does anything much, except go out for coffee or to a private job once they have clocked in. Often, though, they return in the afternoon when anything they do in the office is on overtime.

The only person who really works is known as the *fanatico*, and it is he with his fourteen-hour day who keeps the whole office going. Indeed it is amazing how often in Italy one finds the *fanatico* holding everyone's conscience on his shoulders, whether in schools, in hospitals and universities, or in government offices. Often his motives are a source of perplexity: is he playing father to another family of colleagues? Or does he in fact earn more, although he has no time for lucrative work on the side? Perhaps he really enjoys being the pillar of the establishment and blaming his colleagues for their sloth. I often wonder what would happen if all the *fanatici* in Italy went on strike. Perhaps new ones would arise and take their place, like a bees' hive adjusting the balance of workers and drones.

However, the problem is not only the people who work in the bureaucracy. It is also the way previous autocracies have emphasized the need to control everything. *Controllare* and *sistemare* (to organize) are among the common Italian verbs. Mussolini said it was impossible to govern Italy. Organization is based on mistrust and a presumption that

Italians are essentially anarchic, when, really, people treated like children behave like them.

As no fewer than three mayors of small towns have explained to me, this is one of the basic reasons for so much delay. Take, for instance, a new project for a municipal building. First the Commune has to be sure that its construction does not violate any law and, second, that it is worth doing. Once this is done, the project has to be approved by the Communal Engineering Department. However, the same process has to be "controlled" at regional level in the same detail, and returned to the Commune with variations. Variations on the variations then have to be sent back to the Regione for approval.

This process can go on for years until, with high inflation, the original costing has to be reconsidered, which may mean starting at the beginning again.

As most universities depend directly on the State, a law has to be passed if any extra staff are appointed to a department, and if a teacher is being subsidized to go on a course abroad, authorization has to be signed by the Minister himself.

An Italian's reaction is interesting when you tell him that the British have no identity cards. At first, he won't or can't believe it. Then he asks: "But how, then ...?" – and stops suddenly when he realizes that he doesn't quite know what he wanted to ask. What he was probably considering was how you know that Englishmen exist, or how they themselves know they exist, if they haven't some piece of paper to prove it. But appreciating that this instinctive reaction is ridiculous, he then probably wants to ask how you "control" people without proof of their identity. How can you be sure that people staying in hotels or being checked by the police are really who they say they are? Then, though, he suddenly realizes that there aren't many occasions when it is helpful to identify yourself, and that in the situations where it would be really valuable, such as robbery, murder, rape or escaping to Switzerland to avoid gaol, the system is not really very effective. He then begins to wonder why identity cards do exist in Italy, unless of course he himself is a bureaucrat, in which case he changes the subject because he knows that they are justified largely because they provide a living for thousands of his colleagues.

In Italy, you have to renew your birth certificate every three months because you might have died in the meantime and someone else might pretend to be you. In order to enrol a child at school you have to obtain a certificate of residence, a certificate describing the numbers and professions of your family, a birth certificate, last year's tax return and a letter from your work-place, stating your hours of employment. All these different documents are obtained from separate offices and must be collected personally. With queues, or rather crowds, it may well take a morning for each of them.

In order to obtain an X-ray, you have to get a certificate from a doctor, go to the local health authority to have it stamped, and then go to another office to pay for the stamp. In order to work as an English teacher, a foreigner has to go to six different offices several times in order to satisfy the requirements. Procedures vary from region to region: in Turin you are not allowed to work until you have permission, but you cannot apply for permission until you are working!

One reason for this is to increase revenue. All dealings with a government department have to be done on what is called a *carta bollata* – a stamped piece of paper. This costs the equivalent of just over a dollar per lined sheet, and will be refused without compensation unless it is written on every other line, with definite margins and without anything crossed out illegibly. The system was introduced by a Duke of Savoy early in the eighteenth century as a form of petition which had to be paid for. Until education for all was started in Italy after the Second World War, it also meant that the large illiterate majority had no possibility of getting in touch with government. In 1982 it brought in no less than the equivalent of a million dollars.

One effect of this diversity, of the need for "control", of the multiplicity of laws, of the checks and balances, is that bureaucrats often do not know whether what they decide is legal or not. I heard an amusing example of this when a friend wanted to send a wallet as a present to her nephew in America. She decided it would be best if she insured it, and in the post office the clerk told her that she shouldn't tie up the parcel with string: it had to be sealed. So she went to three shops, all of which had run out of sealing wax. In the end, she got some from a friend and put two seals on. However, returning to the post office, she was told that was not enough: she had to have no fewer than seven. So she took the parcel home again. Unfortunately, there was hardly room for all the sealing wax, and when she returned to the post office, the clerk told her that she must also put a special seal on the wax, or what proof would there be if the parcel were opened illegally?

By this time, she was furious. However, she complied and finally delivered the packet into the clerk's hands. Two days later, though, the postman delivered a parcel at her home. To her amazement and fury, she discovered it was her nephew's present. The postman told her that the parcel was still not in order, and that it looked as though it never could be, so they thought it best to send it back to her.

My friend decided to complain to the director who, surprisingly, was pleasant and apologetic. He summoned the clerk and told him that he should know that there was a regulation which for some reason stated clearly that insured parcels could not be sent to America. The wallet should be sent as a letter and it was not necessary to register it. Under the director's eyes, the unfortunate clerk was compelled to fetch an envelope, unpack the wallet and place it in the envelope. In the end, the parcel actually arrived.

As everywhere in Italy, the question of which party you belong to is also important in the bureaucracy. Although recruitment is by way of public exams, a job is also a reward for services rendered. It is also a means of supporting party workers, who, paid by the government, will spend a proportion of their time helping those who favoured them.

This sprawling loose labyrinth conceals all sorts of other activities: bribery, for instance. If it is impossible to get anything through rapidly, a citizen is tempted to pay for speed, or create a network of mutual favours. In 1984, Giuseppe Azzaro, the Vice President of the Christian Democrats in Sicily, shocked everyone in an interview in *La Repubblica* by saying that the price of every administrative contract in Sicily is increased by 10–15 per cent to include what is called a *tangente*, or pay off, to officials. As Indro Montanelli pointed out in his newspaper *Il Giornale*, corruption involves party funds as well as individuals: "The single individual when he has scraped together his little hoard of ill-gotten gains, even a big hoard," he writes, "calls a halt to his activities and perhaps even goes into philanthropy. Not so the thief acting by proxy for his party. The Moloch to which he is tributary is never satisfied."

As has already been noted, the party in Italy is like a big family, to which loyalty is owed before the State. Although, unlike Britain, the government grants funds to parties in proportion to votes obtained at the last election, further cash is always needed to satisfy voracious supporters, or finance more votes.

In Italy, it is easy to be reminded of Tolstoy's dilemma: how can you love the whole world while also loving your family?

In most Mediterranean countries, the idea of earning money for a large firm, or a big abstract organization such as the government, and not extracting as much as possible for your nearest, seems cold, almost unnatural.

A lot, also, has to do with whether anything can be done to clean things up. I remember a shopkeeper I know being fined the outrageous sum of one and a half million lire (the equivalent of $700) for failing to report the sign he had placed, four years earlier, outside his shop. When he went along to complain, the official told him that if he brought 300,000 lire, or a fifth of the sum, and gave it to him personally, he would tear up the charge.

What should he have done? In an ideal society, he would have denounced the official, or taped a compromising conversation. This, though, would almost certainly have been countered by others who had the same practices and interests, working in the same office. Public opinion would have been indifferent or, at most, people would have thought him a little mad. He would have made enemies, wasted a lot of time, perhaps have provoked revenge, and all the time he was being given an opportunity to save over a million lire! It may be reprehensible, but it is hardly surprising that he reacted by putting the sum in an envelope and delivering it next day!

Perhaps the increase of scandals in the last few years is a sign that opinion is beginning to turn against dishonesty in the public services. At least it is making Italians shake their heads and produce disapproving noises at actions in which most of them would have participated, or at least taken for granted, ten years ago. Now, at least, magistrates are beginning to charge some of those believed to be corrupt.

Probably this change is a symptom of the country's adaptation to becoming so rapidly the seventh industrial power in the world. Only the Industrial Revolution produced a largely honest civil service in Britain. In Italy people are coming to realize that an industrial society needs a well-run, flexible bureaucracy in support, and that results, not personal gain, are required.

A lot of the corruption comes from the fact that salaries in the bureaucracy are low. It does not make so much difference that pensions give security: since 1979, you can include any years you have worked for a private firm in your pension count, which for women is only nineteen years and twenty-four for men. As you can leave school at fourteen, it means that theoretically you can get a pension when you are under forty – in fact in 1983 the newspapers tried to discover the youngest pensioner and found she was thirty-three!

The immense government deficit must also be demoralizing. One is amazed in the Rome and Milan metros to find that the Italian talent for design seems totally lacking, with bare neon lights, black rubbery floors and drab wall-covering, until one realizes that this is not the product of exuberant Italian enterprise but of local government offices probably full of shuffling, blinkered penny-pinchers.

The total number of government employees, excluding teachers and the armed forces, was precisely 2,712,401 in 1982 – one in eight of the total Italian work-force: roughly a third of the number employed in industry and slightly more than those on the land. Almost four fifths are from the South and it is ironic that the heirs of the conquered Bourbon state now administer United Italy, revenged perhaps for Garibaldi and the defeats inflicted on them by the pale Piedmontese.

Apart from the few *fanatici*, government employees operate lethargically* in a tangled system from which they cannot be dismissed, a system riven by party divisions and corruption. Until recently there was actually a Minister for the Reform of the Bureaucracy, but the post was discontinued as no Hercules was found to clean the Augean stable.

Until the bureaucracy is modernized and reformed, laws will have as much effect as water in a maze of porous irrigation channels, and the Italian government will continue to resemble a brain in a paralysed body: perhaps imaginative, dramatic and original, but with very little command of muscles and nerve ends.

---

* Legislation tends to be applied rigorously at the beginning and then forgotten. An example of this was a law of 1982 compelling restaurants to give an official bill with tax included, to customers who could be asked for it within a certain radius of the restaurant. At the beginning, one restaurant was fined 27 billion lire (11 million dollars) for failing to comply! Now receipts are given less consistently as fines are rarer, and you can sometimes pay less if you say you don't want a receipt.

IV
THE ECONOMY

Background – State Industry and Taxation – Present Attempts at Reform – Private Industry

BACKGROUND

With a population of fifty-seven million, Italy has few natural resources, except its people. It has random supplies of lead and zinc in Sardinia, and practically no coal. It does produce a third of the world's mercury but has little else. There have been discoveries of oil and gas which, however, contribute only a small proportion of total requirements. The mountain ranges in the north provide opportunities for hydro-electrical plants, but only 6.8 per cent of electricity consumption is covered by these.

In the late nineteenth century and at the beginning of the twentieth, Italy did develop a number of industries which were to flourish: among them Pirelli (tyres), Fiat (cars), Olivetti (typewriters and computers). However, with a long peninsula divided by mountains and history, and a strong religious and agricultural tradition, Italy seemed unlikely to compete with the bigger industrial powers, with their manufacturing traditions, their resources of coal, their backing of sophisticated financial structures, their reserves of specialized labour.

Yet suddenly, in the ten years' boom between 1957 and 1967, Italy became the seventh industrial country in the world. Production increased by 91 per cent – more than any other European country. Italy was in the same position as South Korea or Taiwan today, or perhaps Great Britain in 1800. Labour was cheap. The new factories were operated by people who had come off the land and had, therefore, a tradition of hard work and the patient perfectionism of the peasant who is also a craftsman. There was also enthusiasm for this new form of economic activity which allowed earnings and opportunities undreamt of for thousands of years. It was possible to learn from the mistakes of the pioneers of the Industrial Revolution, and build pleasant, often beautiful factories, away from the smear of coal which disfigured so many of the early manufacturing towns in Britain.

The peasant sense of independence also meant that as soon as a worker had learnt his trade, he set up his own business, thus increasing industrial production. Financially, too, there was the support of the massive loans, grants and investments which, starting with Marshall Aid, characterized American financial policy in Europe and Japan after the war. As other countries grew richer, the demand for Italian goods also increased, particularly as she could undercut prices with the reserves of labour which flowed up from the South, or from the farms of Central Italy.

Increased wealth also began to percolate southwards, partly because of the large government aid programmes, and partly because the four million workers who emigrated, particularly to Germany and North Italy, sent back their savings to the families they had left behind.

Just as the first phase of this industrial revolution had been rapid, so the next stage developed abruptly. If Italy could have grown in isolation, she would probably have found her own organic solutions. However, she turned a movement which had been developing slowly for years in older industrial countries almost into a revolution: the precipitous demand for a more egalitarian distribution of wealth, for more social services, for more opportunities for everyone, for better education, and for an efficient government to be the vehicle of these reforms. Whereas the student revolution in Paris in May 1968 produced little more than a tremor in other countries, in Italy it started a decade of unrest and conflict. This, coupled with the disastrous consequences of the increase in the price of oil in 1973, produced many of the problems which affect the Italian economy today.

I remember in 1967 reading a book by an Englishman who tried to explain the way Italian employers treated their workers as proof that the Roman tradition of slavery had never really been broken. Although everyone shared in the new prosperity, workers' interests were secondary to profits, to display, to re-investment. Family loyalty also meant that it was taken for granted that everyone outside these nuclei could be exploited in the interest of immediate relatives or colleagues. Trade unions were weak: anyone could be dismissed without difficulty. In big organizations like Fiat, little time was spent on considering the problems of the Southern workers pouring into Turin in their hundreds of thousands. An outline welfare state existed, inherited largely from

Fascism, but, as for thousands of years, care of the worst off was left largely to the Church.

Industrial exploitation in Italy can never be compared to the horrors of nineteenth-century industrialization in Britain, or even in Germany and France. But then, despite the takeover by workers of factories in Turin after the first war, and the partisan movement in the second, there had never been a great workers' movement such as developed even in Spain and created general awareness of the possible consequences of extremes of wealth. Everything was tempered by the fact that an Italian could always break away and form his own business. Or he could supplement his wages by making motorcycles in his back garden, or helping at his wife's shop in the evenings. Given that it was primarily a family economy, individuals could earn less, because they were part of small communities where everything was shared. Of course, Italy had the biggest Communist party in Europe, but then it co-operated, albeit uneasily, with the Christian Democrats, and while it could protest it was not a part of government.

Everything, though, changed with the mass movements, starting in 1969. As always, the government gave way, and rigid laws were passed. The first was the "Statuto dei Lavoratori" (the workers' statute) of 1970, which applied to any concern with more than fifteen employees. Union representation had to be accepted and the new law also made it very difficult to dismiss workers, allowed employees to have ten hours of meetings a year in working time, and increased the likelihood of absenteeism by paying those who were ill from the first day. In the heated atmosphere of that time, these perhaps reasonable provisions were used as an arm against employers. In 1973, there were almost as many strikes, totalling 156 million days, as in Britain. Wages inevitably began to rise and between May 1973 and May 1974 they went up by an average of 26 per cent.

This tendency was supplemented by another rigid provision, unique in Europe: the "Scala Mobile", which sounds like a term from opera, literally means the "moving staircase" and is a way of indexing wages to inflation. It was started originally in 1945 and, in the years of the boom and of relatively stable prices, was an effective way of adjusting wages automatically, without disputes. However, as inflation grew, the Scala Mobile fuelled it. Every three months, the price changes were examined of a "basket" of goods – which are hopelessly out of date as even today they include the cost of a cap, when caps are rarely worn, and of Nazionale cigarettes which hardly now exist. The number of corresponding "points" in the increase of salaries was then decided on. The problem here, of course, was that businessmen tended to increase their prices in anticipation of this automatic rise, and the OECD calculated that wages were responsible for roughly 40 per cent of the price rise in Italian manufactured goods between 1977 and 1979.

STATE INDUSTRY AND TAXATION

Over the years, inflation has been raised further by increased government expenditure, particularly in the sector of State industry. It is often not realized how much of Italian industry belongs to the State, and yet the reason for this is not ideological. Neither Communists nor Socialists support the principle. Indeed its only political justification, in Italian terms, is that it provides innumerable opportunities for political nominees and, often, "perks" for the parties which control it.

The first of these State holdings, called IRI (the Istituto per la Ricostruzione Industriale), was set up in 1933 in the middle of the Depression. Its original purpose was to rescue three major banks which had embroiled their customers' money in widespread investments that were now going sour. It took over these investments and by 1936 had a considerable holding in telephones, ship-building and steel. After the war, IRI took part in the boom and was responsible for starting a new steel plant in Taranto in the South and for sponsoring the superb autostrada system (5,900 km). Just outside Naples, it completed the Alfasud car factory in 1968. Because IRI was government controlled, it directed much of its energies and finance to the South where, by the end of the 1970s, it had contributed almost 38 per cent of new manufacturing jobs, while its share of the total Italian manufacturing force was 6 per cent. Among many other organizations it now controls are the airline Alitalia, the three official television channels, RAI, and Finsider, the national steel industry.

Another agency, ENI, was set up in 1953 to concentrate on the utilization of oil and other primary sources of energy. Led by the dynamic entrepreneur Enrico Mattei, who was killed in an air crash in 1962, it established AGIP, the Italian state-owned petroleum company, and expanded into many other fields. It now has 120,000 employees. Yet a third agency, EFIM, which operates in a wide variety of manufacturing enterprises, was set up in 1962.

Unfortunately, all these State holdings were badly hit by labour troubles after 1969 and the increase in the price of oil in 1973. On government instructions, they took over "lame ducks". A typical example was the chemical company SIR, based in Sardinia, which went bankrupt in 1976 with 2,600 employees, and was absorbed by ENI. As a high official of ENI told me, a national enterprise in Italy could never be as efficient as private companies. For one thing, the usual party politics interfere. Between October 1981 and March 1983, ENI had no fewer than four presidents and each of them brought his own team of directors and staff. The third and probably the ablest, Umberto Colombo, was moved to the nuclear energy agency, ENEA, because the Socialists insisted he should leave ENI, and this alone produced a two-day debate in Parliament and a vote of confidence.

In 1984, IRI, ENI and EFIM lost a total of almost three thousand billion lire (one and a quarter billion dollars).

Apart from these losses, the State seems to subsidize almost anything. There are between fifteen and seventeen million social security pensioners, many of whom are "invalids" who simply have to get a doctor's certificate to qualify: there is one village in the South where 80 per cent of the inhabitants are "invalids" and one wonders where those who have to push them around come from. Industry is helped by what is called "Cassa Integrazione", which means that laid-off workers are "temporarily" unemployed and the State pays 80 per cent of their salaries. Continually, in Italy, one is surprised by the way anything worth doing, from theatre to festas, is funded, maybe by the Commune or the Region or the Province – but in the end it all comes from the Treasury.

If expenditure is lavish, taxation has many loopholes: it was recently calculated that if all the evaders were made to pay, government income would increase by no less than the equivalent of seventy billion dollars. On the cover of the magazine *L'Espresso* in April 1984, a pirate-like figure with red nose, bleary eye and small sharp teeth is portrayed sailing away in a boat called "Evader 84" which is full of lire.

There are legal ways of avoiding taxation: you can split the profit from your firm among all your family, including grandparents and uncles; or, given that there are eight rather vague classifications of IVA (VAT), you can usually get away with buying in a high category and selling the same goods in a low one, thus gaining taxation credit.

Fraudulent evasion is less clear but its extent is indicated by published figures for declared income in 1983. These show that workers taxed under IRPEF, the Italian equivalent of Pay As You Earn, pay 70 per cent of all direct taxes. Their average income for 1983 (8,632 lire) was actually higher than that declared by contractors (7,274 lire), who very often employ them, while private businesses admitted to even less: 5,100 lire.

As a result of excessive expenditure and insufficient revenue, the deficit which the Italian government needs to cover through borrowing is enormous: now a total of 450 billion lire (200 billion dollars). Annual borrowing in 1983 was 93 billion lire or about 40 billion dollars – an increase of 26 per cent over 1982. The interest paid on this amounted to no less than 9.3 per cent of the country's entire gross domestic product – double that of the UK and Canada, and much more than that of any other industrial nation. The International Monetary Fund calculated that no less than 51 per cent of private savings was absorbed by the government's need to borrow, thus reducing the amount available to the private sector and forcing up the price of money.*

At the same time, unemployment in 1984 was running at about 12 per cent. The country, warned the governor of the Bank of Italy, was on the verge of economic collapse, and the sudden devaluation in July 1985 gave credence to his gloom.

As always in Italy, though, there are many uncertain factors. In the first place, unemployment is not as stark as elsewhere because families help each other (see p. 168). In the second, all the statistics exclude the "black" economy of small family businesses which, according to Umberto Agnelli, make up 30 to 40 per cent of the economy. They flourish partly because those with fewer than fifteen workers are exempt from the Statuto dei Lavoratori, partly because they don't pay much tax. Officially, Italy seemed to be rushing towards the chasm but in fact its economy is cushioned by illegal activities.

PRESENT ATTEMPTS AT REFORM

Nevertheless, something had to be done. In 1983, a meeting of four of the leading journalists of *La Repubblica* had made ten recommendations. Among them were proposals for reforming the financial system of the government, creating a new agency which would find jobs and training for the unemployed, and suggestions for controlling salaries so that they did not rise ahead of inflation, and thus increase it.

Already, at the end of January 1983, an agreement had been reached between unions and employers, reducing the Scala Mobile by between 15 and 18 per cent. In return, the government promised to freeze charges on public services such as electricity and gas to the inflation target of 13 per cent. It also relaxed some of the restrictions on industry,

* When the prime minister, Minghetti, first balanced the budget of the new Italian state in 1876 he was so moved that he wept when he announced it in the Chamber. Now, no one would believe it.

such as the obligation to choose unskilled labour sent by the employment exchanges. Now, firms could actually recruit half of their intake of new labour from people of their own choice.

In 1984, the Scala Mobile was reduced by a further three points. However, in this case it was done arbitrarily by the Craxi government without consultation. The result was a one-day general strike and obstruction by the Communists in the Chamber of Deputies, which delayed the passing of the measure for four months.

Then, in October 1984, Visentini, the Minister of Finance, put forward a new measure of reform. He proposed taxing small businesses, and punishing evasion above 50 million lire ($20,000) by prison. The reaction was tremendous, with shop-keepers striking and organizing mass processions in protest. Even the Communists gave this proposal only half-hearted support as many owners of small businesses vote for them; while the MSI (former Fascists) proposed 2,000 amendments in order to delay.

Why, asked the owners of small businesses, should we be taxed on the same level as those in offices and factories when we have to take risks which employees don't have? Indeed, the danger here is that it is from the very sector which assures Italian prosperity that money will be channelled to the State which, almost certainly, will use it inefficiently for personal enrichment or for party benefit – a basic factor lying behind the distrust which leads to tax evasion. Nevertheless, the Visentini measures were passed.

Another step which might reduce government debt has been the attempt to sell off 49 per cent of many of the companies owned by the big State holdings, although government would still be in control. A further one is the limitation of pensions and benefits so that no individual can receive more than the equivalent of $10,000.

All these measures may reduce the public debt and thus lower inflation, which already in 1984 had begun to descend towards the planned single figures. However, it is important to realize that anything achieved will be applied only in part. One reaction to the attempts to tax small businesses was an interview in December 1984 in the newspaper *Corriere della Sera* with an official in the Department of Finance. Much of the opposition, said the interviewing journalist, came from those who feared that their income would be estimated by employees of that department, because they would have to give them a *bustarella*, or bribe – a suggestion which was denied by the official.

Sometimes modern Italy is reminiscent of France before 1789 where vested interests and bureaucratic entanglements were so strong that the only way to bring about reforms was to sweep everything away, and start at the beginning again. However, although the French monarchy, too, was undermined by an immense deficit, the large Italian middle class have a moneyed interest in tranquillity, rather than tumult; while the people themselves realize that it is compromise that has taken them so far in such a short time.

Meanwhile, industry is as flourishing as it can be in a world recession. There were 64,000 new businesses in 1983, as opposed to 35,000 which closed down. As Umberto Agnelli said in an interview, "Past experience shows that Italian society knows how to fight back when times are hard." That, surely, is the key to everything.

PRIVATE INDUSTRY

I never realized the effect of dust on a computer head until I visited Olivetti, and saw a chart which showed that a speck of dust is about ten times as thick as the gap between the head and the disc. I was led in a white overall through a room where disc containers were being completed; then to a compression chamber with two doors like the exit of a submarine under water; through another door, into the compression chamber, where white figures were polishing discs under strong inhaling machines which sucked up any dust that might have survived this process.

In the vast hall of the production centre, where simple wires are turned into computers, workers were practising the *isola* (island) system which they say Olivetti invented in 1975, and which Volvo and other firms have imitated. This system abolishes the assembly line and means that little groups of workers co-operate together on each stage of production, thus avoiding monotony.

In 1978, Olivetti seemed like yet another firm which as a lame duck would be taken over by IRI to add to the government deficit. They were losing $10 million a month. Then a professional manager, Carlo De Benedetti, took over, reduced employees by 8,000, upped expenditure on research and development to $30 million in 1980, and increased revenue by 21 per cent in 1983 and profits by 40 per cent.

Apart from its computers, Olivetti is one of the leading producers of office machines in Europe. They were the first to manufacture the electronic typewriter in 1978, and have now sold over a million and a half. They have always been interested in international tie-ups as a means of sharing research and technical know-how. In 1984, they made an agreement with AT&T (American Telephone & Telegraph), which bought a 25 per cent share of their firm. The agreement also provided for co-operation and research in office automation, which will lead to important developments in new machinery combining telecommunications and computers.

After visiting Olivetti, I went to the Fiat factory of Mirafiori in Turin and watched cars being assembled, mainly by robots. In the engine department blunt-nosed machines carried the engines from one bench to another, even steering faultlessly into an alcove so that they could move on to a conveyor belt. Other robots, which looked like long-nosed dragons, protruded their snouts into car interiors, emitting sparks. Entire chassis were moved round a vast floor, like slow-motion bumper cars which managed to avoid one another. The only manned assembly line was for the fixing of back windows. Men and middle-aged women prepared the frames, fixed the windows and secured them; 20 per cent of the workforce are now women.

As with Olivetti, the turn-round in Fiat has been remarkable. In 1979 the company lost an estimated 200,000 cars through strikes. In the previous six years, there had been twenty-nine terrorist attacks against Fiat employees, with four killed. In those days, a worker turned out only 11.2 cars per year, while Opel employees produced 29 and Toyota 43.

In October 1979 everything changed: sixty-one militants were sacked for proved cases of intimidation, vandalism and sabotage. The following year, the new managing director, Cesare Romiti, decided to lay off 23,000 workers, who were placed on Cassa Integrazione. As a reaction, the factories closed for thirty-five days – an age in Italy, where strikers receive no pay from their unions. This strike was broken by an unusual event: "The March of the 40,000," as it is called – a silent procession through the streets of Turin by middle managers and workers. As Giorgio Benvenuto, the leader of one of the more moderate unions, said: "It was a dangerous indication of the incapacity of the unions to represent everyone."

Now, Fiat has recovered. Since the 1981 loss of the equivalent of 120 million dollars and of 35 million in 1982, Fiat Auto has been in profit. It now produces thirty-five vehicles per worker annually, and lost less than a day's production of vehicles in 1983. It is now the sixth largest company in the world, and the biggest car producer in Europe with more than 12 per cent of sales. In Italy it has increased its share to 55.4 per cent of the market. Here, it is favoured by a far-sighted mutual agreement with Japan, brought about in 1953, whereby both agreed not to export cars *en masse* to each other's countries. Thus Japanese imports are limited to only 2,200 cars a year.

In January 1983, Fiat also launched its new small car, the "Uno", which was voted the car of the year by the European car writers and sold 325,000 units in the eleven remaining months of the year.

All this has been achieved, too, by aggressive cost-cutting. In 1983 Fiat withdrew from the American market, where it sold only 12,000 cars a year, and from South America – with the exception of Brazil. It has cut down suppliers from a thousand to six hundred, which has slowed the price increase of car parts, and has also reduced the number of its basic car chassis from thirteen to six, thus simplifying production.

Fiat is the largest firm in Italy, with interests in almost everything from Ferrari and tourist agencies to bio-engineering and building aeroplanes. "If Fiat sneezes," they say, "the Italian economy catches a cold." The effect on Italy of this recovery and, particularly, the end of the thirty-five-day strike was momentous. The demonstration that unions were no longer all-powerful, as they had been for the previous ten years, affected every large industry. A manager in Phillips (Italy) gave me figures for his firm: the percentage of absenteeism went down from 17.5 to 11.2; and the items produced per worker per year increased by 26 per cent. This, however, was partly the result of reducing the total workforce from 10,131 to 8,480.

Further south, in Umbria, I was taken round the Buitoni chocolate factory, which like Fiat and Olivetti started as a small family firm, in true Italian style. Now, it is part of CIR, a holding company of De Benedetti's, and it also produces spaghetti and tinned foods, exporting 30 per cent of production to the United States.

To my surprise, there seemed to be few people working in the large, high-ceilinged workshops. Sacks of cocoa from the Ivory Coast lay in the store room and, nearby, a single workman was churning a great mass of unsugared chocolate in a vat. However, all round, machines were clicking, carrying biscuits which were covered with successive layers of chocolate, wrapping up Baci di Perugia (literally, Perugian kisses) in silver paper with deft movements.

My companion explained to me that three years ago, the situation was very difficult but that now things were going well. They had got the older and less efficient workers put on Cassa Integrazione and, with more machinery, had increased production by 30 per cent. Before, unions had even objected to a person being moved from one machine to another, but now they were less rigid and realized that everyone would be out of work if the firm did not survive.

In Italy, as in France and Spain, unions are divided on political lines rather than professions, so you do not get demarcation disputes. Also there is no closed shop. The biggest union is the Communist CGIL, the next the CISL which originally was Christian Democrat, although today there are also many other points of view. The smallest is the UIL, which is Socialist and Republican. They were united into one group until 1984, when they fell out over the reduction in the Scala Mobile, which the CGIL objected to and the others did not.

Strikes do not normally last long, for, as one union leader explained to me, it is easy to cripple a factory simply by getting those workers making one part of a product to go on strike while the others are still "working", to be followed by another strike of those working on another vital part, and so on. In this way a lot of damage can be done with workers losing only a few hours' pay. On the railways, for instance, a region will go on strike for twenty-four hours followed by another, so that although only one area is on strike at a time, the whole network is disrupted. Unions are permitted to strike for political reasons by a law of 1974 which, as a Left-wing jurist said at the time, meant that Italy was now "a democracy of the workers".

Although unions are now more reasonable, this does not mean that small groups do not strike at short notice. Immediately the holidays start, life-savers remove their swimsuits and don normal clothing until they receive a rise. Or, as happened in the summer of 1984, three people who were responsible for signing a document allowing incoming aircraft to refuel decided not to do so, holding up Fiumicino Airport in Rome for days.

Nevertheless, Italian industry has, by and large, got over the crisis of the '70s. This has been done by decisiveness, adaptability and inventiveness. An example of this determination to survive is the motorcycle industry: Italy is one of the few countries whose motorcycle industry has not been knocked out by the Japanese. In a parking place about half the motorcycles are usually Italian, some made by the fifty small firms which still survive, most by one big manufacturer: Guzzi.

Guzzi's main factory is on the shores of Lake Lecco, near Como; lying on a slope with a view of the lake, it looks from outside like some sprawling bungalow hotel in the sunshine. Signor Ermellini of public relations told me that they had beaten Japanese competition partly through quality, cheapness and styling. They had concentrated on the high c.c. machines which the Japanese didn't make. Also they had been helped by the fact that the public had grown to appreciate their motorcycles over the sixty years since they started, and wanted to buy Italian. In 1966 the firm had had a crisis because the public no longer wanted the utilitarian machines they then made, and the cheapness of cars had been competitive. So they sold out to a company called SEIMM, redesigned more sporting machines, and extended the sales organization, particularly abroad. Now they manufactured about 40,000 machines a year, of which 40 per cent are exported. "When things are going badly," said Signor Ermellini, "is just the time to take risks and invest in new things. It's too easy to be hypnotized by possible disaster, like a bird by a snake!"

It was necessary, too, to be flexible. In 1974 they had formed closer links with European motorcycle firms to stave off the Japanese threat and share the manufacture of components. They had written inviting the chairman of Norton motorcycles in England to take part, but he had answered: "I am for free competition." Next year, Norton went bust.

It is this Italian nimbleness which has allowed them to survive, despite far greater problems at home than most industries have to deal with. In Germany the share of industrial production in the economy has gone down from 38 to 32 per cent, and in Japan from 36 to 31 per cent since 1970. In Italy, it has remained constant at 29 per cent.

Of course, in terms of development, the prospects for the economy fluctuate as they do everywhere: in the June 1984 edition of *The Economist* Intelligence Unit review on Italy, possibilities were said to be boundless, with a forecast of a 7 per cent growth in exports. By September, though, everything had changed, and there was an expectation of a growth of almost nothing. This was confirmed by the panic devaluation of the Lira on July 22nd 1985.

As in most industrial countries, the Italian economy hangs on a number of pegs: the level of wages; the size of the government deficit; the rate of inflation and, therefore, the cost of exports and of borrowing money; the degree of interference and competence of the State. Underlying this is the fact that industrial exports only just balance the importation of oil and gas, which have to be bought in increasingly expensive dollars, and that there is a big deficit on agriculture. The situation is precarious and foreign trade in the last few years has been in deficit.

Nevertheless, nothing in Italy is what it seems. Underneath statistics is the successful "black" economy and, probably most important, the resourcefulness, hard work and inventiveness of the Italians themselves. Adaptability, after all, is an Italian tradition. Here is Francis Haskell writing in similar circumstances about the economic situation in the sixteenth century:

... the long tradition among Italian businessmen of accommodating themselves to new circumstances succeeded in overcoming these setbacks.

When the demand for woollen cloth tapered off in Monza, the cloth makers turned to the manufacture of felt hats. When Turkish pirates interfered with trade by sea, the Venetians and the Anconitani opened overland routes to the East through Split and Ragusa.... When in the early 1590s the whole Mediterranean basin was struck by a whole series of crop failures, the grand duke of Tuscany sent ships to buy grain in Poland and the Ukraine – at no small profit to himself and to the Florentine bankers who helped finance the operation.*

The duke of Tuscany and Turkish pirates no longer exist, but the modern Italian way of dealing with economic problems is probably not so very different.

* From *The Italian World*, edited by John Julius Norwich.

V

THE FAMILY

Links – Family Industry – Family Values and Attitudes to Children – Sex – Feminism and Homosexuality – Sense of the Past – Death – Class-consciousness and the Generation Gap – Youth and Protest – Unemployment – Drugs – Petty Crime

LINKS

We waited for Ausonio's family at Civitavecchia. They had been away for the "White Week", skiing in the Alps above Turin. They had taken a cheap package trip, organized by a union, although Ausonio was anything but a supporter of trade unions.

The train arrived and a sudden, jostling torrent of blue and red anoraks, of skis held at all angles and looking like pieces of flotsam and jetsam, poured into the piazza outside the station. For a moment there was total confusion. There was shouting, embracing: "Mamma!" "Giorgio!" "We'll be seeing each other!" "Ciao! Ciao!" Hands were held and then released reluctantly. Even men clasped one another, thumping each other on the back.

Noise subsided gradually as if the curtain were about to come down on the end of an opera.

We drove back with Paola, Ausonio's wife, and she told us that the skiing had been fun. However, she had gone mainly for the children. She would have been quite happy to stay in Viterbo where they lived. Her family were there and her mother was still alive. Then there were her friends and she enjoyed the charitable work that took up much of her time. Travelling was all right but it made her restless: she kept on thinking of home.

Family closeness means that Italians are personal. In planes they will applaud the pilot if he makes a good landing because he is not part of the mechanism of a flight but an individual who has brought everyone through the hazards of air travel. He should therefore be applauded in the same way as an opera singer who gives pleasure.

Often bewildering for the Anglo-Saxon visitor is the naturalness with which Italians touch each other. Usually it is simply an extension of the physical warmth and affection of the family. If you go, as I did once, with your tie blown untidily over your shoulder to pay your bill in a bar, the girl at the cashier's desk may well reach over and adjust it as a matter of course. If you go to a barber to have a trim, as I did in Naples, you may suddenly find that your eyebrows are being sheared and that the scissors have found their way into your nostrils to snip at superfluous hair. The question of physical privacy is irrelevant here: you have given responsibility to the barber and if he thinks you look ridiculous with bushy eyebrows and hair sprouting from your nose, it is up to him to put it right. Once I was in a bar and the lady in charge noticed I had a trouser leg caught in my sock. "Pull your trouser down!" she said in faltering English.

The way men embrace each other without self-consciousness can also be surprising. Living in a northern country must, in turn, be strange for Italians because of the withdrawal of touch. I remember an Italian student at International House in London wondering if the reason Englishmen recoiled from touching or embracing each other was due to excessive consciousness of sex. Perhaps he was right. Certainly the fact that we are less demonstrative within our families could mean that touch is associated more with sex and less with warmth and spontaneous friendliness.

The reason for this family view of the world probably lies in the fact that until recently Italy was a predominantly agricultural country. As in Britain before the Industrial Revolution, most people lived on the land, or in small country towns or villages, dependent on co-operation and loyalty to each other for the little prosperity they enjoyed. Social life revolved round a community whose members had known each other all their lives. Very few people needed to travel unless poverty forced them to emigrate.

Although Italian industrial development started in the north at the end of the last century, 40.8 per cent of Italians still worked on the land in 1950. It was not till the boom of 1959–62 that Italy really became a significantly industrial country. In any case, the drift from the land was predominantly to small family industry where the pattern was not so different. Even today, in the 1980s, it has been calculated that 65 per cent of Italians are still dependent on a family economy.

After the Second World War, the real opportunities came with economic development and easier money. The peasant was poor, hard-working, used to abstinence, to surviving. Money was important to him because he had so little. His life had made him tough, resourceful, adaptable, in the tradition of relatives who had started the great emigrations which continued from the 1880s to the 1960s.

Near Montefiascone on the border with Tuscany, I talked with Signor Capelli, a man who had built up a large hotel and restaurant, starting after the war from almost nothing. He told me he had been in the air force during the war. Afterwards he had bought a small plot of land with the savings he had made, and some time later had extended it. Life had been hard – fourteen or fifteen hours a day – but he had put money by. He bought another piece of land, and the idea had come to him of starting a small drinks and sandwiches stall to take advantage of the tourist trade. By this time he was married and his wife helped him. They added on a small dining room and he got help with loans from the local authority and from the banks, and also built a few bedrooms. Everything went very well. The road outside was broadened. The number of tourists grew. "I thought," he said solemnly, "why not a bigger restaurant? Perhaps more rooms for passing guests!" As he spoke, his eyes shone as if he were re-living what to him had obviously been an imaginative experience which then had come true.

"Nearby was this quarry with stone that I liked," he went on, waving at the pink-grey blocks of stone in the wall. "So, I bought one of those *motocyclette* trucks and brought all the stone down from the quarry. Many journeys. And trouble. There were jealous people about. But I got the family and some friends to help. And we built all this...." He looked about him as if he still couldn't believe it. "We put stone on stone; we borrowed machinery; I got a friend to do the ironwork. Isn't it beautiful? Now, from April to October, we are crowded out. And we have parties coming at Christmas – a hundred and fifty people last year, and we have another cook to help my wife – the one who made the *zuppa inglese* you have just eaten! And we are very, very busy."

He told me he was sixty-two, but that there was still a lot to do. He had bought a patch of land near Lake Bolsena. And a motor-boat. Next summer he was going to turn it into a camping-site and a picnic area, and the motor-boat would be hired out, or used for water-skiing. "And when do you think you'll retire?" I asked cautiously.

"Retire?" he exclaimed as if I had named some rare disease. "Retire?" He took off his cap and scratched his thick, black hair. "Though perhaps one of my sons will take over sometime. Then I can go and start something else!"

In some ways, there are parallels with the closeness of the Jewish family. Thus, before the French Revolution, the Jew was the property of a foreign prince, allowed to live only in his ghetto. With the exception of Piedmont and the Veneto, the Italian too was dominated from the sixteenth century by foreign dynasties and foreign troops. The only strength both groups had was through family unity.

Jews were allowed to live only through usury. Italians, also, have a tradition of banking which is the oldest in Europe, starting in Piacenza in the twelfth century. Indeed, during the Middle Ages Lombards and Florentines were the moneylenders of Europe, and it was on their commerce and banking that the splendours of Venice and Florence, Genoa and Pisa were built.

More recently, the great emigrations of both Italians and Jews occurred at the end of the nineteenth century and the beginning of the twentieth. It was necessary in both cases to reinforce the bonds of family in order to overcome difficulties in new countries where the reception was sometimes hostile. Although there are many differences, both the Jewish and the Italian family have needed to be close in order to survive, and neither has had much reason to trust those outside their immediate community.

Leonardo Sciascia, probably the best-known contemporary Sicilian novelist, writes: "The family is the State for the Sicilian. . . . Perhaps he will become excited by the idea of the State and will go out to lead the government. But the exact definition of his rights and duties will be that of the family."

Renata Gauer, a German sociologist married to an Italian and researching contemporary family life in a Calabrian village, told us: "It is difficult to limit research of this kind because in Italy the family extends everywhere."

In spite of the differences between South and North and, indeed, between individual regions, one thing in common is this closeness of family ties. There may be stronger patriarchal and matriarchal bonds in the South, but as an Italian economist has written, "Italy is a father of a family going out to work each day." This idea of a prosperous family economy is one of the most difficult things to understand about Italy because it is not easy to quantify. Statistics may indicate that the economy is in a state of crisis – indeed *la crisi* is one of the Italian's favourite words. Scandals may erupt as frequently as boils on a beggar's back. Governments may fall soggily every few months. Yet Italy remains as prosperous as ever, with more expensive dresses visible on her streets, more cars, more restaurant meals per head, more holidays by the sea or in the mountains, more second homes than any country in Europe.

The National Statistics office, ISTAT, continually produces gloomy tables of decay and decline. But most of these figures cannot by their nature include everything. An economist I know once told me that the government had reckoned there were seventeen thousand firms which were not registered, and fifty thousand which paid only half the taxes that they owed.

"But how can the government know that?" I asked, whereupon he looked surprised, and changed the subject. Italians love statistics. Someone has asserted that there are 850,000 wild dogs in Italy and has even published tables showing the proportion of these to the total dog population in each of the twenty-two regions. No information on how the beasts were counted is forthcoming. The magazine *Europeo* even produced statistics in August 1984 for the places where Italians made love most frequently. The orthodox won with 78.2 per cent for bed, followed by a car with 12.4 per cent. At school rated only 0.2 per cent and on the stairs 0.5 per cent.

Some time ago, an historian called Dard, writing about the *sans-culottes* during the French Revolution, said that true research was difficult because "the People have no archives". The same could be said about Italians and the family economy.

FAMILY INDUSTRY

We met Stephen Tobin by a newsstand in front of the Pitti Palace in Florence, and drove out into the Tuscan countryside which must be among the most beautiful in the world – perhaps because it blends the intimate with the extensive. If you are in a valley, everything is close and small. The rough stone farmhouse seems a solitary refuge from everywhere and everyone. Then you climb a hill, and the countryside is fringed by a distant ridge on one side, or broken by small, round hills, where the sloping rows of vines look well combed, and olive trees are dots on the grey earth, and cypresses are like dark spires.

For those who have had the Bible endlessly intoned at school, olives and wine seem the essence of richness. In any case, the Tuscan landscape is already familiar as a background in paintings of Virgin and Child, of a transfixed San Sebastian, of a Crucifixion, so it seems to have something of the Holy Land.

We were driving out to a village called Certaldo for strictly practical reasons: to visit a shoe factory. Stephen is employed by an American agency which researches into the style of shoe most likely to succeed on the American market. Once this has been decided, Stephen visits some of the hundred factories in Tuscany and gets them to make the required number of shoes on time.

Certaldo itself is a beautiful town on a ridge with a castle and a street of medieval buildings and a thirteenth-century church. Boccaccio was born here and his house was the one building hit during an air raid in 1944. However, it has now been rebuilt as an exact replica of the original.

The factory is in the lower, modern town. Inside it was light and cool with only a dozen employees, seeming more like a workshop. At this time of year, in October, five hundred shoes were produced each day, Stephen told us. Most of the different parts were made by women working at home. The factory was thus really an assembly plant.

"But why isn't everything done in one place?" I asked. "Wouldn't that be easier than sending vans round to collect all the parts?"

"No – it's cheaper this way. People prefer to work at home. Also, if they're independent, they aren't actually employed by the factory."

"What's the advantage of that?"

"Well, it's a bit complicated. But if they're employed here, the factory has to pay an additional 42 per cent of gross salary for social security. Then, of course, there's also the Statuto dei Lavoratori!"

"And they avoid all that quite legally?"

"Yes – and then there's the Scala Mobile, which means raising wages every three months whether or not your firm is doing well."

"So if everything were manufactured within the factory – ?"

"It would go bankrupt. The Americans would never accept the prices. They'd buy in South Korea, or Brazil."

I talked with Signor Mori who, with his partner, Signor Spino, had started the factory eight years previously. His workers were well off, he said. Most came to work in their own cars. He pointed at a man who was retouching the finished shoes, and told me that he had now saved enough to buy three flats. He lived in one; his parents with the rest of the family in another; and his grandparents in a third.

Mori himself had started his business from his savings while working in another shoe factory. A lot of workers had done that – learnt all about the profession, saved up, and then started on their own. "Others spent all their money on cars and girls," he said. "I lived with my parents and saved everything I earned."

"And are you paying back your parents what your upkeep cost you?" He looked perplexed. "Pay them back? Why? It's all in the family."

Later, near Arezzo, I visited a small factory that made gold chains. It was owned by Signor Gori and his wife. From outside, it was like a fortress, with heavy bars at windows and doors and a camera poking out above the entrance.

Inside, a few machines stood on the linoleum floor. Gori picked up a shabby, oblong container like a bit of stained tubing which was used for heating and melting the gold. Afterwards, the metal was stamped into narrow, flat bars which were punched out to make chains. The remaining gold scraps fell into a plastic wastepaper basket. It all seemed so casual, with none of the sheen which might be associated with working in gold.

In a little side room, Gori poured gold beads into my hand. Then silver, like drops of mercury. One dropped onto the floor and rolled under a cupboard. I started anxiously. "It doesn't matter," said Signor Gori firmly. "It will be recovered."

He told me that he had seven workers and that, as with the shoe factory in Certaldo, a lot was done by people in their own homes – particularly polishing.

The gold industry itself had started in Arezzo after the last war with one firm which was now the biggest in the world. Since then, independent workshops had multiplied, as they had in Certaldo: those employed acquired the skills and then started their own firms, as Gori had done. Now, there were no fewer than 400 factories in the Arezzo area, producing jewellery, gold bracelets and chains, which were exported all over the world. The local bank vaults were full of gold because everything had to be manufactured to order as the price fluctuated so much.

Machines too were produced locally, and new inventions were being made the whole time and developed in small workshops. This created a parallel industry and, at the same time, improved and speeded up the manufacturing process. Gori himself had just paid the equivalent of $6,000 for a new soldering machine which he demonstrated proudly.

As we left, we were asked to scrape our shoes on a grille. "That's for gold dust," said Gori, also brushing my clothes thoroughly. Even the water was filtered, and the floors swept carefully every day. As a result, no less than two kilos of gold and twelve of silver were recovered each year.

I visited other small factories which followed a similar pattern. In Varese, in the north near Lake Como, I called on Giuseppe Villari, a man in his early forties who designed and made machinery for producing plastic containers. He, too, had worked for another factory – in his case as a designer. Then, in 1973, he had decided to set up on his own. A partner would of course have made it easier from the financial point of view. But, said Signor Villari, "Anyone who has a partner has a boss." Much of his production was exported to France. A few years ago he had packed a bag and gone to Grenoble, in search of business, speaking his bad French. There he had met someone who had agreed to orders which covered 30 per cent of his production. Then he had gone to an international trade fair as an experiment and someone had snapped up his entire production for a year.

His problem, he said, voicing the complaint of all Italian entrepreneurs, was the government. The Scala Mobile with its three-monthly inflation-linked rises meant that costs were continually increasing. In February (1983) it had gone up the equivalent of about $12 a month for everyone. This also meant that wages were being equalized more and more. Because you never knew what inflation was going to be, you didn't know how much salaries could go up. By raising wages for skilled workers you might easily find yourself priced out of the market. With the system as it was, unscrupulous employers were tempted simply to pay workers extra under the counter.

In Meda, north of Milan, I visited Signor Longhi, who now has three factories. His father was a carpenter and he was orphaned at fourteen. He then became interested in devising machinery for making furniture, and his career grew from there. Now he exports 12 per cent of his production, particularly to the United States, Arab countries and Japan.

In 1980 he had a financial crisis and has slowly climbed back. "Competition," he told me, "is like a Ferrari race. Everything has got to be right from the start." His factories too, although bigger than the other ones I visited, rely on workers producing parts of furniture in their own small workshops. "It is natural," he said, "for Italians to want to work for themselves."

He too complained bitterly about lack of official co-operation, in this case in the Commune of Meda. Ten years ago he had bought land on which to site one big factory, which would be more convenient than three separate ones. However, over all these years, the Commune, which had agreed in principle to the idea, still could not decide whether to give him official permission to go ahead. The trouble was the deadlock caused by different political parties who continually obstructed each other.

This type of small factory, manned by a few individuals, or small groups working at home, flourishes particularly in what is known as "The Third Italy" – a term used to mark out the area that is neither North nor South but lies in central Italy and in the eastern part of the plain north of the Apennines. If you drive along two hundred miles of motorway from Pavia, south of Milan, to Bologna and beyond, you will pass small factories one after another. It is reckoned there are 150,000 in the province of Emilia Romagna alone.

However, small family enterprises abound all over the peninsula. Thus any visitor to Naples is struck by the stalls on the pavement, by the steps used as a shop, covered by every conceivable object from picture frames to lampshades, by the crude signs advertising umbrella repairs or even a hospital for dolls.

According to Teresa Gorman writing in the *Daily Telegraph* (6.4.83), "Naples, with no registered glove factory, exports more than five million pairs of gloves a year." A fascinating book by Luciano De Crescenzo, called *Napoli di Bellavista*, illustrates and comments on a number of other Neapolitan professions: the lady who goes to private houses every day to comb hair and relay gossip; the open-air chiropodist whose patients have their ingrowing toenails trimmed as they lean a foot on a metal table; the man who will repair a broken zip, or a tear in your trousers, while you wait – not to mention the fortune tellers and the man who hires you an invalid chair with someone to push it, so that as a "cripple" you can get the best view at football matches, however fit you may be!

Further south, there is perhaps as much individual or family initiative but it tends to be confined more to agriculture, to illegal activities on a large scale, or to the "disposal" of government aid in the form of pensions and subsidies. There does not seem to be the same desire to start small industry. In Basilicata, after the earthquake of 1980, 75 per cent of government funding was allotted to the stimulation of small industry. However, up to 1983 there was little interest and only seventy enquiries had been received. Southern villages, particularly in Apulia, seem quite different from those in the North. You wonder what that difference is and then you realize that there are only residential houses and quiet streets, without the buzz of small commerce.

Another indication of this contrast is the absence of co-operatives in the South. These were founded over a hundred years ago by Andrea Costa Masarente in Bologna, and in the North provide an ideal balance, particularly in agriculture, between the small family enterprise and the need for expert marketing and exporting.

In Parma, we visited one of the big cheese co-operatives. The prospectus mentioned that in his latter years Molière had subsisted almost entirely on Parmesan cheese, and that Boccaccio had mentioned it in the *Decameron*.

At the dairy, we were told that the farmers bring their milk in every evening and morning. Both consignments are poured into great metal vats and heated to 33⁰ centigrade. Then, rennet – described in the prospectus as a natural extract from the stomach of a suckling calf – is added, and curd is produced. In a large, spotless shed with the early morning light pouring through the big windows, we watched as men reached down into the vat with paddles and brought up great wads of cheese.

We then went through to the storehouse which was a rodent's paradise. Twenty rows of cheeses, separated by shelves of wood, rose to the ceiling, looking, with their round polished rinds, as if they might well be used by Scotsmen for curling on ice. An illustrated notice, showing a man being struck by a cheese on the back of his neck, warned against getting too close. Between the two rows, an automatic polisher was working, clasping a cheese affectionately in metal arms and then polishing it with black-haired brushes.

These cheeses are kept for eighteen months and have to be eaten within the next half year. In each of the vast sheds there are between a hundred thousand and two hundred thousand. Each one is tested regularly by a man with a small hammer whose job it is to go round tapping them in turn. The resulting sound will tell him whether they are in good condition or not.

The co-operative itself is run by a council elected in an assembly which includes all the three hundred members. No one is allowed to resign from the co-operative unless everyone else agrees, or unless they are expelled – which again requires a unanimous vote.

After costs have been deducted, profits are distributed to members in proportion to the quantity of milk they provide. As the co-operatives themselves are not profit-making, they are helped by the government with cheap loans and tax deductions. Members, therefore, get a good return from participating.

Most co-operatives also belong to what is called a *Consorzio,* which, in this case, is a voluntary association of twelve hundred cheese-makers who represent over sixty thousand dairy farmers. (For wine, see p. 35) Founded in 1928, the object of this Consorzio is to give the monitoring and technical advice needed to maintain standards. As cheese similar to Parmesan is produced in eight other countries and sometimes sold with sawdust mixed in, it is essential to have a body which guarantees both name and quality.

Apart from these general forms of marketing and selling, individual approaches also abound. Many businessmen, like Giuseppe Villari in Varese, simply pack their bags and go abroad to seek an individual purchaser. Other forms of co-operation also exist. In Varese I came across a school of English run by two brothers, George and Charles Crowhurst from Britain. Their Italian wives are sisters and the two Englishmen have lived in Italy for almost twenty years. Apart from teaching English, they have also developed an "Executive Club". Members meet every fortnight to discuss in English their experiences in trying to sell their goods abroad. A monthly bulletin on up-to-date world economic news is also produced. Most important of all, though, is the way the Crowhursts act as brokers. As English is the universal commercial language, they ring up firms abroad on behalf of their members to find out if there is any demand for specific goods. As a result of these activities, the Crowhursts recently pulled off the unusual coup of arranging for the export of three thousand plastic globes to Sri Lanka for use in geography classes at State schools.

However, much of the drive for small family industry or agricultural enterprise comes from the transformation of the *contadini*, or literally peasants, in the last thirty years. As long ago as 1915, D. H. Lawrence wrote in his *Twilight in Italy*: "The peasant is passing away, the workman is taking his place. The stability is gone.... And the new order means sorrow for the Italian more even than it meant for us. But he will have the new order."

It is this released energy of the countryman which provides the fodder for every industrial revolution. How long, though, can it last?

Obviously, much depends on the international situation and the government's ability to contain inflation which could eventually price Italy out of international markets. In Bologna I went to see the director of the Banca Commerciale in an office which was all sunlight with the shapes of tall towers hovering beyond the window-panes. The director was pessimistic. The economic crisis of 1975 had not affected the region because it did not hit small firms. Now, though, an increasing number of these were in *crisi*. Exports were holding up but earnings were lower because prices had to be kept down. One difficulty was that loans were too expensive: overdrafts varied between 18.75 and 25 per cent. The director calculated that sixty times the number of firms were now in trouble than had been the case in 1970.

Later I talked with an elegant, exuberant lady who had worked in the textile business for thirteen years. She had never known it so bad. At Carpi, a textile centre between Parma and Modena, the boom seemed over. According to her, the unions had launched a campaign against people who did piecework at home, with the result that more and more was done in the factories so that costs had gone up. Firms in Germany which used to import large quantities of Italian textiles were now finding it cheaper to buy the copyright of Italian designs and set up their own manufactures.

Signora Cortaldo, head of a leading family fashion firm in Florence, confirmed this. She herself sells a lot of her designs to Japan and gets a commission on articles they produce as Italian goods are now too expensive. The Italian economy benefits in the sense that money comes into the country in this way, but the amount earned is less and the result is disastrous in terms of unemployment.

An example of a local product which has already decayed was provided by a visit to Scacchi's, near Como, who manufacture silk foulards with admirable efficiency, taste and economy. In the factory, a few workmen adjust machinery which produces vibrating cascades of red, blue and green silk thread. However, although Scacchi's sales are good, the silk itself is now imported. Before the war Italy was one of the largest cultivators and in 1973 still produced 19,000 kgs of cocoons, but now the breeding of silkworms is almost extinct. Wage increases and rises in the cost of living have made the operation uneconomic. Strangely, Scacchi now import a lot of their silk from China, and re-export a good proportion of their finished goods back round the world to Japan.

The real challenge comes from similar family economies in the Far East, in Hong Kong, Taiwan and South Korea. In 1982, Italy had 39 per cent of the trade in shoes imported into the United Kingdom. But over the last few years the South Korean percentage has risen very fast and if it continues in this way is likely to overtake the Italian, because Korean shoes are cheaper if not better made. In 1984, I bought an Easter egg in Milan containing a small rubber ball which could have been manufactured anywhere without difficulty but which had a bold label "Made in Taiwan". Harbinger of the future?

However, it is unlikely that the Italians will allow themselves to be outdone in this way without a long struggle. Through hundreds of years of tormented history, and natural disasters, they have learnt how to survive. An example of flexibility was a textile manufacturer I met in Sardinia who told me he could no longer compete with the South Koreans in cheap cloth for everyday use. So his firm had switched into marine clothing for yachtsmen and sailors, and they were doing very well. Certainly the urge to succeed is still there. Poverty and desolation are still recent memories, spurs to energy and effort.

The crucial question is how long this energy, this sense of enterprise will continue in future generations. I discussed this with a young man who had resigned from his father's flourishing business in carburettors, an enterprise founded by his grandfather. He now kept bees on a manor house near Milan, running it as a business although he didn't need to. First, he showed us all the processes of honey-making and how the most productive flowers were cultivated. Then he told us how the Italians were not fond of honey, regarded it in fact as something to be taken in hot milk mainly as a cure for a sore throat. Then obliquely we talked about his personal situation and he said with a smile: "We have a saying in Italy: the grandfather founds the business, the father enlarges it and the son spends!"

For the moment, anyway, Italy is fortunate in its fragmented economy, which in fact may even replace the monotonous inheritance of the big factory.

To Anglo-Saxon eyes, however, there is much that is suspect. Because of our own history, or the version that has come down to us, piecework is associated with exploitation and the sweatshops of the early Industrial Revolution, symbolized by Thomas Hood's "Song of the Shirt":

> With fingers weary and worn,
> With eyelids heavy and red,
> A woman sat in unwomanly rags
> Plying her needle and thread.

Now, of course, she would not be in unwomanly rags but would probably be working for a holiday abroad, or a new car. Yet there may well still be exploitation. Whatever we may think of unions, the deliberate attempt to avoid their presence raises suspicions; while the fact that tax evasion seems easy in these small, fragmented yet prosperous industries may seem scandalous and anti-social.

However, Italians have rarely been able to afford principles before survival. If government or the unions interfered to a greater extent, there would probably be less income for taxes to be paid from. As Einaudi, the first President of Italy after the war, once remarked: "If Italians paid all their taxes, they would have to find 110 per cent of their income!" That was in 1948 and since then many additional exactions have been imposed with strange-sounding names like IVA and SOCOF, IRPEF and IRPEG. Because Italians are known to be equivocal in their approach to taxes, these are set at a level which assumes anyway that only a small proportion of them will be paid.

In any case, Italy cannot be assessed simply through foreign eyes. Values, and attitudes to government and trade unions, party politics and festas, need also to be looked at from the point of view of people in farmhouses in Tuscany, offices in Bologna, perhaps from a group of chairs on a pavement in Naples, or a few rooms in a crowded tenement inhabited by Sicilian emigrants in Turin.

FAMILY VALUES AND ATTITUDES TO CHILDREN

Saint Nicholas performed the miracle of resurrecting three boiled children, which can presumably be construed as giving them the greatest gift of all. In the eleventh century his bones were stolen from Myra in Asia Minor and brought to Bari where they now lie in the church named after him. For this reason, parents in Bari also give presents on the saint's day on December 6th, although this practice does not occur elsewhere in Italy.

Father Christmases do, however, abound – in fact my small son ceased to believe in him when we went into a restaurant in the Piazza Navona in Rome and no fewer than six Father Christmases came in, and discarded beards and capes prior to eating.

In Bari, and all over Italy, presents are given at Christmas as well. A story by Italo Calvino about Marcovaldo, a countryman who comes to live in the big town, satirizes the Christmas present scene.

Marcovaldo is sent out disguised as Father Christmas to present gifts to important people. Among others, he delivers a parcel to Gianfranco, the son of a Commendatore, and brings his own son, Michelino, along.

"You see, Gianfranco!" the governess says, "Santa Claus has come back with another present!"

"Three hundred and twelve!" the child sighs without looking up from his book. "Put it over there."

Michelino is so sorry for the bored child that he goes back and wraps up a hammer, a catapult and a box of matches which he delivers. Gianfranco is delighted: he smashes his presents, shoots at the glass balls on the Christmas tree, and ends up setting the house on fire.

To his amazement, Marcovaldo finds that the director of his firm is also delighted. The incident has given him the idea of "Destructive Gifts" which he now manufactures with great rapidity. "The important thing is that the Destructive Gift serves to destroy articles of every sort," explains one of the directors of the firm. "Just what's needed to give the market a boost."

After Christmas, there is January 6th, the day of the Kings. Although the custom is beginning to die out in Rome itself, presents are dropped down the chimney in many parts of Italy by the Befana – an ugly witch-like woman, whose name is a distortion of "Epiphany". In parts of Lombardy presents come from the Infant Jesus – as always in Italy there are regional differences.

However, it is the First Communion which is really the great day in a child's life. After the ceremony perhaps a hundred guests will sit down to a feast in a restaurant and each will bring a gift. The child, at nine or ten, will be the sole centre of attention, the recipient of more presents than he or she knows what to do with.

"For many parents it is a compensation for their own poverty in childhood," said Margherita Ciacci, a professor of sociology at the University of Florence. "Those who were reasonably well off before the war are less generous, more careful."

Renata Gauer in Calabria confirmed this, saying that too many of the families she had researched also made their children over-eat and gave them the most expensive delicacies because they remembered their own hunger before the boom of the late 1950s.

Certainly, as I know from personal experience, Italians really seem to love children. When we lived in Rome our identity was determined by Jimmy, our three-year-old blonde son. In the *quartiere* we were known only as "la mamma e il papà di Jimmy". Even men would pass their hands through his hair in the streets murmuring "biondino, bellino". I have fond memories too of staying in a hotel in Alassio before the war, when I was a boy of six. "Bambini" – the very word evokes concern, and indulgence: when my brother and I fled our Italian governess at bedtime, we would be given *zuppa inglese* and marmalade omelettes in the kitchen and then hidden in the pantry when she came down to look for us. It was very different when we settled only twenty miles away over the French border at Menton. There, children were brought up with tight discipline, excessive authority and very little tenderness.

On the whole, the offspring of Italian families seem lively and well balanced. At International House in London, Italian students of both sexes seem the most enterprising and independent of all. With or without much English, they will soon visit the sights, discover the night life, make friends. At the same time they are hard working and very lively. In fact, if a class is dull and apathetic it is always a good idea to transfer a couple of Italians, because like pepper and salt they give it flavour and a dynamism of its own.

Perhaps it is just because the Italian family is essentially an economic unit which has a definite object – to increase wealth – that it seems to have created this balance between co-operation and individual energy, independence and authority, affection and lack of possessiveness, which is an ideal in any society or working group.

The father is respected insofar as he goes out to work and supports the family successfully. The mother, at least in the recent past, is at home and the children's affections and sense of security centre on her. Both do their best to ensure that the children are polite, study hard and do not disgrace the family with the neighbours. However, they seem to enforce this because they feel it is desirable, not simply because they need to show they are in command. On the whole, they accept the fact that children are lively, noisy and fun loving, and give them considerable independence so long as they keep within these limits. The result is that the children return the affection and are loyal. Rarely do you hear negative remarks about parents from Italians, as you do in so many northern countries. Children soon become aware that if the family is to become more prosperous and more highly esteemed, co-operation is necessary. In some ways it is the primitive phenomenon of everyone going out to hunt as soon as possible, while learning that working together is essential, or the cave will be empty and everyone hungry.

It is always interesting to watch an Italian family together. One I remember, in a train in Sardinia, consisted of a young mother wearing a blue anorak and long gold earrings and two little girls who moved around the carriage asking questions about the towns we passed. The little girls talked without shouting and moved without barging into anyone. They were perhaps four and six years old. The mother did not shout at them and tell them to sit down. She smiled and just answered their questions without self-consciousness. One of them had a miniature windmill on the end of a stick, consisting of a blue plastic bow which turned when she thrust it through the air. She went out into the corridor to run with it and put her tongue out at an old lady dressed in black who was standing outside the compartment. The old lady objected not because she was personally offended but because this was not a pleasant thing to do. Indeed, she was obviously used to little girls who put their tongues out at old ladies, and talked as if it was the sort of thing she herself used to do when she was six years old. The little girl meanwhile zoomed up and down the corridor with her miniature windmill, and finally ended up in the old lady's compartment talking earnestly to a nun who was sitting opposite. In turn, the old lady settled down in our compartment and a conversation ensued which included the child of four. Indeed, what I like about Italian families is that children are not regarded as appendages, but as individuals who have certain tendencies because of their age and are certainly no less important than adults. Everyone is going through their life cycle in different states of dependence and independence, but nobody should therefore be ignored or pushed aside, or regarded as a nuisance simply because they are young or old.

The phenomenon of the family as a team continues into adulthood, partly because everyone is probably working together, and also because of the shortage of accommodation (see p. 222). This means that sons and daughters all over Italy tend to live with their parents until they get married. A rather cruel joke observes that Christ was probably Italian because he lived at home until he was thirty, presumed his mother was a virgin, and she certainly believed he was God. Generally, though, there seems to be little discontent. At Bologna, Professor Pierpaolo Donato told me that they had recently had a questionnaire among the students at the university on their attitude to parents. Were they too permissive or too authoritarian? A large majority had said that their parents were neither, and that in fact the balance was just right.

One example of this is the Italian's horror of corporal punishment. Renata Gauer, telling us about her research into Calabrian families, said they might fight and even bite each other in a rage but that there was no physical punishment as such.

In the appendix of an interesting social survey by Professors Donato and Ardigo on a small industrial centre, Montegranaro, in Le Marche on the Adriatic coast, there is a detailed questionnaire with answers from three different adults: a craftsman, a student and a sales representative. The questions are about three phases of their lives: childhood until twelve, adolescence until eighteen, and adulthood until twenty-five. The answers, therefore, are more relevant to the '60s and early '70s, but they do give a limited insight into the attitudes of some adults of the '80s. On punishment, there is mention of going to bed without supper or being made to eat standing up. In one case, for arriving late in the evening the "punishment" consisted of getting an envelope with money in it and being told to go and eat at the inn. Spontaneous blows were given by a father and, once, a kick from a mother because the child got dirty.

Perhaps because the family in Italy is essentially an economic unit, Italians also give the impression of being purposeful and realistic. There seems to be less personal questioning about the path to be followed, and whether this or that is ethical or not, than among those whose culture has been influenced by Protestantism.

Because families were, until recently, large, Italians usually seem at ease with people. There has never been the detachment produced by boarding schools, and classes have been mixed since the last war. By the time they are adult, Italians have usually gone through the gamut of close emotional experience: the squabbling, the loving, the confiding, the envy, the spontaneous joy, and the disappointment. Between the sexes there seems to be little shyness. Big, close families bring familiarity and knowledge.

Italians appear to have been little touched by the sublimation, the mooniness and the sentimentality of Romanticism. Foreign travellers may regard Italians as "romantic", but this does not mean they feel it themselves. Barzini, in his excellent book *The Italians*, brings out their realism and earthiness with the story of an English family in Italy who do everything they can for their maid when she becomes pregnant. However, the neighbours all presume that the Englishman is the father. Why else would he do so much for her? In the end the English have to go back to their country because they are blackmailed by the maid's family who expect a permanent arrangement for mother and child.

Except in Sicily, Italians had little experience of feudalism with its code of honour, its chivalrous knights, its damsels in distress. Indeed it is amusing to imagine Don Quixote as an Italian. He would certainly not have been deluded enough to confuse giants with windmills or to attack harmless wineskins. Probably he would have stayed at home to make love to Dulcinea if he found her to his liking.

Italians seem free of inhibitions or considerations which could brake their active, extrovert lives. True, they give great respect to abstract ideas and most of their politicians tend to speak more of philosophy than of concrete programmes. This, though, is part of their classical past, which still pervades the schools but often seems merely a kind of cap doffing – like the respect paid to graduates who are addressed, particularly in the South, by titles such as *dottore, professore, ingegnere* and even *geometra* which means "surveyor". "What shall I call you when I introduce you?" asked an Italian friend as if in doubt about my very existence. "Will *professore* do?"

This attitude often produces respect for intellectual authority or status, particularly if it is foreign, which is almost a genuflection. As an instance, an eminent British doctor I know was invited with all expenses paid to come out and give a lecture at a conference at Ancona. It was almost entirely an Italian audience. "I don't speak any Italian," he told the organizers. "Will the audience understand English?"

"Oh, probably. Some of them. But please don't worry!"

When he gave his highly specialized talk, he could see that most of the faces in front of him were blank, if intent. At the end, though, he received thunderous applause. This mystified him until it was explained that he was being applauded essentially because he was an eminent foreign doctor who had given up his time to come all the way out to Ancona to speak to them. It was an honour. The conference must be good if he was there. It had been a great event. Understanding what he said would have been an advantage, of course. But it was not the real point!

Although many of their values seem perplexing to us, Italians are strong, perhaps because of all the disasters that have afflicted them. They seem to have few of those guilt feelings about trade, bred from the inequality and misery of the Industrial Revolution. In other European countries, industrial wealth has often produced ugliness: the Black Country in England, the Ruhr, the industrial areas of northern France. In Italy, on the other hand, Venice or Florence, Bologna or Naples, Modena or Lecce have so obviously become beautiful cities because they were rich. In any case, it is probably pleasanter to be rich by the Mediterranean than round the North Sea. Money ensures that sisters or brothers, parents or grandparents can enjoy the sunshine, the beaches, the wine, the ski slopes, the interminable sociability. It ensures, too, a sense of success and the pleasure of showing others what has been achieved in an ostentatious society of competing families.

The Church itself makes this materialism easier in the sense that it willingly takes care of the burden of spiritual self-questioning. "Work is easier," says the craftsman in Donato and Ardigo's questionnaire, "because with God at one's side one works more happily." Practising Catholics are now a minority of only 30 per cent in Italy. However, whether he goes to church or not, Catholicism is still part of the Italian's psyche in the same way as lungs or a kidney are part of his body.

Italians, after all, have lived with the Church for more than sixteen hundred years. There have been political conflicts involving the Church but no long religious wars similar to those during the Reformation in Northern Europe. Even the conflict between Guelf and Ghibelline in the Middle Ages did not concern religious belief but more the question of whether Pope or Emperor should exercise temporal power.

Even today, only one per cent of Italians are Protestant, and those mainly in the Alpine valleys in the north where the Waldensian Church is heir to almost a thousand years of "heretical" movements.

The Church in Italy has always been ostensibly wealthy.* St Peter's

* As long ago as the fourteenth century, Datini, the merchant of Prato, saw no conflict in writing "For God and for Profit" at the top of each page of his accounts books.

in Rome seems more a palace than a place of worship, and in the last decade the most spectacular news emerging from the Vatican apart from the attempted assassination of the Pope has been the way it has been deluded by the bankers Sindona and Calvi.

The Italian, therefore, can live in a tradition which does not induce reflectiveness or soul searching. Goethe, travelling in Italy in 1787, made many observations which still seem valid today. On his way to Perugia he met an officer in the Papal army who, noticing him lost in silent thought, said: "Why do you think so much? A man should never think! Thinking only makes him grow old." And then: "A man should never think about one thing only, because he will go crazy: one should have a thousand things whirling about in one's head."

Certainly one thing still apparent today is the Italian's ability to absorb himself or herself in the present. If you descend the escalator in the metro in Rome or Milan, you will find it blocked with people standing on both sides. All would probably agree that in order to catch the train as quickly as possible it would be more sensible to leave a side free for those in a hurry. However, everyone is absorbed in the immediate moment, chatting, looking at people's clothes, wondering about relationships. Why should they organize the present for the future, particularly in such a trivial situation?

However, when they get to the bottom, they are in a different "present". The platforms are near. A train may be about to come in at any moment. Crowds are gathering and, if they do not place themselves in front, they will be unable to squeeze in. So they run, they jostle, they push forward without irritation or hostility, because they accept that this is part of everyone's daily life.

Or go driving with an Italian. Although he may not be in a hurry, he will delight in speeding as fast as he can without causing a crash. He will protrude his car into every opening, go through red lights if he is sure another car is not crossing his path. He does not consider the possibility of being burnt, or lying broken in a hospital bed, or harming someone else. He is exuberantly concerned with getting the most out of "now" and is confident that other drivers will have the same quick reflexes as he has, confident that they too will know how to survive.

Or remember the festa in Gubbio (p. 47). The Ceri are transported at great speed through the crowded piazza. No path is cleared for them by officials, but as the Ceri approach people "arrange themselves", as the Italians say, and a way opens as in the Red Sea.

Then there are the boys in the bell tower two hundred feet above the square. One of them emerges, kicks the bell and, as it swings down again, retreats, to come out again and give it a further push.

In most other countries the crowd would probably panic. Some would be trodden underfoot. Others might be crushed under the half-ton Ceri. Meanwhile, the parents of the boys in the belfry would probably collapse with anxiety, shout to them to come down at once, and later complain to the municipality that this was scandalously dangerous and should be forbidden.

The Italian boys' parents, on the other hand, are probably proud to see their sons up there, rotating a 400-year-old bell so dexterously. The drama, the enjoyment of the moment are too great to allow them to think of possible disasters. The boys, in any case, are no longer babies and so long as they are pleasant and polite and do not create *scandali* they are old enough to decide for themselves.

Perhaps it is just because the Italian has great confidence in his ability to cope with the moment that long-term planning often seems irrelevant. In Italy, organization so often seems a game, a chance for animated discussion and self-importance, the pleasure of working out a *sistema* for its own sake, an opportunity to be imaginative, to embellish, to fantasize.

A friend of mine in the British Council attends occasional meetings at the Ministry of Education in Rome and described how these are voluble, lively and argumentative. However, at the end what has actually been decided is unclear. Then minutes are sent out to all who attended. These bear little relation to what was discussed. In the end, those in charge make their own decisions, and work into the small hours in order to implement them.

In Florence, we had drinks in the Piazza della Signoria with a girl who worked in the cultural department at the Town Hall. This was Thursday and she was helping to organize an exhibition in the Sala d'Armi which was due to open on Saturday.

"It's hopeless!" she bewailed, looking down miserably. "Everything is so chaotic. We planned to have neon lights attached to the walls but now the inspector from the Beni Culturali* says that we can't touch the walls because the building is historical. And the police won't allow lorries outside because it's a no-parking area, so we can't unload any of the exhibits. It's a shambles! Everyone is at cross purposes and it's all because the Christian Democrats are now in charge at the Town Hall. Before, when the Left was in power, everything worked beautifully."

"But will the exhibition open on Saturday, then?" I asked.

* (See p. 60).

She looked at me in surprise. "Of course!" And she went on to say in matter of fact tones that they were going to hang the neon lights from a special wooden structure that was being constructed so that the walls were not damaged, and they were going to work all night because the lorries could then park outside. "After all, it's advertised everywhere," she said. "Of course it'll open!" And it did.

This ability to resolve everything at the last moment, to organize on a personal level rather than through abstract planning, this absorption in the present shows two things. First, how the values of the small family community are still applied to relatively large structures, often giving an external sense of chaos and disorder. And, secondly, how successful it is in generating the vitality, the hard work and the freedom to be ingenious and creative of the individual Italian.

To the outsider, it is one of the mysteries of Italy: how, amidst all the apparent disorganization, it continues to survive and even to go forward. Indeed, an article in *The Economist* in July 1983 which outlined all the fearsome predictions and evidence of disaster was ironically called "E pur si muove!" – "And yet it still moves!"

SEX

In his book *Italia* Enzo Biagi has a chapter entitled "We speak so much about sex!" In it, he states that in Italy the importance of sex is recognized officially: while there is no compensation for an eye blinded in war, 97,000 lire is paid for the loss of both testicles.

Whether officially or not, Italian men have had a high reputation for their courtship and love-making, probably since the time of Casanova. In a novel by a Sicilian duke, Alberto Denti di Pirajno, there is a conversation about a newspaper in "Nordland" which has published an article warning their women to be careful. An Italian translates it aloud to friends in a bar:

> The sunny South is as tempting as the Garden of Eden. The men are gentle savages with velvety eyes, infectious smiles, lithe grace of movement and ravishing voices.... But beware of the wicked spell of the South.... Men down there have no inhibitions whatsoever, they are urged by unbridled, primeval instincts that place them on the level of animals on heat.

This article, comment the Italians, will simply provoke the girls to come in still greater numbers. "They quit their country and their families and rush into this shabby little town, lodging even in stables and pigsties if only they can be munched up by one of our wolves."

Certainly, a major attraction is the romanticized view of Italy: the sunlight, the wine, the gondolas and horse buggies – of which last few actually remain. Also, the magic associations of names: Capri, Sorrento, Venice, Garda, Como, Elba. The sense of the Mediterranean too: the olive trees and vines by bays of warm, blue water. Added to which is the fact that Italians are undoubtedly a beautiful race. Dominique Fernandez, a winner of the Prix Goncourt, talks of "Italianité" in a recent book *Le Promeneur Amoureux*. He defines it as "an affectionate rapport with the world, this indefinable quality of perception and sensuality which is perhaps due as much to the beauty of the countryside and of Italian men and women as it is to the earthy generosity of the eye which knows how to look, and the hand which knows how to touch".

Another factor is the boldness of the Italian male, although this also expresses itself in terms of snatched bags or wrenched gold chains in big cities. In Rome today, the traditional pestering of foreign girls would seem to have abated a little from the days when our female teachers would come back to International House as if pursued by swarms of wasps.

Because they are direct, communicative, and absorbed in immediate objectives, Italians tend to be open and unashamed about their motives. In the holiday town of Rimini there are, apparently, "seduction competitions" among the young bloods: six points for a Spanish girl, five for a South American, four for a French girl, three for an Italian, two for a German, one for an American, and none for a Scandinavian or British girl! As a respectable doctor said to me: "We can't make love to all the women in the world but at least we can try." However, as with males in any society there is also the element of bluff and display. Peter Nichols in his book *Italia, Italia* illustrates this when he writes about the holiday husbands left in the cities by their families who have gone to the seaside. They celebrate their "emancipation" by discussing with friends all the liaisons they are going to form, or already have, and then go off sadly to bed by themselves.

Although love is freer and easier everywhere now, most young Italians probably still get their first experience with a prostitute. There are supposed to be a million of these. Once, they were organized in brothels which were medically inspected. The girls moved from house to house every two weeks, and brothels were an established element in the life of every town and most small villages. However, in 1958, a Senator Merlin, who had once been a teacher, managed to get a law passed which made brothels illegal. The girls were left to "arrange themselves".

The law did not forbid soliciting and today you can see girls leaning casually against cars (rather than lamp-posts) at all hours of the day or evening, or driving round picking up men, or waving at single men in cars. Or, as you drive along main roads, you see a cluster of women at the side, sitting round a fire, forming a mobile brothel *al fresco*. At night, the flames light up tousled hair and drawn-up skirts. Travellers stop as they might in Britain at a Little Chef, and enjoy love amidst the bracken or in the backs of their cars. In Italy, as we have seen, the car is among the most popular places to make love: with the housing problem and most single people still living with their parents, it is the modern equivalent of the *garconnière*, or movable love nest. No wonder, as I was told in a class discussion in English on cars and traffic problems, "a man does not feel a man in Italy unless he has a car."

According to an article in *Due Più*, which is a serious monthly magazine on sexual problems, "the prostitution of transsexuals and transvestites is producing ruthless competition to female prostitution". This is endorsed by Luciano De Crescenzo in *Napoli di Bellavista*. He shows a photograph of two women round a fire with, at the side, a placard which proclaims: "Puttane Vere!" or "Real Whores!"

The article in *Due Più* goes on to describe how the prostitute is changing status. There is still the idea of her as a lost woman, unfortunate and exploited. Yet outside the more traditional towns, she often comes from the middle class and has made a deliberate choice of career. "What will be her future," the writer asks, "once her trade has become recognized as a profession like any other?"

Indeed, at the first National Congress for the Civil Rights of Prostitutes, held at Pordenone in north Italy in February 1983, one of the major organizers said: "We demand the same rights as other people. We are women, we are workers, and we want to be recognized." Another speaker expressed a willingness, unusual in Italy, to pay taxes but only so long as prostitutes were put on some sort of legal footing. Many of them, it was also stated, had had to make this choice because they came from a broken marriage with children, and no alternative jobs were open.

Gigolos, on the other hand, who because of Italian charm and reputation must find their lives fairly straightforward, are not so vocal – perhaps because, like most men in Italy, they have little to complain of. An article in the weekly magazine *Oggi* indicates that for one of them at least, love is no labour. Giovanni Rovai is now sixty, and has written a book called *Gigolo*. He is shown at a celebration, a wine glass in his hand, a cake on the table before him, surrounded by young beauties who for some reason all look very dreamy. Giovanni wants to open an Institute for Amatory Arts in Rome and has been a gigolo since the age of fifteen. He has never had any other job and has had no fewer than four thousand women, an average of two per week. At Viareggio where he practises his profession, he has even been given a "diploma di merito" by some of the holidaymakers. "Graceful gentleness has filled his days," it runs. Love, says Giovanni, is the whole reason for living and he is glad he has spent all his time giving pleasure. The photographs show him wrinkled with thinning hair, but smiling and slim. At the time of the article he was just off to London for a "commission", which he hoped would allow him to buy an overcoat with the proceeds.

Giovanni is sad about the future because he feels that love no longer exists. Men only think about power and money. They are too exhausted most of the time. Women, he says, once looked for love. Now they are hesitant and no longer give themselves with trust.

Maybe Giovanni is only talking indirectly about how old he is. However, sexual attitudes have certainly changed in Italy in the last few years, as they have in most industrial countries. For one thing, the pill is available everywhere and the whole ferment of the '70s has revolutionized mores. Results can be seen in the Eurostat figures for 1981. Population growth has sunk to 1.5 per 1,000 people, which is almost as low as Great Britain and much lower than France. At the same time, abortions are the second highest within the EEC and illegitimate births are therefore low, with only 4.3 per cent compared to 12.5 per cent in Britain.

Indeed, I was told in Turin that one hospital there gives a warmer welcome and better facilities to women coming in for abortions than it does to those who are going to have a baby. Apparently some middle-class women tend to regard a baby as on a par with any other expensive possession: "Oh well, I decided to end my pregnancy because we want to go on holiday to Kenya this summer. It's a pity, but I can always have one next year, unless of course we decide to buy a new car."

Both the pill and abortions have meant that traditional attitudes to chastity are disappearing, although in a country as complex and varied as Italy, and with an issue as personal as this, it is difficult to generalize. Traditional constraints must still be strong as new developments are so recent. When I visited the immigrant Italian community in Bedford, it was interesting to hear the Italian priest say that he thought the community had not been much affected by the free thinking current in England since the war. He had tried playing a tape giving sexual advice to those getting married as he could not very well advise them himself.

However, he had had to desist as there were strong objections.

As recently as 1974, the Italian High Court gave a judgment in which it was stated that "the cunning concealment on the part of the wife of loss of 'integrity' can constitute a grave injury to the husband". While in a book, *I Sultani*, Gabriele Parca states that among the men he questioned, who were all between 20 and 50, 66 per cent said they had gone virgin to the altar.

Although the South of Italy has changed greatly in the last twenty years, traditional thinking still seems stronger than in the North. An example of this was the story told by a friend in Naples about a Southern girl who was teased mercilessly by other women in a Northern hospital because she admitted to being a virgin at twenty-seven!

In Florence, Margherita Ciacci told us that research showed that established families tended to be less worried about their daughters than those who had only been prosperous since the war. Both might take a daughter's boyfriend along on holiday, but while the first group would accept their being lovers, the second would supervise them closely, and make sure they were not alone together.

Certainly, the 30 per cent who remain practising Catholics must be influenced by Pope John Paul's adamant refusal to countenance any variation on the Church's teaching on chastity and contraception. However, here again we are faced by Italian flexibility and spontaneity. I remember having a discussion with two young female teachers about how difficult it must be for Italians to confess when figures showed that contraceptives were widely used. "Oh, no," one of them said. "At confession we tell the priest what we want to." The other nodded.

Interesting here is Professor Donato's research into attitudes of women in the city and province of Mantua in north Italy. In the late '70s, he conducted a survey of 600 women. Of these only 23 per cent were against abortion under any circumstances. While of the 254 practising Catholics who were asked about their attitudes to premarital sex, a large number (147) were in favour of it "when one is in love, or when one wants to".

The point, probably, is that given the pill and free abortion, sexual freedom is no longer a menace to the family structure which itself is the key to Italian thinking. The days are over when a girl might bring back an extra mouth to feed without a husband to give economic support, because there is always an alternative.

With divorce, on the other hand, it is different. Despite the almost 60 per cent support for it at the referendum in 1974, and the fact that it has been legal since 1970, the Italian divorce rate is the lowest in Europe, apart from Ireland where it is forbidden. In 1981, only 13,000 couples were divorced in Italy, compared to 150,000 in Britain which has a comparable population. One reason, obviously, is that Italian bureaucracy makes it more complicated. It is also slower: five years of separation are necessary first, if both partners agree to divorce, and seven if one does not. However, since 1972 there have also been only 26,000 separations. Luca Goldoni, a well-known Italian journalist, says it is because Italians do not believe in resigning. "To resign from matrimony," he wrote in the *Corriere della Sera* in March 1983, "is objectively more complicated than to change political party. In addition to the children, there are long-formed habits, the domestic topography, the view from the window. We are also separating from a host of friends, from a part of our own lives."

In any case, there is a considerable amount of tolerance, of laxity within marriage, at least outside the South. Barzini tells the story of the husband who knows that his wife's lover, surprised the previous evening, is hidden under the bed. So when coffee is brought in the morning, he pours out a cup and courteously places it on the floor!

The welfare and advancement of children comes first, as always. A young friend of ours who is married with children told us: "I would prefer my husband to be unfaithful to getting a divorce. It would be too much having to live alone and support myself and probably the children. I'm sure he'd never pay me anything even if the courts granted me alimony. And the upheaval! We Italians don't expect people to be virtuous – only sensible! After all, we are brought up on Original Sin. We don't have the rigidity, the pride and subconscious Protestant rectitude of the North. I would expect discretion and would, of course, create hell if I found out. But I would never carry it too far."

And would she, herself, be unfaithful?

"Well, you know, I might be. On a journey or something. But never here. It would get round town too fast."

FEMINISM AND HOMOSEXUALITY

What is important is that women's attitudes to men in Italy seem to be changing fast. In the Fascist era, women were regarded as mothers whose duty it was to produce soldiers and workers for Mussolini's State. Now, as Biagi points out in his *Italia*, they demand satisfaction from men. Biagi quotes Giorgio Rifelli: "Until yesterday the sexual life of the Italian male relied on two premises: conquest and possession. Today what happens? Women have discovered eroticism and therefore aspire to a share of pleasure. But with emancipation they have also acquired the right to confrontation. This means that for their mates it is not enough to act. They also have to get involved." It will be interesting to see how far the Italian male loses panache and boldness as women themselves become more independent and more emotionally demanding. A psychiatrist, Dr Marco Cecchini, told me that the growth in the number of transvestites was largely due to this. Brothels had been the real confirmation of man's domination over women. Now, men who are not necessarily gay often prefer to go out for an evening with a transvestite who, while he has a feminine appearance, is not so different from themselves.

Recent films have introduced this theme directly or indirectly. In Antonioni's *Identification of a Woman* (1982) the main character, a film director, falls in love with an elusive woman who evades him because it seems she has a lesbian lover. A girl who attracts him by a swimming pool tells him she prefers sex with women because they are more *morbide* – the Italian for "soft". In despair, he goes off to Venice with a woman who wants him and finds that with her he is impotent. In this atmosphere of threat, almost of paranoia, he is lonely and isolated in what seems a dream-like female conspiracy to exclude him as a forceful, self-centred man.

In Naples my wife, Brita, went to see Lina Mangiacapra, the feminist film director, and founder and organizer of the annual festival at Sorrento of the "Cinema al Femminile". In 1983 she won the Premio Fondi, which is a national award for film-writers. She is particularly interested in rewriting myths and fables from the woman's point of view, as she feels that they have been moulded in the past by men. Thus, in her re-interpretation of Cinderella she makes her much more independent and not solely interested in the Prince. As a film director, she also complains that most films are directed by men and the film festival at Sorrento is a way of encouraging more films about women, and directed by them.

Unlike many feminists, she is against men only when she feels they are imposing their own point of view, or vision of the world. Her ideal, as she said to Brita, is a civilization where women have a sense of their own dimension and can express their own consciousness as freely as men. She doesn't believe in one-parent families; children need both father and mother with neither sex monopolizing self-expression, or muting the other.

In an interview in March 1983 for a newspaper, the *Corriere del Ticino*, entitled "But why have women given up their dreams?" she said that much of the fervour of the '70s has passed. There is a new generation now, more interested in spectacular than in real problems. Before, there was a belief that the world could be changed. Now that faith no longer exists.

Indeed, the very success of women in Italy in the '70s has perhaps made feminism less relevant to new generations. Before 1969, adultery by women was a crime, with stiffer penalties than rape. The psychology behind this was based on the idea that a man "owned" his wife. Rape was temporary possession of the female body, while adultery was theft not only of the body but also of allegiance, of the whole woman, love, "soul" and body.

Now, finally, Italian women are legally on a par with men. In 1971, they obtained equal rights over children. In 1977, a law was passed giving them equality at work, the same pay, and retirement rights at sixty. Also a wife now has personal ownership of any property she has brought to the marriage, while those working in the civil service can get a pension after fifteen years if they have one child. Maternity leave is also good. Five months' paid leave and a further six months unpaid are available, with the right to return to the same job afterwards.

Professionally, too, women are involving themselves to a greater extent. After the war, there was one female engineer and two women lawyers in Milan. Now 9 per cent of magistrates and 21 per cent of doctors are women; while from the universities in 1982 a third of those who graduated in economics, 10 per cent of engineers and two-fifths of those who passed out of schools of law and social studies, were women.

In Milan, Federica Olivares, a graduate in economics, has started a club called "Donne in Carriere" (Career Women), and estimates that there are 280 women managers in Italy. In Rome, Anna Maria Marmoliti, who works for the Central Committee of the Socialist Party, has started a "Club delle Donne" which has 800 members, and which in 1983 began the presentation of eight annual awards to outstanding women in the arts, management and the professions.

An article in the weekly magazine *L'Espresso* in August 1983 discusses the approach which women should have in roles which hitherto have been the domain of men. "The aggressive woman, typical of feminism, is out of date," says Lietta Tornabuoni, a journalist who writes about women's fashions. "A woman's appearance should reassure. Even if inside she is made of steel, the appearance should be of honey."

In Turin, women have also managed to establish their rights within the unions, particularly at Fiat, as we were told by Carla Brivello, an active feminist and a librarian at the university. Women have their own section called "Intercategoriales" which meets separately and they are allowed time off for these meetings. They also have a representative in a number of factories, who works to ensure that women are not discriminated against as far as new jobs are concerned. Now that 40 per cent of the entire Fiat workforce are women, the company recently had to alter their premises to accommodate this increased number.

However, Carla confirmed that the struggle is harder than it was in the full flush of the women's movement a few years ago. True, 50,000 women attended an anti-rape demonstration in Rome in February 1983, and a successful international conference was held in Turin in April 1983, with 600 delegates. Nevertheless, the recession and family loyalties mean that women still yield first place to men as far as industrial work is concerned. Many factories prefer women as part-time workers in a time of high unemployment and women will accept these opportunities rather than insisting on full-time work. Some women, Carla said, don't even apply for the dole, out of traditional resignation and self-respect.

Feminism, with all its achievements, has also been affected by *il riflusso* – a term used to describe the ebbing of the tide of forceful social protest which, in contrast to the flood of the '70s, seems now to be receding.

This is also true of the gay movement, although in Italy there has never been a law against homosexuality, and the age of consent is the same for both sexes at sixteen. "Homosexuality has never been a problem in Mediterranean countries," said Zeffirelli, the film director, in an interview published in *Advocate*, an American gay magazine, "also because no one talked about it!"

In Turin, I went to see Angelo Pezzana, the only person who has been elected to the Italian Parliament on a gay ticket for the Radical Party. Near the Piazza Castello in the historical centre, Angelo owns a large bookshop, the Luxemburg. He himself is in his forties and speaks excellent English.

Turin, he told me, is the city in Italy where there is most tolerance. This is partly because there has been a campaign for more information about gays ever since 1971 when *La Stampa*, the Turin newspaper, published an anti-gay article. As they refused to accept a reply, Angelo Pezzana and his friends created *Fuori*, a cultural homosexual magazine where they could publish what they wanted. A thousand copies were distributed to friends in ten Italian towns, and for six months it was sold on bookstalls.

Then, in 1979, the Fondazione Penna was started, named after a homosexual poet who is not widely known but has been praised by Moravia and Aragon as one of the best poets of this century. Its object is to distribute unbiased information about homosexuality all over Italy, and according to Pezzana it is this diffusion of information which will do most to reduce prejudice.

A recent survey undertaken by the Foundation shows that almost 60 per cent of Italians believe that homosexuals interfere with children, 53 per cent that they are violent, while 73 per cent of parents regard a homosexual child as a "misfortune". The survey also showed that the further people live outside the big cities, the greater are prejudice and ignorance.

Otherwise, there is little to fight against specifically. In the north of Italy there has been help from municipalities of the Left. In Bologna, premises have been given to a gay centre called Club 28 for debates, exhibitions, concerts and dances. While in Turin the Foundation is subsidized by the cultural department of the municipality.

However, the real problem is the Church. "The Pope expects us all to live like monks in total chastity," complained Pezzana. The resulting crisis of conscience is a torment to believing gays. A friend of his, Ferrucio Castellano, who was a strong Catholic believer, had committed suicide because of this, a few weeks previously.

However, here too things are changing gradually. In various towns, such as Turin, Assisi, Padua and Mestre, groups have been formed by individual priests who fight against the prejudices of society. The real enemy is hypocrisy. In an editorial in the only national gay magazine, *Babilonia*, a journalist, Felix Cossolo, has put the blame on gays themselves. He has criticized their timidity, their reluctance to "come out", their acceptance of a life where they go to gay bars at night and then assume respectable guises in business or the professions during the day, joking about the girls they have had.

As Angelo Pezzana commented sadly, "In Italy, you can be happy. But still not gay."

SENSE OF THE PAST

In an Apulian village we talked with a wheelwright. By the side of an empty piazza he had a shed full of metal scraps, while outside there were two old horse carriages with crumbling paint and pitted black leather seats.

On one side of the piazza was the façade of an old church with nothing behind it. Near it was a long wall with feeding stalls for horses and a row of tumbledown buildings with ragged roofs.

"There used to be a great horse fair here," said the wheelwright, waving his hand round to circumscribe the piazza. "It was the biggest in the *paese*. People came from all the neighbouring towns. Rich people with their families to buy horses and carriages and goods of every kind. They stayed opposite. There! It was a hostel famous all over the countryside. Crowded with important people it was. There was endless talk about buying and selling. Gaming. Great festas. Now it's all gone!"

"But anyway you've got the memory!" said Brita.

"How d'you mean? I'm only sixty! I wasn't alive then!"

"You weren't? But you describe it as if you remembered it vividly."

"How could I?" said the wheelwright, not a little piqued. "It was two hundred years ago!"

James Morris in his admirable book on Venice describes the way his housekeeper, Emilia, talks of everyone giving money for the Church of the Salute in gratitude for the end of the plague. "It happened just three hundred years ago," writes Morris, "but so strong is the sense of family in Venice, and so compressed are all its centuries, that Emilia half believed she had contributed a few lire herself."

Interestingly enough this sense of the past and of tradition does not seem to obstruct the way Italians take easily to modern ideas. Perhaps this is because their history has been one of continual change, adaptation and survival. Since Machiavelli looked back on the Romans as models there has been no obstructive fixation on a Golden Age to imitate and be anchored to, and an Italian will often explain modern events in terms of general historical causes. Rarely will you hear an Englishman talking about the undoubted effect on his national character of the rise of Protestantism. Yet Sicilians will tell you of the way the Arabs or the Normans have affected them and often when talking to Romans you expect emperors to emerge from the Palatine at any moment. I even remember a discussion with a girl in Perugia in which she said that the trouble with the city was that it had been taken over by the Romans from the Etruscans!

In Italy, there has been no real barrier separating past from present, no equivalent to Stephen Spender's remark that for him the division was the French Revolution: he always imagined that before it everyone wore fancy dress. One reason, almost certainly, is that large-scale industrial development has been so rapid and confined to only a few northern cities. Anyone over thirty can recall customs and ways of living which indeed may still continue in many parts, and which stretch back to the beginnings of European civilization. Another reason, surely, is that so much of the past is still visible, and not only in distinguished tourist centres. In the small town of Castro Villari in Calabria, you can still mark out different conquerors clearly by their buildings. Starting at one end of a ridge is the Church of Santa Maria del Castello constructed originally by the Normans. Then there is the gloomy prison, barred at the windows, which was erected by the Angevins and is still used. Then the Palazzo Capelli which was built in the time of the Bourbons and is a private mansion now used on the lower floors as a school. In front of this stretches a tree-lined avenue created by Napoleon and beyond is the rest of the town, built mainly in the nineteenth century. Then, way over the plain, is an immense concrete factory at the foot of the mountains. With its flashing lights and tall chimneys with wisps of indolent white smoke, the whole solid structure in that wild landscape looks like a creation of space invaders, assembled at random in the place where they first landed.

Instead of ages accumulating one on top of another, as they do in Rome, history in small Italian towns tends to stretch out horizontally. The variety of regions and landscapes and of the people themselves is multiplied by reminders of so many historical ages that one seems in Italy to be living on a large number of different planes all at the same time.

This was illustrated in a day we spent in and around Viterbo, north of Rome. First, we wandered round the medieval city and noticed a large open fireplace by the side of the street. We were just discussing whether it had been used as a communal street warmer on cold nights, when a man approached and explained that its function was once to warm the sentries who guarded the palace opposite. He introduced himself as Alberto Tuchetti, a sculptor in copper, and pointed to his studio at the top of one of those stone towers which were erected in so many towns of central and northern Italy (see p. 30).

Many of the buildings around us, he explained, were linked by stone staircases, or joined by corridors inside the arches which spanned the street. The covered way where we were then standing had once been part of a long gallery which led down to the battlements. Outside, the buildings remained as they had been in the Middle Ages. However, the way they were occupied changed the whole time, like different colonies of bees' nests in the hollows of an old tree.

"Have you seen the *cammamienti*?" Alberto asked suddenly. These were old Etruscan roads which had been dug twenty or thirty feet below ground level. Covered by the overhanging trees of what had then been forest, they had allowed the Etruscans to travel without being seen. One *cammamiento* stretched forty kilometres from Viterbo to the sea. "Why don't we go and look at it?" suggested Alberto.

As we walked to the car, Alberto told us how the Pope had taken refuge in Viterbo from disturbances in Rome in the twelfth and thirteenth centuries. Once, there had been three thousand chapels in the city as each cardinal built one for himself, and they had accumulated over the hundred years of papal rule. There had been many sieges too. Once, the starving inhabitants had saved what little food they had and fattened up a cow. They then threw it over the battlements to pretend to the army outside that they had plenty to eat. Discouraged, the besiegers departed.

As we drove out, Alberto showed us how parts of the city walls were literally layered with history, with the big blocks of Etruscan foundations, a Roman stratum above, and on top the medieval battlements.

We came to the *cammamiento*, which was just the beginning of a narrow road with great walls of earth on either side, and cavities where tombs perhaps had been. We got out of the car and walked. It was dark, with trees swaying over in a tracery of branches, and an occasional stump where one had been broken off by the heavy snowfall a few weeks earlier. There was silence except for the wind rustling the trees above. It was only a sunken road but it was evocative. Now it was metalled but it had been used for about 2,500 years, and it was easy to imagine the Etruscans walking and riding along the forty kilometres to the sea under this tunnel of branches.

Because so little is known about them, I find Etruscans attractive, mysterious figures, easily evoked by their sculpture and tombs – or even their *cammamienti*. They seem vague and shadowy. Their language may well resemble the sounds of the countryside: the chirp of crickets or the whisper of leaves. Romans are definite, prosaic: they wore breastplates or togas, spoke Latin, carried short swords. Etruscans seem to flit between trees, or commune in undiscovered tombs. Indeed, there is an Italian writer who has claimed in books and a television programme that he has met and talked to Etruscans!

We went up a rise and heard suddenly the clop of horses' hooves. We looked questioningly at one another and then back down the *cammamiento* which was hidden now by overhanging branches. Then from below two horsemen appeared, trotting gently along as they chatted quietly, seeming to belong to any century, any race.

That afternoon we drove out into the countryside with an old friend, Ausonio Zappa. We stopped at Tuscania, part of which was destroyed by an earthquake in 1971. An ex-student of Ausonio's was deputy mayor, and we called at his house. Great embraces and thumpings and expressions of delight ensued. When they were over, we went down the garden which ended at the top of a short cliff. There, said the deputy mayor, pointing over the damp hills in the drizzle, were the ruins of the castle which Barbarossa the German Emperor had destroyed in the twelfth century during the wars between Pope and Emperor. That on the large hill was the Church of San Pietro, with two towers at the side. Originally, the church had been built on the site of a Roman temple whose pillars could still be seen in the crypt. In fact it had influenced all the churches in Christendom because it was the first to be built with an aisle and two naves.

The towers themselves were all that was left of the old town of Tuscania before it had been transferred to the present site.

Nearby was also the restored church of Santa Maria Novella whose roof had collapsed during the 1971 earthquake, during which the stone rosette at the end of the building had fallen out and been shattered. Inside, there was a stone papal throne and later, when we visited it, Ausonio, who had once studied for the priesthood, had the satisfaction of sitting on it.

Fascinated and a little bewildered by so many facets of the past, we then went to the town library where we met Franco, the mayor, a youngish man with a cap. At his bidding, the girl in charge fetched various oblong containers and spilled thirteenth-century bulls out onto the table as carelessly as if they were newspaper cuttings. "Look," said Franco, pointing at one which had a great red seal and writing which reminded me of Magna Carta. "Celestino IV. And that one, Innocent IV!"

We walked through the building which had originally been the hospital and were shown a Romanesque chapel which had been turned into a small concert hall and art gallery. Lights hung down from the high arched roof and there were attachments round the smooth stone walls for paintings. "Before the earthquake this was a ward," said Franco; "all the walls and ceilings collapsed. But the structure stood firm. Suddenly we found that this chapel had existed all the time and we hadn't known it was here." It dated probably from the twelfth century and the crumbling of the false internal covering had killed six old patients.

We walked over to the Clarissan Convent of St Paul. On the way Franco told us that he had heard last week that another Etruscan tomb had been discovered and robbed by the *tombaroli* – the name describing those who make almost a profession of finding and emptying them. "The trouble," said Franco, "is that the government pay only a few thousand lire for each object found and foreigners pay millions of lire!"

We went up a narrow alleyway, past a wall with a few barred windows and Franco hammered at the door of the convent. "Chi é?" asked a voice in the darkness beyond a grille. "Sono Franco!" replied the mayor.

"His sister is the Prioress," said Ausonio. Soon, she appeared, greeting him affectionately, teasing him because the Christian Democrats were doing badly and saying he should do more to strengthen them if the Church was really going to be defended. After more banter, we said goodbye and walked back while Ausonio told me that the Clarisse were the female equivalent of the Franciscans, and that their rules were very strict. The convent had been built in 1259. A hundred years ago, he added, St Joseph had visited a stricken nun in her cell, and cured her of her illness.

We said goodbye and drove on to Ferrento. The drizzle had stopped. Damp, green fields sloped up from shallow valleys, or covered flat stretches on the top of small hills. I wondered how many Etruscan tombs still lay undiscovered.

When we got to Ferrento it was dusk. On one side of the road was a deep valley and patches of dark wood spread out on the hills beyond. Over the valley stood two massive crumbling towers of masonry, the last remains of the walls of the city where Otho, one of the three emperors who competed for power after Nero's death, was born. On the other side of the road was a theatre standing almost alone. "It is supposed to be one of the best Roman theatres for its acoustics," said Ausonio, and we took it in turns to stand on the stage and declaim.

The rest of the city is still buried. Beyond the theatre is a brief Roman street with marks of chariot wheels, and on one side they have begun to clear a hypocaust and tessellated pavements. From there, you can see the way the fields have covered the remains. Cows graze at a slightly higher level, and from the banks of earth that separate the excavated area thick slabs of stone protrude. Pompeii, Herculaneum were destroyed by ash and lava. Ferrento is interesting because it was shattered by the coming and going of invading Goths and Lombards, Franks and Byzantines. It was abandoned, and a medieval town was built nearby. Then it was simply buried and lost for centuries.

As I stood with the valley and the crumbling towers darkening in the dusk, I felt amazed that what had been a large town could simply be covered by drifting earth and grass and grazing cows.

For Italians it must seem representative of the instability of their past and by inference of their present. When exploring foreign countries it is easy to forget the unconscious assumptions of those who live there, bred into them by the surroundings they are brought up with. The experiences of this day of ours with its extraordinary tracery of different epochs which still – apart from Ferrento – were part of everyday living in the 1980s, could also be undergone almost anywhere else in Italy.

Even the big cities still display different civilizations. Industrial Milan has a centre which is recognizable in terms of different epochs: the narrow streets round Via Manzoni, the Austrian feeling which remains, the piazza in front of the medieval cathedral, the busy street which until recently was the moat before the city walls, the Sforza castle which represents the last time it had its own duke.

Behind one graceful and regular façade of the Piazza San Carlo in Turin, with its galleries and central statue of Victor Emmanuel II on horseback, you come suddenly on a city of glass which would grace New York.

However, it is in the small towns, where most Italians live, that there seems to be least distinction between past and present: in the north, round Modena and Vicenza; all over Tuscany and Umbria; the little mountain villages of the Abruzzi; Erice and some inland towns in Sicily which seem almost untouched; the crowded villages, often with Greek names and dialects, in Apulia, in the heel of Italy; villages such as the one we visited in Calabria where they have spoken Albanian since their ancestors fled the Turks after the sack of Constantinople in 1453.

In many countries, history is rejected or found tedious because it seems to have no relevance today. To most Italians it seems to be a cause of neither wonder nor rejection, but simply something that is there.

DEATH

This lack of wonder applies also to Italian attitudes to death. In Sicily, on the Day of the Dead – our All Saints Day at the beginning of November – presents are carefully wrapped up in splendid paper and given to children from dead relatives. "We do it," explained a Sicilian friend, "to make the children feel that those who were close to them have not really gone away, to ensure that they do not forget them. Now of course," he went on with a laugh, "they don't believe it as we did. But they still want the presents!"

In 1983 on the Day of the Dead, we found ourselves at Monte Cassino, where one of the fiercest battles of the Second World War was fought. The cemeteries of the Poles, Germans, French and British who with the Americans and Italians fought in this battle are spread out along the valley below Monte Cassino, which, founded as a Benedictine monastery in 529, was destroyed by American bombers in 1943.

The British cemetery has white crosses and stone pilasters, engraved with names in gold of Canadian, Indian and British fallen. It is set in a simple green space surrounded with trees. The Polish dead lie beyond Monte Cassino in rows beneath a great cross, paved out on a large, sloping, green field. The German cemetery has small marble crosses set in rows round terraces which are framed by low walls on a hill. Unlike the gentleness of the others, it looks somehow like a fortified bastion with its hard stone curves overlooking the plain, and its regularly planted cypresses standing to attention.

The Italian war cemetery is further away on the road to Naples but we stopped at the local one, a small enclosure by the side of the road. Here, two men were selling candles brashly at the entrance, while inside little groups were laying chrysanthemums on the tombs. Some of these were inserted into walls, with names inscribed on plaques, while for those who could afford it little chapels had been built, where whole families were buried. In the sunlight, groups of two or three busied themselves replacing flowers, raking gravel, or simply staring intently at the name of the person they had lost. As had happened for hundreds of years, a community was coming together on a definite day to commemorate those who had died.

In contrast, the national monuments to international wars, lying in the valley with the mist swirling down from the hills, were almost empty of visitors. There were testimonies: a votive lamp which had been given by Pope Paul VI to the German cemetery; a stone plaque which stated that the people of Cassino had contributed to the setting up of the British cemetery. In the German one, we met a boy who had travelled hundreds of miles to put flowers on the tomb of a boyfriend his mother had had before he was born; we also talked with a couple from Naples who were visiting the grave of a soldier the husband had known during the war, who had been knifed by the partisans.

Of course, distance and the fact that the soldiers died over forty years previously had their effect. Nevertheless, the contrast between empty stateliness and the long lists of names in gold on the one hand, and the

Italians busying themselves silently with the annual tribute to their dead seemed significant.

Perhaps because of families that until recently were very large, Italians are used to death. Infant mortality is lower than it once was, but it is still second highest in the EEC, coming after Greece, with 14.1 deaths per thousand. A friend of ours from Naples pointed out how different attitudes were in Britain: "In England, I was shocked," she said, "to feel that death was almost a taboo, something that shouldn't be talked about, something regarded as morbid."

In Italy, it is surprising how many corpses of saints are exposed under glass. In Modena Cathedral you come across the figure of St Germanius. You look at his sumptuous robes and suddenly become aware that under the mitre a skull is smiling. In Gubbio, the preserved body of San Ubaldo lies above the altar of his church. While in Viterbo, there is Santa Rosa, a young girl who died in 1250. She stares up from her glass-topped case, her teeth solid and prominent, her bony feet protruding from the bottom of her robe. Her skin is dark, but that is only because she was scorched in a fire some years ago. In fact, said the nun in attendance on her, it is amazing how supple her limbs still are, after more than seven hundred years. Before a festa, her robes are changed and it is possible to move her arms into or out of the sleeves without difficulty. "She is like a young girl," said the nun, "alive but unconscious. In a way you feel sorry for her lying there and expect her to wake at any moment and float away in clouds of glory."

Perhaps, though, the most extraordinary example of casual exposure of death is at the Capuchin catacombs of Palermo. When we visited them on a Sunday morning, they were officially closed. However, there was no difficulty in getting in. We went along a corridor, then down some steps and there, ranging along the walls, were thousands of dusty, fully dressed skeletons, suspended from cords round their necks.

The whole exhibition is divided into sections: "priests", "professional people", "women", and also "children" who were often dressed in tattered first communion dress. Some still have crinkled skin or wispy hair on their craniums. Some have top hats or bonnets, and tilt slightly towards each other so they seem to be whispering together, with their jaws hanging open in various expressions of protest or surprise. Once they all had glass eyes but these were taken by American soldiers as souvenirs during the last war.

This kind of interment was forbidden by law in 1881. Nevertheless, the prize exhibition is a little girl with smooth cheeks and auburn hair who died on December 6th 1920. Amidst the dusty, ragged skeletons she has a strangely normal and honeyed expression, and in the tourist literature is known as the Sleeping Beauty.

Several methods were used to preserve the corpses: a bath of arsenic which petrified them, or a calcium solution which covered them with a thick, protective layer. Some were operated on by specialists who removed everything that was corruptible, leaving only skin, muscle and bone. Another method was to leave bodies to dry in an alcove or in the sun.

The reason for this practice is obscure, but probably, like the presents on All Saints' Day, it was a means of keeping more closely in touch with dead relatives, who at least were visible and tangible, dressed in their finery. Lady Blessington described in 1823 a ceremony held once a year in the church of Santa Chiara in Naples, which perhaps illustrates how it also was in Palermo:

> The subterraneous chapels are guarded by soldiers. The altars are arranged in the usual style of those in Catholic chapels; innumerable torches illuminate the place; and an abundance of flowers and religious emblems decorate it. Ranged around the walls, stand the deceased, unhappily disinterred for the occasion and clothed in dresses so little suited to their present appearance that they render death still more hideous. Their bodies are supported round the waist by cords, concealed beneath the outward dress; but this partial support while it precludes the corpse from falling to earth does not prevent it assuming the most grotesque attitudes.

Lady Blessington was also horrified by the vaults in the cemetery where in an unsentimental, practical way, the dead were thrown and then covered in quicklime so that after a time their bones could be burnt for fertilizer. "The depths of ocean were a better grave than this den," she wrote, "where death, while robbed of its solemnity, is rendered more ghastly, more terrific, and more revolting by its victims being thrown into disgusting and obscene contact, to rot and mingle their putridity together."

Today in Naples, and in many other parts of Italy, a body is left to decay in a tomb for two years. Then it is cleaned, often by the nearest relative if he or she has not got the money to pay someone else to do it. The bones can then be placed in a smaller space in the overcrowded cemetery. Every so often, relatives will go back to clean the bones once more and to replace the shroud, as if they were doing the laundry for someone still alive.

As always, customs and attitudes are different in the north of Italy. However, if you go to the great monumental cemeteries in Genoa or

Milan with their palatial tombs, their sculptured angels, their ostentation in stone, you also feel the dead are not forgotten – even if they are remembered by their glorification rather than their corpses. To a foreign visitor these may seem typical of the Italian love of display, of a tradition which goes back to Hadrian's tomb in Rome which was large enough to be converted into a papal fortress; or more recently to "the wedding cake", whose white marble is superimposed on one end of the forum to commemorate Victor Emmanuel II, the first king of Italy.

However, in its own way, this commemorative attitude to death is also part of the family pattern. Just as most Italians want to do as much as they can for their children so they want also to buy the most splendid tomb they can afford for someone close to them who has died. The visual memory of the dead is needed as a reassurance that they have not disappeared completely. Just as the past is part of the present, so the death of people close to you does not mean they are totally separate.

CLASS-CONSCIOUSNESS AND THE GENERATION GAP

Except between families and groupings there are few frontiers in Italy. Snobbishness exists as everywhere, but role play is more important than any innate sense of superiority. If you are the boss of a firm you will probably treat your employees in a rough, authoritative way because you are in charge, and that is the fact of the matter. When, though, you are outside your firm you may defer to other forms of power. There is no equivalent of the British fee-paying public schools, or of Oxford, Cambridge, or the Ivy League colleges. There is no class in a permanent, innate sense. The desire to communicate penetrates most hierarchies, and it is interesting the way so many meetings end up as bawling matches.

There has, of course, always been a strong middle class, ever since the days of the mercantile city-states of the twelfth century. The Florence of the Medici excluded nobles from the self-government of the city. Later, from the sixteenth century, the aristocracy were not Italian, but mainly ruling foreigners. Even the Doges' Venice was an oligarchy rather than an aristocracy, and it was the Austrians who between 1815 and 1866 offered titles to the great families which, in many cases, were rejected. After unification, it was not until 1922 that a definitive "Debrett's" of the Italian nobility was drawn up. Now there is no monarch, no court and, except in Naples, no equivalent memories of Versailles, Potsdam or St Petersburg.

"Aristocracy – what a vague term!" said Prince Ruspoli in an interview in 1983. "It includes people who are so diverse: gentlemen and ladies who are scattered everywhere, who have only a little in common. It's a class which does not exist."

There is the same lack of division between old and young. Talking of social provision for the old in Italy, Professor Antonini, head of the department of gerontology in Florence, said in an interview in 1983: "Up to now there hasn't been the need, given that family life has been sufficient guarantee for the care of old people." Because parents have lived so much for their children, it would be socially and personally unacceptable for sons and daughters not to look after them in turn when they are old. As the whole family usually live together until sons and daughters are married, they get used to sharing a home as adults. Later, when one of the old couple is widowed, it may well be a godsend for him or her to stay in the young couple's home when they are out at work, or to contribute financially from a pension or savings.

In an article in the *Times Educational Supplement* on an exchange organized between schools in Camberwell Grove and Florence, Tom Baldwin commented on the surprise of the English girls at finding grandmothers in so many of the homes they stayed in, and also at the fact that they "actually seemed to have a prominent part in decision making".

Change, however, is inevitable. For one thing, old people everywhere are living longer. For another, the low birth-rate also means the number of old people is increasing, and that with smaller families there must be fewer young people able to lodge and help their elders. As one of the schoolchildren's reports in the International Year of the Aged states: "Twenty years ago, the family was patriarchal. Old people had a definite place, were respected and were sure of dying in bed, surrounded by sons and daughters. Now, instead, they are often alone and when they are fortunate and still live with their families, their sons and daughters no longer have time because they work."

In Palermo, I discussed this with Bishop Giallombardo who is in charge there of the Church's "human" projects. "There are so many problems now," he said. "Yesterday, I was called by a lady who works and yet has to look after her old mother of eighty. She said she couldn't go on. What would I advise? I had to tell her she shouldn't give up. Her mother wasn't ill or anything. What could I offer her? The trouble is that the will to look after old people is less."

In 1983, it was calculated that 19 per cent of old people in Italy live by themselves. There are hospices for the old, pleasantly called "houses of rest". However, these vary greatly in number and quality, depending on the town they are in – as so often in Italy. Inevitably, the problems are greater in the big towns such as Turin, Rome, Milan or Palermo. In Milan a priest told me he knew of several old people who lived in rooms at the top of buildings where there was no lift: some were incapable of going out for food because they couldn't climb stairs. He and a group of volunteers brought them food and visited them regularly. But he wondered how many suffered alone without any help, apart from that given by neighbours.

In many northern towns there is a well-developed service for old people. In Trieste, near the Yugoslav border, two out of five inhabitants are pensioners because recession has hit the town particularly badly, so young people have left to work elsewhere. Among facilities are two special centres with library, reading room and a place to show films. There are discounts for old people on buses, and at cinemas, and cheap lunches are provided. The municipality also organizes holidays to the sea or mountains, free laundry and a subsidy with a maximum of 200,000 lire ($80) to those in need. Home help is also available.

In Trento, services are similar and anyone who has a pension of less than 400,000 lire ($175) a month can get a grant which brings it up to that figure.

These of course are towns which were under Austrian rule until 1919 and have welfare schemes similar to those of northern Europe. The further south you go, the weaker the central organization and the more the family takes its place, particularly as far as looking after old people is concerned. However, throughout Italy, as we have seen, there is no dearth of welfare benefits and almost a third of the adult population receive an old age or invalid's pension.

One interesting development for old people is what is called "The University of the Third Age" – to translate literally. The idea for this originated in France and has now spread to about fifty cities in Italy. In Palermo, I climbed a broad stairway, with the cracked, blotched paint usual in aristocratic mansions which have been turned into public offices. On the first floor, there were the reception area and big lecture room of the university, which had just been set up. The organizer, an energetic man of sixty-five, told me that anyone over forty could sign on whether he or she had educational qualifications or not, and that the average age of those who attended was fifty-five. Courses, as at other universities of this kind in Italy, were predominantly on subjects of local interest. In Palermo, apart from simple medicine and first aid, they included Pirandello, Sicilian literature and the Mafia.

A lecture was given on each subject once a week so that "students" could attend all the available five courses. Lecturers were teachers from Palermo university who gave their services free, while each of the fourteen trustees contributed the equivalent of $50 to the general fund. Fees were minimal: the equivalent of $12 entrance for a four-year course and $20 a year. At the end, a certificate was given, based not on exams but simply on attendance. There was no compulsory reading: a book list and duplicated notes were provided – it was important that the people should get what they themselves wanted from the course.

In France, the whole organization is much more selective and academic. Characteristically, the object in Italy is not to exclude anyone, or to embarrass those who have little educational background. In fact, what would in Britain be called Adult Education is being exalted by the name of University, and run through voluntary help rather than by the municipality.

However, an additional service has also been set up, called "Tribunal of the Third Age", which consists of three retired magistrates and four members of the course. These meet once a month on Saturdays and deal with complaints from old people about transport, water supply and administrative services, giving advice and putting pressure on the local authority where necessary.

Whatever the actual effectiveness of this organization, it is an interesting attempt to solve the dilemmas which countries with weaker family ties have been confronted with for some time and have usually tried to solve institutionally. In Italy it is still difficult to do this because institutions so often don't work effectively and, in any case, centuries of family organization make people reluctant to depend on anything colder and less personal. Professor Antonini stresses the need to allay the fears and sense of isolation which old age can bring in modern times. "The best social worker," he says, "is always a relative."

He also attacks the modern idea of dividing life into phases with the assumption of slow decline after retirement. After all, an old person costs the equivalent of $400 a month in a home and $80 a day in hospital. This money, in his opinion, is best spent in ensuring that old people can remain part of the community as long as possible so that the slow decline that leads to residence in a home or hospital can be delayed.

In Palermo, Bishop Giallombardo emphasized that, however well designed and comfortable it may be, a home for old people is bleak unless there is a family atmosphere. One way of achieving this is to pay the transport for old people to go back to their families during the day and use the residence only to sleep in. This happens now in practice and with the solidity and strength of the Italian family structure behind them, many old people involve themselves at home.

If social organization gradually takes over, even in the South, my guess is that the cohesion and warmth of the family unit will express itself in any new developments.

Of course, some Italians challenge this and even deny family influence altogether, because they regard it as something primitive, particularly if they come from the North, are ashamed of the South, and aspire to be "modern" – which for them implies the kind of quick-speed, egotistic hedonism they feel is typical of the United States and Northern Europe. Also, if they really are to the Left, rather than just having tribal affiliations, they quite correctly regard the family as being the principal obstruction to the "impartial" rule of institutions.

However, there is an old Italian song of the 1950s which expresses one of the precepts on which Italian society is based:

> Io ti do una cosa a ti,
> Tu mi dai una cosa a mi.

In English, this means: "I give you something to you. You give me something to me." After all that Italian parents have given their children, it is unlikely that their sons and daughters will not return it in some form – whatever shape society may take.

YOUTH AND PROTEST

"We really felt betrayed," explained Giancarlo. "All the promises of liberty, of democracy which we had grown up with since 1945 had come to nothing. There were just these corrupt old men shuffling along in power, in politics, in the universities, in industry. They controlled everything, made personal fortunes, had no sense of responsibility in their jobs, were clever only in knowing how to protect themselves. We wanted to sweep them away, build a new, clean Italy, an Italy to which the young could give their energy, their idealism, their imagination. We would talk into the small hours round café tables about politics and the ideal society. About America, embroiled in Vietnam, and what a dirty world it was. We were so intense! I remember asking a girl to come dancing after one of these meetings, and she was shocked. 'This isn't the time for triviality!' she said. 'We have so many things to talk about! So many things to do!'"

The student revolt in Paris in May 1968 probably had little lasting effect either in the rest of Europe or in America. In Italy, though, it was a trumpet call and started a chain of events which convulsed the '70s. Unlike France, students and workers co-operated in demonstrations, strikes and sit-ins. Unlike France, the Communist Party sided actively with the dissidents. Unlike France, there was no strong Presidential executive capable of quieting the unrest, or leading it down different paths. Unlike France again, there was also a strong party of the Right in violent conflict with the Left.

Starting with bombs in Rome and Milan in December 1969 which killed fourteen people and injured a hundred, the decade was characterized by street fighting and a series of outrages, culminating in the explosion at Bologna railway station in 1980 which killed as many as eighty-five people and injured two hundred.

Industry, meanwhile, was afflicted by innumerable strikes and sit-ins. "If the Italian industries managed to survive the '70s, they can only improve in the '80s," wrote the manager of a branch of a multinational in north Italy in a 1982 handout to foreign customers.

Indeed, the 1970s in Italy can be said to have achieved as much as many revolutions, yet without guillotines or, paradoxically, a real change of government. New legislation introduced the welfare state in medicine, social security and trade unionism. It was established that taxation should in principle be related to income, and divorce and abortion were legalized.

Like most revolutions this one may seem ultimately to have changed very little except on paper. Many of its measures were hasty and ill thought out, with consequences which are difficult to deal with. However, it has changed perceptions and defined new attitudes and has brought Italy closer to its industrial neighbours over the Alps. It has also shown that central government in Italy, perhaps because of its relative irrelevance, can survive radical change, can, python-like, absorb and digest almost anything, and yet always return to its original shape without changing the pattern on its body.

Paradoxically, this survival was due mainly to the attitude of the Communist Party, the largest in Europe, with almost a third of Italian votes. Berlinguer, appointed General Secretary of the Party in 1974, was convinced by the overthrow of the Allende government in Chile that a government of the Left could achieve nothing if only a small majority of the nation – and that the poorest – was in favour.

In the municipal elections of 1975, the parties of the Left reached their highest level of electoral support and captured control of many of the major cities, such as Naples, Rome, Milan, Florence and Turin. However, in a country where voting is theoretically compulsory, the

Communists, Socialists and Social Democrats, who would form an uneasy coalition at the best of times, attained a bare majority of only 51.3 per cent. To take power, Berlinguer realized, would be to arouse the opposition of international finance and of powerful national vested interests which might rally to an unscrupulous rag-bag of Fascists, Monarchists and disillusioned Christian Democrats who, aided by American finance, might seize power, as in Chile.

Berlinguer chose what came to be called "the historic compromise": the Communists would support the government in Parliament. In return, measures of which it approved would be introduced. The result was a flow of radical legislation. But what of all those young people of whom Giancarlo was an example? Although the Communist Party supported them in their demonstrations and protests outside Parliament, the historic compromise seemed yet another manoeuvre, typical of that fudging and kaleidoscopic shifting which, in principle, was what so many young people were protesting against.

One result was increased activity by the Red Brigades, which is a general name covering a number of terrorist groups, all working together to destroy confidence in the State. Founded in 1970, they used indiscriminate killing, "knee-capping", bank raids and kidnapping to create a sense of fear and anarchy. Italy had never had a successful revolution, which could have modified or weakened the old ruling class. It was better, therefore, they argued, to clear everything away and start anew.

Less clear was what would happen if the State did collapse. The Red Brigades, presumably, would take power and create a Left-wing government whose outline was uncertain, but which would be "just", "pure", "incorruptible" – in short the kind of puritan utopia of the virtuous which has resulted in brief, bloody autocracies like those of Robespierre, or Pol Pot in Cambodia.

The young men in the Red Brigades justified their actions because in their eyes the State itself was a source of violence and, indirectly, of murder. This is illustrated in *The Death of Men*, a novel by Alan Massie who lived in Rome during the '70s. In the book Tommaso, a young marquis who has joined a Red Brigade, argues that the money spent on an autostrada because it would gain votes and fill politicians' pockets is itself murderous as the money could have been spent on cardiac or dialysis centres. "So someone whose life could have been saved is dead because of this cynicism, and others are dying because that road has been built. So who is the worse killer? That politician or the boy – maybe me – with a machine gun?"

It has often been said that the Red Brigades were influenced by Catholic tradition and thought, and that they were an alternative form of expression of disillusioned Catholic youth. Renato Curcio, their founder, had a Catholic boarding-school education and was a member of the Catholic student movement when he joined the first faculty of sociology in Italy, at Trento, in 1964. This was founded by a Christian Democrat, Kessler, and one of its projects was to bring Catholics together to examine what had gone wrong in Italy. Curcio, however, soon transferred his interest to Marxist politics, took a prominent part in the student revolts of 1968–9 and was the original founder of the Red Brigades. Captured in 1976, he is now in prison in Palmi in South Italy. When Aldo Moro was captured and killed, he pronounced from prison that "this act of revolutionary justice is the highest act of humanity possible in this class-ridden society".

This kind of sententious jargon, highly moralistic, whose values seem upside down, reminds one of Jesuitical sophistries. Denouncing something or someone is common in Italy. Often you wonder how it is that you always seem to meet the few who don't give or take bribes, as any discussion about politics usually involves attacks on corruption. Until of course you delve deeper, as I did one evening in Aosta when having a drink with a Christian Democrat pastry cook, a Communist ski instructor and a Socialist plumber. After the usual denunciation against those who don't pay their taxes, it became clear that the plumber was often paid by individuals without an official receipt, that the pastry shop didn't find it necessary to record all its income and that the ski instructor was paid on the side for private classes, which of course he never declared.

This is not so much open hypocrisy but more a question of playing different roles at different times, without consciously putting them together. It stems probably, like Red Brigade jargon, from the dichotomy between the Church pulpit and what happens in the market place. It is also sectional: thus if you are robbing for a political party, or your family, or a cause, you are justified, even if everything goes into your own pocket. Like that extraordinary incident on the boat from Naples to Ischia, which was boarded by pirates who stole the wages of hundreds of poor employees, which were being transported to the island: "Don't worry! We are proletarians!" were the last words of a pirate to the captain, as they departed.

Perhaps the most perverted example of this doctrinal obsession was the Red Brigade murder in January 1983 of the lady who watered the flowers and checked in the parcels in the prison of Rebibbia in Rome.

The gang, consisting of two boys and a girl, captured her and took her to a house where they went through a ritual "trial". For, as she was on the staff of a state prison where Red Brigade captives were held, she was an "enemy of the people".

A photograph of her shows a hunched woman of fifty-seven in a shabby coat, looking down at the floor with her hands clasped hopelessly on her lap. She sits under a banner inscribed with phrases such as "Power of the Armed Proletariat". A tape of this "trial" reveals the story of the "accused". She was given work in the prison, almost as a favour, because her father, who was a plumber on an invalid's pension, died and she had no means of support. The pomposity and sense of power of the "judges" comes out clearly during the interrogation, which reveals that the woman had nothing to do with prisoners, that she couldn't get another job because of her age and arthritic condition, that just after her father's death she had no income at all and survived by cadging meals off relatives.

When she breaks down and cries, her interrogators tell her that she needn't think they are going to be moved by her tears, and there is the sound of a shot. "Proletarian Justice" has been done. Later, the three "judges", who were all in their early twenties, were arrested when robbing a post office, and one of them broke down and sobbed.

The year 1980 was among the worst for terrorist outrages, with 122 people killed, but since then Red Brigade activity has been decisively reduced. In 1981, the number of those murdered dropped to 31, and in January 1983 a statement of surrender was issued from the prison where Renato Curcio and other terrorists were held. It admitted that "the cycles of revolutionary struggles in the beginning of the 1970s, based on the wave of workers, and radical student movements, have substantially ended".

Rightly, Italians are very proud of this. They balance it against all the scandals and disasters of the last few years and point out that they dealt with the Red Brigades without it affecting their democracy. How was this achieved? Partly by a law of "penitents" which allowed a reduction of sentences by three-quarters for those who gave evidence. Help was given to those who then wanted to flee the country – although the brother of one penitent, Patrizio Peci, was killed in revenge: a moving photograph shows the ex-terrorist at the graveside looking down at the ultimate consequence of all the murders he committed.

Another measure was the setting up of special anti-terrorist units which resulted in the freeing of the American general James Dozier in January 1983. Dozier was the first foreign victim of the Brigades and had been abducted from his house in Verona six weeks earlier, and smuggled up to a first-floor flat in Padua, concealed in a trunk. In a brilliant operation, the "leatherheads", a special group of police, burst into the flat, released him, unharmed, and captured five terrorists and a mass of documents and information.

As a result, the courts in Milan, Rome and Turin have been full of sullen and defiant youths, enclosed in cages like animals in the zoo, clasping the bars, chatting, listening, even copulating: at least one pregnancy has been initiated, concealed behind the massed bodies of the accused.

In January 1983, fifty-nine terrorists were found guilty of the murder of Aldo Moro in 1978 (see p. 11), and in December 135 were tried for other murders – although among this number only nine received life sentences because so many had given evidence. This mildness provoked a storm of protest among those related to victims, and among the public at large. However, the clemency was also a sign that terrorism was no longer so greatly feared. In March 1983, a poster appeared all over Rome, showing terrorists on trial, snarling like savages, while inset below was a group standing round a victim who was lying in his own blood. Underneath, were the words "Democracy has been saved!"

At their peak, the terrorists were estimated to have had about 1,000 armed participants and perhaps 10,000 helpers. Four hundred gave evidence against their comrades, and the trials summarized the tragedy with accounts of casual killings, of parents unaware that their sons were terrorists, of people bewildered because their relatives had been killed for no apparent reason. Indeed, perhaps the most terrifying thing about it all was the difficulty in understanding it. There seemed to be no positive political motivation, no national or religious creed, but simply the urge to eradicate. It was like the actions of people under a malignant spell in a horror film. Why should the cheerful postman who delivered the post at the house of a student of mine every morning turn out suddenly to be a member of a Red Brigade?

In Bologna, I went to the Institute of Sociology in the university, up the broad stairs and under allegorical paintings on ceilings to talk with Professor Pierpaolo Donato who felt that the Red Brigades were now not only dead but, more important, "out of fashion".

In 1968, he told me, young people really had believed they could change things politically. Frustrated fanaticism had led not only to the Red Brigades but also to the Right-wing Black Brigades. However, already at the Communist Conference in Bologna in 1977, students had begun to show social rather than political interest, concern for what in

Italy are called the *emarginati* – literally those "on the fringe": handicapped people, the old, the mentally ill, the drop-outs.

Now, in the '80s, even that has changed. Young people are more "American", intent on pleasure, on material acquisition, on personal success. Their political interest tends to be limited to local affairs and local elections, rather than national issues. The nature of their personal relationships is also of great importance. Donato compared them to a river flowing underground: because they are more concerned with each other and what is immediately around them, it is not so easy as it used to be to know which way they are going.

Gigi Dall'Aglio of the theatre group Collettivo di Parma confirmed this in his interpretation of the *Hamlet, Macbeth* and *Henry IV* which the group put on at the Riverside Theatre in London in 1983. To him, the three plays illustrate – among other things – the changes of attitude which he himself has seen in Italy during his own lifetime of thirty-five years. *Hamlet* represented the belief that words could change things; *Macbeth* was murder, squalor, fear – the whole period of the outrages, the Red Brigades and youthful frustration. While *Henry IV* exemplified the present alternatives: either the escapist clowning of Falstaff, or the resigned acceptance of a political status quo which it is impossible to challenge, in the shape of Henry IV and Prince Hal.

In Bologna, I also went to see other university teachers. One of them, when accompanying me out, pointed at the walls round the central lobby. "A few years ago, these were covered with inflammatory posters and graffiti," he said. "Now their blankness, their emptiness shows how students no longer externalize!"

In a disjointed fantasy film called *Sogni d'Oro*, distributed in 1981, Nanni Moretti satirizes the way Italian youth have changed. In one scene, Michele, a film director who lectures at university, gets his whole class to stand and repeat the refrain: "We are shit!" – like robots. In a fantasy sequence a rival director is shown creating a strange cabaret out of an anti-Vietnam procession with a group of workers and students shouting slogans, carrying posters and clenching their fists, while at the same time they move absurdly in time with the dance music, as if they were not in control of their bodies.

Italians now in their thirties often speak nostalgically about the '70s, rather as the old Fascists talk about the war – as if it were an exciting, worthwhile battle which they had lost. "I remember going to one of those demonstrations which now take place so rarely, in the piazza in Milan, a few months ago," a signorina in her thirties told me. "It was rather like that poster on Woodstock ten years later, with all those middle-aged people shouting old slogans, singing the same political songs, behaving as they did in their early twenties – enacting something which has no reality – only nostalgia."

Now a research project by Alessandro Cavalli from the university of Pavia concludes that modern youth no longer feel they have a social role and therefore get involved only in whatever they are doing at the immediate moment. He compares this absorption to a digital watch where time appears as a sequence of present moments, as opposed to the more old-fashioned clock-face where the present is marked as part of a circle, which includes present, past and future. To the question he posed to adolescents, "Which of the following activities have you taken part in during the past week?", the most frequent answers were as follows: watching television, taking a *passeggiata**, listening to the radio, records or tapes, reading, looking at shop windows, going to a bar, and finally, some form of sport.

However, the echoes of protest still continue, and one of the interesting aspects of walking through Italian towns is the way you come across little groups of students who have set up a few crates covered by a blanket, with pamphlets and posters denouncing the arms race, or drugs, or missiles, or who ask everyone to sign a petition to increase pensions.

The installation of Cruise missiles in Comiso in southern Sicily has also stimulated opposition among young people, with processions organized by the Communists who are the only major party supporting unilateral disarmament. In October 1983 there were processions against Cruise all over Italy, consisting largely of students and secondary-school children. One evocative poster showed a forest of matches with one that was lighted poised just above them.

In Palermo, a leading Communist official told me that more than a million votes against Cruise had been collected in Sicily alone. Emulating the Swedes, it was planned to have a chain of people holding hands over eighteen kilometres near Comiso as a protest. The installation of Cruise in Sicily, the official said, not only put the people of the island in danger but also represented a threat to Middle East countries like Libya, since Sicily's geographical position made it a natural link between the rest of Italy and countries round the Mediterranean.

However, it is characteristic of the political situation in Italy that protest is associated so obviously with the Communist party. Indeed,

---

* A communal stroll usually taken on the main piazza of a village, or town.

how can there ever be any pretence of political objectivity when
everyone knows that things are only achieved by banding together in
strong protective groups and sniping away at the others – not
necessarily because one disagrees with them but simply because they are
rivals for power and patronage?

Because Communists are the only supporters, the suspicion that
Moscow is behind the movement is even greater than in most European
countries. Italians, too, are very much aware of their dependence on the
United States and there is the feeling expressed by a worker living near
Comiso which was quoted by Campbell Page, the *Guardian*
correspondent, that "Dollars are better than Peace". In any case, the
missiles are in Sicily, which to many Italians is almost a foreign country,
far from the centres of population and power. "At worst," joked a
northern Italian, "it could be a way of getting rid of the Mafia, once and
for all!"

UNEMPLOYMENT

Another concern of youth, also common to the whole of Western
Europe, is unemployment, which in September 1983 was 11.6 per cent
of the working population – identical to that in Britain. However, as
has been said, it is particularly important in Italy to beware of official
figures. The year's conscription for everyone over eighteen makes the
comparative situation worse in Italy, as does the system of Cassa
Integrazione (see p. 107). There are also about a million university
students and, as a professor in Cosenza university told me: "Many
students stay on because they can't get jobs. In some ways our university
system is just a way of postponing the dole."

However, every Italian situation is paradoxical. In some universities,
such as Bologna and Urbino, students come up from the South to enrol,
precisely because they know that during the summer they can earn
handsomely in the holiday resorts on the Adriatic coast, such as Rimini.
Their savings allow them to live at university for the rest of the year,
independently of their parents. Many other students attend university
while they actually have jobs. Indeed the whole system is "very loose" –
as one university professor put it. Anyone who has the *maturitá*, which is
the rough equivalent of British A-levels, can enrol and in most
universities can be a student almost for life.

It would also be interesting to know the proportion of unemployed
who actually have jobs. Talking of her neighbour's son, a friend of mine
in Varese said: "Oh, now that he's unemployed, the family bakery is

much more successful as he delivers bread to people's homes which they didn't do before." In any case, dole money is very low – only about 800 lire (30 p.) a day, so no one can live on it. Those who have never been employed receive nothing, so a boy or a girl leaving school has to live off his or her parents, or find a job in the "black economy".

In Potenza, I went to see the general secretary of the local trade union. The offices were in a modern building which was part of an ugly concrete sprawl on the side of a ridge. Corridors were full of men smoking, raising their voices, gesticulating. In Simonetti's office, a poster on San Salvador was in red letters, as if dripping blood. Another quoted a poem by Brecht: "It is night. Couples caress each other in bed. The young women give birth to orphans."

The general secretary was young, fluent, dynamic. "The province of Basilicata has an unemployment rate of 16 per cent – the highest in the EEC," he stated indignantly. "It was all right after the earthquake in 1980 because a lot of labour was absorbed in repairing buildings. But now we have 50,000 without work! It's all the fault of the government for not encouraging new industry!"

However, as so often in Italy, delving produced an alternative version:

"Well, actually the numbers of those without work throughout the year are only a few thousand. A lot are on Cassa Integrazione and then there is special employment."

"What's that?"

"Well, people who may or may not be in work," he said mysteriously.

I asked about young people coming out of school who could not draw the dole.

"Well, most of them are all right. In the summer they help with the harvest and earn enough for the rest of the year."

It is rarely appreciated how much Italy looks after its citizens, as if each region or town were an enormous protective family. Also, given that political parties still rely on buying votes, it is more rewarding, particularly in the South, to subsidize family groups than it is to set up new industry. A factory will probably lose money and employ a limited number of people who will soon forget which party is responsible. As I was told in Calabria, "in the South, we have reached the post-industrial stage without going through the industrial". Certainly, no country in Europe is more prepared for the economic phase we all seem to be reaching: a small automated industrial base and an accumulation of small businesses which together subsidize mass unemployment.

In Italy, though, the subsidy does not seem so much a stimulus to creative leisure as a means of increasing small-scale economic activity. This is taken for granted by Italians in a way that often seems strange to Anglo-Saxon ears – as when I discussed the disappearance of extreme poverty in the Calabrian countryside with an economist:

> No – in the countryside you can be reasonably well off, better now than in the towns. After all, you not only have your dole and probably also a pension but also your earnings from your work and the produce from your patch of land. If you've just left school and therefore have not been employed before, a neighbouring farmer will probably testify that you have worked for him for the legal minimum of fifty-one days. Then you can draw the dole without difficulty. If the whole family are on the dole and also working and also cultivating their land, they can probably save and put some money into modern comforts or better fertilizers, or maybe a little business in a neighbouring village or town. And so it goes on.

Those who are made redundant also get a fixed sum payable by law, called *liquidazione*. This is the equivalent of about a fifteenth of annual salary, which is supposed to be put by and given to the employee when he leaves. The employer of course rarely saves these sums and the result is that employees sometimes get what they want from management simply by threatening to leave en masse and thus bankrupt the firm.

In the case of redundancy, the newly unemployed can use this sum to invest, or start a business.

It is difficult, therefore, to assess the real unemployment figures in Italy. As elsewhere, though, there is obviously a demoralizing effect, making Italian youth less confident of the future, more critical of the objectives of their schooling, and less interested politically.

DRUGS

Perhaps high unemployment has also had an influence on the taking of drugs, which has grown enormously since 1977. Important here is the sense of political futility, at least according to an ex-drug addict quoted in *La Nazione*, a Florentine newspaper, in 1983: "The end of the revolutionary culture gave us a choice which to many of us seemed inevitable: either violent action or drugs." The speaker goes on to say that heroin also seems to have a political justification because it evokes so much middle-class disdain that addicts feel yet more separated from the hated "bourgeoisie".

A report from Censis, a research organization, puts the number of drug addicts at 200,000 at the beginning of 1984, with 1,200 deaths since 1973. Returns from different parts of Italy show that the worst area is Rome and its province, the whole area to the north up to the Apennines, and then east into Emilia Romagna and the Veneto. The South remains relatively immune, with a slightly higher ratio in Sicily, Sardinia and Naples and its province.

The area round Verona is particularly affected because the town is a commercial crossroads with outlets east to Austria and Yugoslavia, north to Germany and Switzerland and west to the big industrial cities of the plain and to France.

In Kenya, of all places, I met an English girl who had worked in Milan for four years helping drug addicts. "It is worse for Italians than for others," she told me, "because their families are close and, whether they go to Church or not, they are supported by their religious traditions. Taking drugs, therefore, means a much greater break than it does for North Europeans who are often isolated already. It cuts them off from everything that has sustained them. It makes them more alone and tottering."

A girl called Manizia Scoglio, talking in the magazine *Oggi* about her ten-year fight with heroin, said: "At the beginning, I was looking for something, and I considered drugs an experiment, at best a means of reaching what I was searching for more easily. Afterwards, however, drugs were the end of my life, the only way of losing consciousness of my despair, of forgetting that I was no longer searching and no longer even capable of looking for anything."

Now, according to Censis, the age of those taking drugs has gone down and the average is fifteen to eighteen years old. In Milan in December 1983, there was a massive demonstration of mothers against inactivity on the part of the authorities. One of their objections was that the only solution was to send their sons abroad to France or Spain where there were adequate centres but where treatment cost the equivalent of at least $150 a month, apart from everyday expenses, which most of them could not afford.

"Drug addicts are despised," said a doctor's wife to me. "It's terrible but people don't want taxpayer's money spent on curing them. Until of course they themselves have a son or daughter who takes drugs. But political parties won't gain votes by urging government action for rejected outcasts. Drug addicts to most Italians seem traitors – they have betrayed all the love and care which parents traditionally give their children."

In Milan, I visited the "Comunità Nuova" which is one of the many independent organizations which try to deal with the problem. I talked to Antonietta Pedrinalli, a social worker who gave me the draft of the 1975 law which is the latest legislation on drug-taking. It establishes that those who take drugs cannot be arrested, but only the dealers. It also provides that private organizations with qualified staff can get up to 75 per cent of approved expenses in State subsidies, and, apart from hospital treatment with the substitute drug methadone, rehabilitation is left to them.

It was a hard battle, said Antonietta. The centre had no authority to compel anyone over eighteen to take treatment. Most of their patients arrived after the "honeymoon period", and lapses were frequent. It was easier now to find heroin. Bars sold it and there were even "drug cocktails". Only a small number of police and Carabinieri had been allotted to drug squads. There were, however, she continued, a few more positive developments. Drug fashions went in waves. Three years ago, a twenty-five-year-old might well take two or three grammes a day. Now the younger addicts from thirteen to eighteen took less. For the moment, the principal drug in Milan was not heroin but amphetamines and cocaine, although thirteen people had died from heroin in the city in the first four months of 1983.

One problem which the Censis report underlines is the way dealers are chosen from among "toxic dependents", which is the term Italians use. As a result, a chain is formed: addicts get the money they need by selling drugs and enrolling new recruits who also join this "devil's circle". As the law of 1975 gave immunity to addicts, pushers carry only a small quantity of the drug on them and it is therefore difficult to prove anything against them.

The real problem in eliminating the drug trade springs from the immense profits which make large sums available for bribery, as became apparent on the arrest of a Carabinieri colonel in Rome in September 1983.

The smashing of the so-called French Connection in Marseilles in 1978 meant that the centre of the drug trade was transferred to Sicily which is now said to provide 80 per cent of the heroin imported into the United States. Gaia Servadio wrote in *The Observer* that whereas a kilo of morphine costs $7,000 in Sicily, a kilo of heroin costs $150,000 on the streets of New York, while the cost of conversion is negligible.

For whatever reasons, it is Church organizations rather than the State which has taken on the major role of rehabilitating addicts. Comunità Nuova, the centre I visited in Milan, is run by a priest, Don Guido Rigoldi, with lay staff, and there are 130 committees throughout

Italy of the Centro Italiano di Solidarietà and Progetto Uomo, which are also run by individual priests.

In Arezzo, the Socialist mayor told me that, although there were hundreds of addicts in the town, only the Catholic societies did anything. The pattern seems to be that the priest inspires, the State pays, and the professionals get down to work.

I decided to investigate further by going to see the Bishop of Arezzo with an English friend, John Donleavy, who helps run the local International House. At the palace, we rang the door bell with, behind us, the Cathedral covered in scaffolding in the sunlight. We were admitted by a tiny white-haired woman dressed in black, who led us through a gloomy hall, darkened by heavy curtains, to a small lift which somehow we all squeezed into. Then we were admitted to a large room where sat Monsignore, looking slightly alarmed at sight of these two foreign intruders.

Desultorily, we talked about the Church and politics and the difficulties of enrolling new priests. Then I asked him what the Church was doing about drugs.

"Oh," he said vaguely, "we have a new scheme." The real problem with addicts, he explained, was that their will and personality had been destroyed and it was necessary to find means of rebuilding them. "So we isolate them in the country for two years. They don't see family or friends. They do manual work and get used to living and working in a community again."

"Are there many centres?"

"Oh, a few. They're just starting."

Six months later, Brita and I were speeding through heavy rain in Palermo, in Sicily, at night. We were searching for one of these centres which, we had been told, was lodged in an old eighteenth-century manor house. We were lost. Around us were blocks of luxurious apartment buildings above plush, lit-up shopping centres. These in Palermo rouse my indignation because they are said to be built from laundered Mafia drug money. Indeed, these new buildings seem a kind of jungle growth: I remember in the Communist headquarters being shown the way new constructions had swallowed up the garden. There was only one large tree left. "We have saved it!" said the trade union leader I was with in a triumphant voice. "Saved it from the Mafia!" – as if these tall blocks with their balconies were part of an advancing army.

Finally, we got to the biggest block of all; there were railings at the entrance and a *portiere* crouched in a steel and metal box. "Where do you want to go?"

"The Drug Centre!" I said boldly.

"Sempre dritto! Sempre dritto!"*

Incredulously, we drove through this valley of concrete, on and on until at the end there was a dark garden and the shadowy outline of a house beyond.

We hooted. A door opened in a rectangle of light with figures outlined against it like insects on a blank cinema screen. Inside, we were greeted by three young men. Alfredo, Luciano and Giorgio. I explained why we had come.

"You are very welcome!" said Luciano, and they began to tell us about their organization called "Comunità Incontro". The Palermo residence had been started about six months previously, with twenty-eight ex-drug addicts who had been on heroin for five to six years. Giorgio himself had started when he was fifteen, influenced by the group he was then part of. Beginning with pot, they had gone on to experiment with heroin. Alfredo had had conflicts with his family and had taken drugs in defiance, knowing it would hurt and worry them. Everyone there had different reasons for starting but most were related to one of these motives.

The centre itself was run by the ex-addicts. They cooked and served meals in turn and kept their own discipline. Every day, except Sunday, they worked on the small farm behind the house, and provided most of their own food.

"You're really like a community of lay brothers?"

"Yes, but we don't have to be Christians. We accept everyone who needs to be here, even if they come straight out of prison."

"And does it work well?"

"Of course there are always problems. But being with other ex-addicts, we have the sense of working together to liberate ourselves. You must remember that once we felt the lowest of the low. Starting this new life has given us some of the self-respect we need. Also, there is the feeling that it is by our own efforts that we are re-creating ourselves."

We were taken round the house. Walls had been repainted and the broken bannisters on the stairs replaced. On the first floor, in a large empty room, members of the community were kneeling on the floor as they glued posters to wooden supports in preparation for a rally against drugs in Palermo. "Three hundred people are coming from our centres all over Italy to distribute leaflets in the streets and to hold a meeting in a theatre."

* "Straight ahead! Straight ahead!"

The posters were sky-blue with three seagulls flying above the words "Libertà nello spazio immenso".

"This is what we are trying to achieve," said Giorgio. "Personal liberty so that we can go anywhere, do anything without looking for an escape or refuge." He started talking about the founder of the community, Don Piero Selmini, who was fifty-six and who knew what hardship was because he came from a peasant family and had suffered as a child during and after the war. In 1979, he had founded the community and now there were seventeen centres with three hundred residents. Don Piero believed it was not enough for society simply to delegate responsibility to specialists like doctors and psychiatrists. People had to be responsible for their own destiny.

When drug addicts first arrived, they were treated by doctors and psychiatrists in one of the community's special centres. But after about a month, when they had overcome their withdrawal depression, they were sent to a residence from which they could only contact their families by phone or letter. It was essential they should be able to stand on their own feet and learn how to work together for the same aims.

"Is it only for men?" asked Brita.

"No. Also for girls and some communities are mixed. There is one for parents and children – the sons and daughters of ex-addicts."

Dinner was at 8.30 and we were invited to stay. Macaroni, bread and cheese were followed by tangerines. I sat next to someone who had been in the Carabinieri for two years but had been dismissed because of drugs. He had had an Australian girlfriend and they had thought of going off to Australia together, but everything had broken up.

I asked my other neighbour about the daily programme. He told me everyone got up at 7.30 and worked on the land from 8.30 till 12.30. In the afternoon they had gymnastics, group discussions twice a week, and then workshop activities: ceramics, woodwork, gardening. They were also training themselves for the time when they would leave the community, and were developing mainly agricultural skills.

"And how is it all financed?"

"Those whose families can afford it pay 10,000 lire [$4] a day. Otherwise, the community is supported by grants and donations. We also earn from our work."

At the end of the table, a young man reached for his guitar. "Every evening we sing. Usually songs we have composed ourselves."

"We have been impaled on the sword of drugs!" proclaimed one song. "We have realized we don't want to die."

It was moving, this community with so little self-consciousness and "prissiness".

As we rose to go, shook hands and thanked them warmly, it was difficult to imagine these healthy, exuberant youths as broken drug addicts. It is significant how in Italy the small community, based on the family pattern of co-operation for survival, is always impressive.

Later, I read in the newspapers how the demonstration in Palermo had been successful and the theatre full of young people and parents. Cardinal Pappalardo had been there and the mayoress, Elda Pucci; however, there had been only one representative from the government, the deputy Mario d'Aquisito. "Only one deputy for hundreds of young people who have come together from every part of Italy!" protested Ugo Minichin, the vice-president of the Anti-Drugs League. "Young people who have come to life once more, both physically and morally!"

PETTY CRIME

In the various publications of Comunità Incontro, I also read that the seven thousand addicts in Palermo need the equivalent of $20 each a day to buy the drugs they need – a total of $140,000 every twenty-four hours, obtained largely through petty theft or robbery. In Italy, as elsewhere, the growth of youthful crime has paralleled the increase in drug addiction. In most big cities like Milan, Turin, Rome and Naples, robbery in the streets is almost a way of life. I remember driving into Turin with luggage visible through the glass top of the boot to be warned by a bystander not to park anywhere. With eloquent gesticulation, he banged his hand down on the glass of the boot as if holding a heavy metal object. Then, deftly, with his other hand he made a snatching gesture above my piled possessions.

Later, we were advised to cover up our radio or the car would certainly be broken into. Fortunately, it is easy to find garages beneath or near hotels which cost the equivalent of £3 or £4 a night.

An interesting symptom of the variety to be found in Italy is the fact that in small towns there is very little danger. "Oh, no, you can leave your car where you like," I was told in Orvieto. "Here we are honest people! Perhaps also" – with a wry smile – "because everyone knows everybody else!"

In big cities there is also the problem of pickpocketing and bag-snatching. In Bari, in Apulia, we explored the old city at midday. From the moment we entered it, there was a feeling of something sinister, of people watching us like cats considering a couple of mice. We asked a boy if there were any restaurants open and he told us they were all closed for lunch. Then we went to a food shop and the owner seemed strangely abstracted, his eyes obviously assessing the fact that my wife, Brita, was holding her bag firmly underneath her buttoned cardigan.

Finally, we entered a piazza where two women were chatting beside a fountain. Suddenly a youth appeared, approached Brita, reached out, and starting tugging at her bag. Brita cried out. I swung a plastic bag at him, and, for some reason, shouted "*Coño!*", a Spanish obscenity, at the top of my voice.

He tussled for a moment and then, unable to detach Brita's bag, loped off like a disappointed bear, while the women at the fountain exclaimed and shrugged their shoulders and looked at us as if demanding tolerance for these quaint native customs. Fortunately, only the strap of the bag was broken and anyway Brita had left most of her valuables concealed in cotton wool in my sponge bag at the hotel.

"The trouble is that most tourists carry all their money with them," the local director of tourism told us afterwards. "It can be as much as four or five thousand dollars, an enormous prize for one bold action."

In Naples or Rome, the danger comes more from youths on motorcycles who grab gold chains, often with lethal effects, or handbags from people walking along the pavement. In Naples, the commonest trick is for the pillion rider on a motorcycle to smash a window of a car and take whatever is immediately available. Or they hunt in pairs with one motorcycle slowing down in front of the car to make the robbery easier. The prefect in Naples has now struck at the root of the problem by ordering the confiscation of all motorcycles with two people aboard, and the chief of police told me that over three thousand arrests had been made for petty crime in 1983. "What else can I do?" he asked. "Of course, I could put 2,000 police on the streets to make arrests at vast expense. But that would seem Fascist and people are rightly against anything which reminds them of Fascism!"

Indeed, this fear of high-handedness is, for good or ill, widespread in Italy. "Problems are like artichokes," the prefect of Naples told me, quoting an eighteenth-century Duke of Savoy. "You get choked if you try and eat them at one go. You must chew them leaf by leaf."

For Italians, drugs and juvenile delinquency are another of the dangers which make up everyday living. They have to be dealt with patiently, almost organically.

How far drugs and delinquency are a sign that the Italian family is gradually breaking up is difficult to say. As always there are paradoxes: youthful crime is often prompted by the family itself, sending out young hunters to garner what they can. Drugs in Sicily, although organized on a vast scale, are still the domain of certain families. Work certainly does not have to be "moral" to keep a family unit together.

To my friend Silvio, in Sicily, the great threat to family values is not delinquency or drugs – it is television. "*Dallas*," he spat, "has done more harm than anything else, portraying a family model of selfishness, violence and individual egocentricity. The opposite of what we want our children or our families to be! And everyone watches it!"

VI
BROADER FAMILIES

~~~~~~~~~~~~

*Mafia: Murder and Clans – Origins and Psychology –' Ndrangheta –
Camorra – Government Measures – Conspiracy Theories*

MAFIA: MURDER AND CLANS

On November 16th 1983, I opened the *Giornale di Sicilia* as I ate breakfast
in a café near the station in Palermo. There were two headlines on page
four. One ran: "Shotgun for a war-survivor." And the other: "They
killed him for his name."

The first referred to the murder of Salvatore Mazzola, a follower of a
Mafia boss who had recently escaped abroad.

The previous day at eight in the morning, Mazzola had left his villa
on foot to go to work at his stables nearby. Suddenly, two gunmen
opened "a volume of fire, perhaps excessive for the elimination of only
one man" – as the newspaper put it. Mazzola fell, peppered with red
holes in the head, thorax and legs. His wife and daughter, alarmed by
the shots, went out and found him. Horrified and weeping, they were
nevertheless determined that the police should not see him in that
condition. So they cleaned his wounds and changed his clothes before
telling the Carabinieri, who therefore arrived ninety minutes later.

This was the second attempt on Mazzola's life within the previous six
weeks. On October 6th, he had been fired at when driving his Fiat 127,
and had only escaped by feigning death. Now he was no longer a
survivor.

The second heading referred to the killing of Benedetto Grado, an
agricultural labourer, seventy-eight, who had been a supervisor at a
large market garden. The murder was also at eight o'clock in the
morning.

A photograph showed a sheet-covered shape on the pavement, from
which shoes protruded at one end, with a half folded umbrella which
looked strangely like a dolphin's head, at the other. Blood trickled

down to a little pool nearby. One of the three women in black ranged against the white wall behind was kneeling. Another stood, leaning against the bricks, while Grado's wife sat crouched on a low wooden chair.

The article explained that Grado was probably killed only because he was related to a Mafia boss, who had recently disappeared. Grado himself appeared to have had no criminal involvement since 1934 when he was sent to the prison colony of Lampedusa, suspected of belonging to the Mafia.

When he was killed, Grado was wearing his son's black coat, which still had bullet holes in its back from the day when the boy was gunned down, ten months earlier. As a final dramatic point, the shots which killed Grado were heard in the church nearby, where helpers were preparing the funeral of Salvatore Zarcone who had been killed the previous weekend in another feud. "One corpse in church and another on the asphalt," as the journalist writing the article put it.

Having finished my breakfast, I walked up to Via Maqueda and noticed a funeral parlour on the corner which announced in faded neon lights that it was open day and night.

In 1982 there were 152 assassinations, including a Communist deputy, Pio La Torre, and the prefect of Palermo, Carlo Alberto Dalla Chiesa, and his young, newly married wife Emmanuela. At least a hundred others also disappeared, probably victims of what Italians call "the white shotgun". This describes murder through casting victims into the liquid concrete which forms the walls of new buildings. Their remains will probably never be found again until discovered as mysterious fossils by future archaeologists, a few million years hence.

The ruthlessness, the tragedy remind one of Shakespeare or other Renaissance dramatists, who often chose Italy for their settings. Giuseppe Ferrara's realistic film *A Hundred Days in Palermo* belongs to this tradition, although it is more of a documentary. It is about the events leading up to the assassination of General Dalla Chiesa and his wife. Carlo Alberto had become famous for master-minding the destruction of the Red Brigades. He was appointed prefect in May 1983, and in the four months before he was killed did so much to counter the Mafia that they had to get rid of him.

His wife, Emmanuela, he married in Palermo itself. In one scene in the film, she goes out shopping with her maid just before the assassination. It is very hot, towards the end of August. In the simmering market, she becomes aware of the meat being cut into bloody slabs. Her glance leaps from one piece of raw flesh to another, while big butchers' knives cut and carve. Some days later, both Dalla Chiesas go to a party given by Sicilian officials who stare and laugh and make ambiguous remarks which would indicate they are plotting their death. A large ice-cream shaped like a naked woman is carved up, distributed and devoured by thirsty mouths.

Emmanuela reminds one of Calpurnia, Caesar's wife, seeing omens of his murder: "And ghosts did shriek and squeal about the streets."

On September 3rd, the couple return home from a restaurant at 9.10 in the evening, escorted only by a thirty-two-year-old policeman who follows them in a blue Alfa Romeo. A motorcyclist with a gunman on the pillion approaches from behind, kills the policeman and then pulps them both with a Kalashnikov. Another car approaches and pumps in more bullets. Then another: the occupant shuffles quickly over to see if they are dead. Satisfied, he drives off.

Then in the silent street, with everyone dispersed and shutters closed like dead eyelids, a woman dares come out. She looks into the car and screams and her man follows her and pulls her away, as if her distress would be interpreted as an affront to that force "without name or colour" – which is how a diffident Christian Democrat politician once described the Mafia.

On a wall of the Via Isidoro Carini where the Dalla Chiesas were murdered, someone scrawled the words: "Here died Sicily's last hope."

The Mafia takes us back to the Middle Ages. Even the recent past reflects events that could belong to the most turbulent days of the great warring barons, or the sanguinary intrigues of the courts of Damascus under the weaker Caliphs. Thus, just after Dalla Chiesa's death, Tommaso Buscetta, who has now become the first Mafia "supergrass", returned to Sicily from America. Ostensibly, his object was to bring the warring clans together. So he invited them all to a "banquet", but of course the food was poisoned. As a result, fifteen members of the Riccobono group, who had been among the most successful survivors in the constant war between the factions, were exterminated.

The war itself heated up early in 1981 when two Mafia leaders, Inzerillo and Bontade, appropriated the equivalent of ten million dollars which was destined for property investment in Atlantic City. With some of this money, they bribed four young thugs belonging to the "opposition" to invite their colleagues to a meeting at Inzerillo's house where they were all to have been killed.

However, the news got out. Bontade was shot down on April 24th, his birthday, while waiting at traffic lights. A few weeks later, Inzerillo was killed. As a result, the four young thugs lost their protectors. They flew to Milan and then to Zurich, intending to make their way to Brazil. However, there they were arrested because they had false documents and the large sum of 120 million lire.

One of them was sent to the Ucciardone, the big prison in Palermo, there to be killed by "unknown" prisoners with thirty-three knife thrusts. The others were released: two of them disappeared and haven't been heard of since, but one was found dead in a burnt-out car in Milan.

The revenge, however, had hardly started among relatives and even friends of the four young thugs. Two fathers were killed: one of them when returning home with his wife and son, the other by two false Carabinieri who made him open his door. Two uncles were murdered. A Tunisian wife has been kidnapped and raped, and the father and brother of another killed. A younger brother was shot in front of a dozen guests. By May 1983, eighteen people had been killed. If the two surviving thugs return – as they will do – the revenge for the revenge will start, and so it will go on.

It is difficult to compare the Mafia with other contemporary phenomena. It is different from terrorism because it is without political idealism. Even today it is not mere gangsterism – in fact it is a relief in Italy to read that a straightforward bank robbery has taken place simply for greed. This means that the money stolen will just enrich a few undeserving individuals. At least it will not be used to fertilize those insidious, venomous plants whose roots already reach almost everywhere.

In the past, it was often said that the Mafia did not exist. Like the wind, it manifested itself without being seen. Indro Montanelli, a well-known journalist and writer and present editor of *Il Giornale*, tells how after the war he went to visit Don Calo Vizzini, the last acknowledged head of the Mafia. Montanelli was put up in a little hotel in the village, where taps only trickled, the blinds could not be moved up or down, and the electric light bulb was so weak that it was impossible to read at night.

After two days Don Calo agreed to see him and, among other things, told him that the Mafia did not exist. After the interview Montanelli went back to his hotel and found that while he had been away, talking to Don Calo, everything had been put right. The taps flowed with hot and cold water, the electric light bulb was the strongest possible and the blind went up or down with a mere flick of the wrist. "The Mafia does exist," Montanelli said to himself. "It does exist!"

The Mafia's real strength is that it is an inversion of the Italian family, with perhaps more loyalty and unity because its members are in greater danger. Pino Arlacchi, in his modern classic on the Mafia, *La Mafia imprenditrice*, shows how a Mafia clan is more successful in proportion to the number of brothers there are in the family and how most of the big clans in Palermo are interrelated, like royals. The only real difference is that the leadership does not go automatically to the heir of the family but to whoever is strongest.

Arlacchi writes of the great advantage the Mafia have in the criminal world:

> The need for secrecy and the impossibility of counting on state laws for the regulation of market forces deeply influence the social and anthropological composition of the criminal world. What better guarantee of secrecy and of mutual trust is there than that between members of the same culture, the same ethnic and regional community and in fact the same family.

An Italian friend of mine who has worked for years in Japan, said:

> With no disrespect to the Japanese, they are strong for the same reason the Mafia are. The Mafia have applied the traditions of their past, such as family unity, loyalty, secrecy, and ruthlessness to their vast commerce in drugs. The Japanese have transferred the blind obedience and all-absorbing co-operative sense of their "daimyos", their ancient feudal tribes, to modern industry. Both are unique because the psychology of the past is not an obstruction. It is actually an asset in the present!

ORIGINS AND PSYCHOLOGY

In Palermo, I met Toby Moore who married a Sicilian contessa when he was in the British army after the war. He told me that her grandfather had been travelling from Palermo to his country estate with a boxful of money on a mule when he became aware of someone shadowing them. Fearful of an attack, he stopped, and he and his servants ranged themselves round the money with their shotguns. "What do you want?" he shouted out in the dusk, at the bare landscape of hills and valleys. A man approached them. "I'm sorry," he said, "but we heard you were travelling with a lot of money and we wanted to make sure you were all right."

Later, his wife's grandfather noticed two people he knew hiding near the wooded border between his estate and that of his neighbour. Next day, he heard that a large number of his neighbour's sheep had been slaughtered. He felt that the reason for this was not his business, and when the Carabinieri arrived he said nothing about what he had seen.

A few days later, the two men came up his drive, leading a beautiful horse. "We'd like to thank you," one of them said. "This is for you."

Some say the Mafia originated during the Arab occupation from the middle of the ninth to the end of the eleventh century. The main argument for this is that the Mafia exists principally in the western part of Sicily which was extensively and consistently occupied by the Arabs. However, De Tocqueville believed that there was another reason: the east of Sicily is dominated by Mount Etna. As a result, few big estates grew up there, and as the Mafia undoubtedly developed partly as a kind of intermediary force between the absentee landlord and his peasants, it did not take root there.

Sicily has always been occupied by foreign invaders and has never ruled itself. In fact, Sicilians never really seem to have wanted native rule. Perhaps there has always been too much jealousy and competition for a local king ever to have been considered. Certainly, on the one occasion when they successfully rose in a national revolt and expelled the Angevins in the Sicilian Vespers in 1282, they chose another foreigner, Peter III of Aragon.

For centuries, therefore, it is likely that the Mafia or their earlier equivalents have represented Sicilian resistance to foreign rule and have themselves often provided a native substitute for government. In the story of the ancestor of Toby Moore's wife, the Mafia were acting, in the first case, as policemen and, in the second, presumably as some kind of punitive rough justice. As Luigi Barzini points out, "a man belonging to the Mafia does not know he is doing wrong. This is approximately the way he sees things. Order has to be preserved. Justice must be assured. Unfortunately, men being what they are, it is often necessary to enforce the will of the Mafia by means of violence. At times, one is also unfortunately compelled to finance the operations of the law-enforcing *cosche** by means of extortion, robbery and blackmail. Do not many organizations fighting an unjust or foreign government do the same?"

By the same criteria, it is also natural to execute traitors and those who help the enemy by giving testimony or by betraying secrets. In the end, after centuries of conditioning, you either involve yourself if you are a western Sicilian or you relapse into bewildered passivity: in 1983, a boy of twelve was hit on his bicycle by a passing lorry and lay unconscious in a street in Palermo for two hours before dying, because

---

* A *cosca* is a group of Mafia families who find it convenient to form an alliance under one "godfather". The word *cosca* means "artichoke" – in other words a lot of different leaves loosely joined in one vegetable.

no one knew whether this was an incident in which they could interfere.

Another factor which helps the Mafia is that it has always been rooted in definite territorial areas. This gives it cohesion and strength. Pino Arlacchi gives an example of this when, after a raid on a savings bank in Reggio Calabria, the criminals responsible were summoned by the Mafia and fined 98 per cent of their booty, which was equivalent to two hundred thousand dollars, for not getting previous authorization!

Indeed, it is important to remember that, however closely the Mafia is linked through its *cosche* and through the massive emigration from Sicily which has created international bonds, it is not a monolithic, closely controlled organization. If it were, it would not be Italian – much less Sicilian or Calabrian. In fact its strength lies in its diversity and in the close-knit cells of its individual families. When it organizes itself on too large a scale and has to bring in foreigners, it fails. It was a Belgian, Albert Gillet, employed as a carrier of heroin, who, when arrested at Rome airport, put the police onto the trail of the heroin "kitchens" of Palermo in 1980. And it was "Doctor" Bousquet from Marseilles who was trailed and led the police to two heroin kitchens – which in turn brought about the arrest of seventy-five of the most important mafiosi.

Another important factor is that the continual dealing with death creates a Darwinian sense of survival of the fittest. Arlacchi describes trivial challenges and defiances between young men which result in what are virtually old-fashioned duels. In a game involving beer bottles, one young man leaves another one out, saying he is just a boy and shouldn't participate. When the other leads the game, he in turn excludes the first one. Tension grows and when the game is finished, both arrange to see each other later. As a result, one of them ends up in hospital, where he tells no one what happened before he dies.

It is "strength" and "force" that are admired: "right" is secondary. Thus in the village of Genuardo two young men were killed by the Mafia boss, Antonio Cassini, because they were threatening his territorial domination. As Cassini had won, the father of the two youths accepted it and protected Cassini by accusing innocent people. New mafiosi groups are set up by the most aggressive and the most murderous. We are in the jungle with males snarling at each other, lowering their horns, not only over the female but also to protect territory and, perhaps in a less animal way, to achieve power and respect.

The energy released in what is virtually a state of war is described in one of those anonymous interviews which so often enliven Arlacchi's book:

> These people are endowed with the most extraordinary vitality. They're never still or at rest. Now they're dealing with business, later they're lunching with friends. Then they deal with more business, then they're visiting a lover ... many of them are polygamous. They have various families and many children. They eat, they drink, they amuse themselves, they kill. They do everything intensely in disorder, without pauses or gaps of time.

Arlacchi also records the answer of a mafioso to a judge who asks whether it is not a pity that Toto Inzerillo (a relative of the Inzerillo shot later, in 1980; see p. 181) was killed so young, at thirty-seven.

> His thirty-seven years are the equivalent of eighty in any one else. Inzerillo lived completely. He had many things in life. Others will never have a hundredth part of these things. It is not a pity dying at that age if you have done, seen and had everything that Inzerillo did, saw and was able to have. He didn't die unsatisfied and tired of life. He died brimming with vitality. That is the difference.

One of the most extraordinary novels about the Mafia is one I have already referred to on page 137. It is called *The Love Song of Maria Lumera* and is by the Sicilian duke, Alberto Denti di Pirajno. It is extraordinary because it reminds one again of the Middle Ages, when barons fight each other, exploit their peasantry, and yet show an inclination towards Christianity – which usually expresses itself at the end of their lives when few alternatives remain.

It tells the story of a beautiful middle-class girl, Maria, who marries a mafioso whom she adores. He is killed with a shotgun when he is driving his car and to everyone's surprise she takes over his *cosca*, establishing her authority and co-operating with other Mafia leaders in cigarette smuggling and the drug trade.

One of these leaders, nicknamed "The One Asleep", is extremely ruthless yet sexually impotent. His aunt is abbess of a convent in Naples, and Maria Lumera corresponds secretly with this lady about her religious feelings. Simultaneously, there are murders, and the dispatch of heroin to America concealed in lemons. Finally, a number of things make Maria certain who killed her husband. She goes to a cottage where "The One Asleep" is staying and strangles him with her bare hands. Then she retires to his aunt's convent in Naples, leaving her "business" to her nephew. The other Mafia leaders come to the ceremony in which she becomes a bride of Christ. They weep copiously because this beautiful and intelligent woman has departed from their midst for ever.

To the modern mind, perhaps the strangest aspect of this story is the combination of crime and religious fervour – another link with the Middle Ages, when this reconciliation was not only commonplace but when murderous acts were frequently carried out in the name of religion.

In an art gallery in Palermo, perched on a little separate platform/alcove at one side, I talked about this with Leonardo Sciascia, Sicily's leading modern novelist who seems to have almost prophetic percipience: his excellent novel *Il Contesto* is a mystery story about a series of murders of judges which happened a few years after the book was published; while *Todo Modo* is about a political group which plots the murder of its leader and was published some years before Moro's death (see p. 11).

About Sicilian religion, Sciascia said, "Sicilians don't really have a sense of Christianity. For them religion is something pagan and, above all, dramatic. It interests them if it fits in with a mood." He also commented on the way the Church had never attacked the Mafia until recently: "The first to describe the Mafia was Pietro Ulloa in 1837," he said. "But it took until 1981 for the Church to recognize that it existed, when Cardinal Pappalardo gave the first sermon attacking the Mafia."

In contrast, Pappalardo's predecessor, Cardinal Ruffini – whose motto, "Hold Firm," is displayed with his crest all over the bishop's palace in Palermo – had written in a pastoral letter that the three worst evils of Sicily were, first, the unjust and defamatory way in which the Mafia was described; second, the publication of *The Leopard* by Lampedusa, and third, Danilo Dolci, the reformer, who has done so much through exhortation and publication to help the Sicilian poor.

"Why have the Church never protested before?" I asked Sciascia.

"Because in Sicily many of them belonged to the Mafia, or at least accepted them as a substitute authority. Now, though, everything has become too fraught and violent."

In *Maria Lumera*, the Mafia bosses feel no guilt about their participation in the drug trade: "... surely they were not responsible for the goons who paid through their noses for a pinch or a drag. Houses were built with rows of windows on every floor, and from time to time, a fool jumped out of one of them and crashed on the sidewalk; but nobody dreamt of laying the blame on the architect."

Arlacchi believes that the Mafia's political links are growing. They have always been able to manipulate votes. Back in 1918, Orlando, the Prime Minister who represented Italy at the peace talks at Versailles, had the Mafia working for him. He was elected for the first time in 1897 in Partinico, a notorious Mafia stronghold which remained his constituency. In his last election battle in 1946, a large canvas sign said "Vote for Vittorio Emmanuele Orlando, the friend of friends!" Everyone knew who was being referred to: the "friend of friends" is what individual members call themselves.

Arlacchi estimates the average election influence of the Mafia in Calabria amounts to about 30 per cent of the vote in small towns and 15 per cent in big ones. This is obtained through economic pressure and by way of *clientelismo*, the term used for the exchange of favours which plays such an important part in Italian life. Arlacchi believes this influence is growing as the Mafia becomes wealthier and more powerful. Interlinking can also be seen clearly in Sicily. Thus at the 1981 funeral of the mafioso Tommaso Scaduto, at Bagheria, there were three mayors and scores of councillors walking behind the coffin. Even more brazen was the 1978 funeral of a mafioso, Giuseppe De Cristina, in a small town called Riesi. Everything closed, including the school and the town hall, and the Christian Democrat headquarters had its flag at half mast.

Certainly, in Sicily there is a feeling of the Mafia being everywhere. They haunt like invisible harpies. Perhaps that is why over the centuries Sicilians have learnt to be silent. Two years ago, apparently, no one talked about them. Now, their new policy of assassinating government officials has made it a more open issue and it is difficult to get off the subject, although you cannot ask certain questions without encountering a wry expression and a shrug of shoulders. As an investigator, writing a book, you may also be interested in the municipality, the lack of water in summer, the agricultural situation. However, it always comes back to that same sinister word.

In Palermo, I talked to a local journalist who said it was unpleasant living in this atmosphere of menace not knowing whom you could talk to, or how what you wrote might alienate someone with a gun. He himself had been rung up and advised to be careful because he had found out that a girl who had disappeared on what was thought to be an amorous adventure had in fact been captured by the Mafia. At the Communist headquarters, I talked to the general secretary who said that at the previous election in June 1983, some of their supporters had been afraid to work and canvass in parts of the city where the Mafia predominated. "They said they had to think of their wives and families!"

On a rainy day, I went to see the mayoress, Dr Elda Pucci, at the Palazzo del Comune which is situated in what is generally known as the Piazza della Vergogna, literally the "Place of Shame". The reason for this name is the large fountain in the centre which is decorated with about forty nude statues of both men and women who are looking with interest at each other. Some of the women use their hands in coy defensive positions which in many cases seems unnecessary as vandals have smashed what might cause them embarrassment.

In the midst of a crowd of clamorous women, I tried to gain entrance to the town hall, to be stopped by an impatient policeman. Finally, I managed to slip surreptitiously into the courtyard which was decorated with palm trees, up the broad staircase, through a large waiting room with black benches round the walls, and into a magnificent suite with high frescoed ceilings, polished wooden floors and chandeliers, which might well have been part of Versailles in its heyday. Then I was admitted into another splendid room, at the end of which sat Dr Pucci, with the statue of yet another nude man at her back, but this time golden, armless, but otherwise intact.

Dr Elda Pucci is single, in her fifties and by profession is a pediatrician of renown. She smiles easily, is precise and seemed very much in control. She was very pleasant to me as a visiting Englishman, partly because she had been invited the following January to London, there to meet the Lady Mayoress and, possibly, Mrs Thatcher.

Like so many Sicilians, she started by attacking North Italian attitudes. In Rome and beyond, the press only talked about Sicily in terms of Mafia, and were only interested in reporting anything negative. They felt Sicily should be grateful for the good the Cassa per il Mezzogiorno had done, which of course was true. But at the same time, so much money had been wasted – enough to put taps of solid gold into every bathroom in every house and factory they had built. Now Palermo itself was being victimized. They had only 4,000 municipal workers compared to double that number in other big cities like Milan or Turin. That was because they had let recruiting get a little behind and then suddenly a law had been passed, freezing all further employment.

But why did Palermo seem one of the dirtiest cities in Italy? I asked. Surely, that had nothing to do with the North! That was because of the unions, she said. People in Palermo had houses that were immaculate inside, but they lacked a sense of community and the realization that the city was a big family.

What, though, of schools in poor districts? Why did so many children leave school before they were allowed to? Why, in such a rich city, was there so much poverty? Why was the eighteenth-century quarter tumbling down?

There was always a problem with taxes in Italy, said Dr Pucci, so there was not enough money for all those things.

Why? Why? – we both knew that the Mafia was the ghost at the feast which neither of us referred to directly. The cleaning union after all was Mafia "protected" and as a result cost the equivalent of about fifty dollars a day per employee compared to the twenty spent by the municipality in Milan.

Also, it was difficult to raise enough taxes because these were collected by private individuals, using a system not unlike that used by the Farmers General in France before the Revolution. It was also said that the town hall had not recruited enough employees partly because they wanted to ensure their own people got in, which made it a slower process than official exams.

Six months later, in April 1984, Elda Pucci left her post as mayor and went back to her patients. She was tired, she told the press, of being used as the "clean face" of a corrupt administration. She was succeeded by another Christian Democrat councillor, Giuseppe Insalaco, who himself only remained in office for three months – and has since disappeared, accused of corruption. Now, in 1985, a government commissioner has had to be appointed. Just as the Church has found it impossible to tolerate an organization which, instead of being the *onorata società*, has become an international industry for crime and murder, so the Christian Democrats, who have been used by it, are trying with great difficulty to separate themselves without losing votes and without too many scandals which might show how involved they were.

How, though, has everything changed? Once the Mafia were both brigands and amateur constables, a symbol of resistance, a substitute for inefficient government. They had their own code of honour, inspired by the chivalry the Normans brought to Sicily, which still lives on in the traditional Sicilian puppet plays based on the adventures of the knights of Charlemagne. Now, the Mafia represents what is almost a multi-national of crime, whose bosses have assets of billions of dollars and a destructive power stretching from Bangkok to Atlantic City.

The Fascists almost eliminated the growth of Mafia power. Mussolini first took against them when the mayor of Piano dei Greci welcomed him and boasted that the Carabinieri were all members of the Mafia. Mussolini didn't like that kind of competition and appointed a new prefect called Mori who fought the Mafia on their own terms. Mori actually challenged a mafioso, Gaetano Ferrarello, to a public duel in the main square of Madonie, the town of which Ferrarello was known as "king". Ferrarello did not keep the appointment. Instead, he emerged from his hiding place in an attic in the police station and said: "My heart trembles! It is the first time I find myself face to face with justice!"

By 1940, the Mafia was under control and its head, Don Vito Cascio Ferro, in prison where he died of a broken heart.

Paradoxically, it was the Allies who gave power back to the Mafia in 1943. Indeed, there is evidence that before and during the invasion the Mafia helped the Anglo-Americans against the Fascists who had come near to suppressing them. Once again, the Mafia was used as a substitute for government and Don Calo Vizzini, its last head, was made a mayor with military vehicles and supplies at his disposal.

During the '50s and '60s the Mafia seemed in decline. These were the years when the South was being transformed, when the autostrada – most of it completed in the 1950s – was breaking down isolation. These were the years of the boom, when money was more important than honour for those who wished to cut a figure. Chilanti, editor of the autobiography of a Mafia leader, *Mafia su Roma*, writes: "Young people from city and country spoke openly about the Mafia; in night clubs, the Mafia were unmasked and mocked at. All in all, there was a great change in people's attitudes."

According to Arlacchi, it was partly this decay that pushed the Mafia towards the acquisition of capital. "For them," he writes, "money and its accumulation constitute the only way of recovering power and self-respect." In Sicily the Christian Democrats had since 1955 established close control over the springs of power. This was the golden period of *clientelismo*, of patronage, and frequently a merging of political and Mafia interests. It was also a time of temptation when large government contracts were allocated, and the Mafia played a prominent part in the building boom.

Other money came from the government through the farmed-out taxation system. The profits of the 344 tax offices, owned principally by five families, amounted to about 10 per cent of total taxation revenue. Also it was possible to postpone the handing over of this money to the government, which meant that an even bigger proportion could be deployed.

Subsidies from Rome to the regional government of Sicily were a further source of capital. Between 1947 and 1971, 830 billion lire, or 550 million dollars, was transferred. Between 1972 and 1976, there was a further 630 billion lire, or 420 million dollars. Because of bureaucratic delays much of this remained unspent* and, to take an example, in 1973 there were 290 billion lire, or 190 million dollars, in bank vaults and credit accounts. With the close relationship between politics, banking and Mafia, this meant money was available for further investment, of which the most profitable was the drug trade.

At the same time, the Mafia itself was changing. Most people had got used to living well, and young students and middle-class people expected a job which often they couldn't get. None of them wanted to go back to the land which their family might own. Some of them were recruited by the Mafia.

It is interesting, too, how the average age of mafiosi seems to have gone down. Thus in a trial of 117 men in 1968, the average age was fifty, whereas in a large trial of 134 men in 1981, the average was thirty-seven. The result has been a further break with the past and a more enterprising and materialistic approach from the new Mafia.

This showed itself in 1975 with the first really large involvement in heroin production when four "factories" were opened at Palermo. Each produced 50kgs a week, or four to five tons a year, bringing in an estimated 400 million dollars after expenses have been deducted.

The next opportunity for expansion was the collapse of the Marseilles drug organization, with the breaking by the police of the French Connection in 1978. Sicily thus became the principal provider of heroin, not only to the United States but also to Europe.

Everywhere, since then, there has been a great increase in demand for heroin, thus bringing in more income to the Mafia. At the end of the 1960s it was reckoned that there were about fifty to a hundred thousand addicts in the United States, which now has gone up to half a million. At the same time, reports have estimated a growth from virtually nothing to 200,000 in Italy and 100,000 in Britain during the same period.

In addition, there has been income from "laundered" investments in buildings, tourist complexes, new projects abroad which not only represent enormous assets but are also useful cover.

It has been calculated that individual mafiosi are now amongst the richest people in the world. Gone is the illiterate of thirty years ago with his dignity, his black clothes and hat, the white stubble on his chin, his measured way of speaking as he sat at a café table in the piazza of his town.

---

* In his book *I Siciliani*, Giuseppe Fava, who was shot by the Mafia in 1984, describes the misery of a Sicilian village, Palma di Montechiaro, with its lack of paving, drains, schools, and its decaying houses, including the palace of the Lampedusas. He then reveals that in the 1960s it was given a grant of eleven billion lire (six million dollars) which was never spent because the local politicians could not agree.

The mafioso of today travels like any rich businessman, has his villa on the French or Italian Riviera, his children at expensive schools in Switzerland, his fleet of Mercedes or Rolls, his smart secretary who arranges for him to stay at the George V in Paris, the Dorchester in London, the Waldorf Astoria in New York.

The Mafia today is even strong enough to take on the government or the Church. In addition to La Torre and Dalla Chiesa they murdered the chief investigatory magistrate, Raffaele Chinnici, in August 1983. A few days before, a Lebanese rang up from Milan and warned the Carabinieri that the Mafia were planning the murder of another government official, this time with a car bomb. When Chinnici left his flat to go to work, a parked car with 200lb of explosive in it blew up, killing him, two policemen and the concierge of his house, and wounding ten neighbours.

No one has yet assassinated a member of the Church, although at the funeral of Dalla Chiesa, where Cardinal Pappalardo gave his hand to no one except President Pertini, a weeping lady was heard to express what was commonly believed: "The next one will be him!" she wailed loudly.

Gestures of defiance against the Church there have been. In April 1983 Pappalardo went as usual to say Mass at Easter at Ucciardone, the principal prison of Palermo, which contained 1,000 prisoners. He arrived in his robes, and solemnly entered the chapel. But it was empty. The Mafia had shown their power over fellow prisoners, publicly defying the head of the Sicilian Church.

I met His Eminence in his palace opposite the cathedral which was built by an English archbishop who was sent as tutor to the Norman king of Sicily by Henry II of England.

The courtyard of the palace was planted with palm trees, and a red carpet with stains on it led up the broad staircase to the main rooms, which were sunlit and cheerful, with tall windows.

When I met him, Cardinal Pappalardo was sixty-five, though seeming much younger, tall with slightly greying black hair. In photographs and in the flesh there is an absorbed expression on his face, a sense of underlying resignation and pain, like San Sebastian receiving his first arrow. He is from Sicily, from Catania and – so his assistant, Bishop Giallombardo, said – is tired of being associated only with denunciations of the Mafia. Like so many people in Palermo, he seemed irritated when talking about local government. The Commune occasionally gave a subsidy of a few millions for a modern art exhibition, or a school of music which the Church had promoted. When we talked about the slum areas of Palermo, he said people didn't want to help themselves. The Commune, which should be looking after practical things, spent all its time bickering about politics.

He looked tired. Palermo is not only damp but also the hottest city in Italy with an average temperature of 28.9° centigrade, rising towards the upper thirties in summer. Suddenly, sitting on the sofa in his reception room, even in November, I had a sense of what it must be like to struggle in this torrid city against sluggishness and apathy. Perhaps the Mafia has survived so long because it belongs essentially to the jungle, because it is forceful and ruthless, cutting through the indifference of people who don't want to be organized but respond only when threatened, or fearful. It was easier for a priest because he had his reward, but what motivation did an administrator have unless he had an inbuilt sense of duty?

Anyway, the war against the Mafia was on. Neither State nor Church could afford to tolerate the power and destructiveness that had grown inside it.

Not only was there the Mafia but also, further north, the 'Ndrangheta in Calabria, and the Camorra in Naples.

'NDRANGHETA

We took the night-boat from Palermo to Naples. At 9.30 in the evening, the horizon was a line of fire as the coast of Sicily began to slip into the distance. The whole shore to one side of Monte Pellegrino burnt with honeycombs of light, where the rows of illuminated windows in tall buildings merged into a glistening, palpitating glow, like a distant forest fire. A full moon rose, crinkling the gentle swell of the Tyrrhenian Sea with silver, while Palermo began to vanish, hovering for a moment just below the horizon like submarine incandescence, or the last reflection of a setting sun.

We were going from Mafia to Camorra, although to say that was simply to be what Southern Italians expected from foreigners: people who were interested only in the sensational, the negative, the sordid aspects of their land; people who were not learned or sensitive enough to notice the beautiful things of which the inhabitants were proud.

As we slept, we sailed past Calabria, land of the 'Ndrangheta – a word stemming from the ancient, Greek-based dialect, still spoken, and meaning "prowess".

'Ndrangheta is an organization similar to the Sicilian Mafia. It too has a vast income from *tangenti* – extortions levied on any business it can "persuade". In Cosenza, on our original journey down to Sicily, we had been told about a recent bomb explosion which had wrecked a factory whose owner had refused to pay.

The 'Ndrangheta specializes in kidnapping, perhaps because Calabria is a mountainous region with Mount Aspromonte rising behind the town of Reggio. "It is an incredibly harsh agglomeration of hill and dale, and the geology of the district ... reveals a perfect chaos of rocks of every age, torn into gullies by earthquakes and other cataclysms of the past," wrote Norman Douglas. "The wanderer finds himself lost in a maze of contorted ravines winding about without any apparent system of watershed."

In Reggio itself, which is the most southern big town in Calabria, and from which you can see the Sicilian coast, we had been told that kidnapping was beginning to include ordinary middle-class professionals among its victims.

"The other day a doctor, who is probably worth four or five hundred million lire [$150–200,000], was kidnapped. We're all beginning to be afraid," explained a friend. "Your family may have to sell house, car, everything – in order to keep you alive."

"But don't the police help?"

"They can't do anything. In 1979, the family of a chemist called Giuseppe Gulli refused to pay a ransom, and went to the police. As a result, Gulli was killed."

In fact, the first kidnappings on a large scale only started in the 1950s and were restricted to the province. In 1979, though, the first kidnapping by the 'Ndrangheta took place outside Calabria. Since then, there have been about seven kidnappings a year, as well as others which are not organized by the 'Ndrangheta – including the abduction of a twelve-month-old baby in December 1983, organized by an engineer in Lucca, in Tuscany.

One married woman, captured by the 'Ndrangheta in March 1983, was carried away from her home in Lodi in Lombardy, travelling in the boot of a Mercedes all the way to Calabria, where she was tied with a metal chain at neck and feet. Another, a general's wife and heiress of a famous jewellery store, was taken with her son and released after thirty-five days and the removal of her son's ears.

Ludovica Machiavelli, a descendant of the philosopher, was kidnapped from her father's castle near Bologna. She told a magazine how she had been trailed by various mysterious individuals for a whole year, and then was stopped and captured as she was approaching home in her Fiat 500. After a long journey, during which she didn't know where she was, she spent a hundred days in a tent which was so low that she couldn't stand up. Often, she had fierce discussions with her captors and told them that her family didn't have any money and that the castle was mortgaged – which the kidnappers refused to believe. Unlike many kidnapped girls, she was well treated although fed on pasta, which she didn't particularly like! Finally she was released for a ransom of two hundred million lire (about eighty thousand dollars), which was much less than had been asked.

Like the Camorra and the Mafia, the 'Ndrangheta also obtains income from new building projects, simply by scaring away competitors. Because it can terrorize its workers and manage not to pay social security overheads, it makes vast profits and squeezes money from every stage of a project. Thus the local bosses, whose share of the operation will be split according to their size and power, will probably own the building and transport companies. They will get their supplies from other groups who either belong to them or are used because they have been terrorized into reducing prices.

Indeed, Arlacchi has shown that the 'Ndrangheta were the only people who really benefited from the well-known fiasco of Gioia Tauro, which is on the south-west Calabrian coast. Financing themselves with the billion lire ($500,000) which they got in ransom after the kidnapping of Paul Getty Jun. in 1973, they took over most of the vast government contract for a new steel works and a large harbour. This was just before the Common Market became aware that too much steel was being produced and persuaded every member, except Italy, to reduce drastically. To increase production, though, was beyond even Italy's talent for evasion.

So Gioia Tauro remains a relic where work is still going on slowly – not so much a cathedral in the desert as a large rubbish dump on a beautiful plain. The town must be one of the ugliest in Italy, built higgledy-piggledy with no civic objective: a labyrinth of dust roads, with half-finished skeleton houses, shabby bars and garages, and concrete bungalows by the sea.

Sadly, you realize what has been spoilt. As you approach the town, the olive trees are thirty feet tall with spreading leafy branches. They are hundreds of years old and interspersed with golden orange trees in a great plantation of lushness. Later, from a soiled, splendid beach, you look over the blue sea at the rocky mountains of Cape Vaticano, and want to weep at our human droppings and waste.

You begin to understand, too, why Italians are so critical of their country. After all, it is only when there is so much beauty and so much potential that there is so much to spoil.

CAMORRA

The boat arrived at Naples at six o'clock. As we approached the bay, Vesuvius was enormous with its two great camel humps on our right. Ahead, houses with closed shutters and shadows under their eaves climbed up to the Carthusian monastery of San Martino, while in the foreground the swollen towers of the medieval castle of the Angevins loomed up, still threatening and self-important, although now used mainly as a deposit for confiscated cars.

The sun was hidden behind the slopes of Capodimonte, and the light was pink and clear with that sense you often get at dawn of everything being washed clean by night. There was no noise, either, except for someone hammering in the docks. The city and bay were immersed in this silence as they must always have been before the advent of the car: when Goethe left to sail for four days over to Palermo, when Nelson's ships were anchored in the bay, when Garibaldi entered after the last Bourbon king had departed to fight on forlornly for a few months, further north at Gaeta.

The difference between Naples and Palermo, between Campania and Sicily, also determines variations between Camorra and Mafia. I once asked a Sicilian why his compatriots had always been ruled by others. "Because we never take risks," he said. Pride and a terror of humiliation make failure doubly feared. A joke told in the North of Italy, which of course is meant to be insulting, is that Sicily is the only Arab country not in a state of war with Israel. Sicilians will talk to you like those other islanders, the Irish, with a memory for past oppressions and evils that is almost as long. "We have the cunning of the Arabs, the strength of the Normans, and the cruelty of the Spaniards," said a Sicilian I had only just met. "And our hands are sweaty, so money sticks to them."

The Neapolitans on the other hand have for whatever reason come to represent the foreign idea of Italians, with their mandolins, their songs, their dances, their wheedling, their delight in the moment, perhaps their fecklessness. "When everyone else is computerized, Neapolitans will be the only ones who remain individuals!" Dr Riccardo Boccia, the prefect, told me. Of them Norman Douglas wrote in his first book, *Siren Land*:

> ... the antagonism of flesh and spirit, the most pernicious piece of crooked thinking which has ever oozed out of our poor deluded brain, has always been unintelligible to them. That is why they remained sober when the rest of us went crazy. There were no sour-faced Puritans in Naples, no witch

burnings, no inquisition – the Neapolitans never indulged in these fateful extravagances; they held that the promptings of nature were righteous and reasonable....

Dr Roberto Pasca told me that in his opinion the Mafia were more efficient than the Camorra, who seem more ostentatious – which perhaps is why more is known about them: I have even come across a map showing the areas controlled by different *mammasantissime*, as the Camorra leaders are called: Bardellino and Zaza, Mazzarella and Cutolo, Alfieri and Ammaturo.

The word Camorra itself comes from the Spanish *gamurra*, meaning extortion money. The society dates from 1842 when three Spaniards arrived in Naples intent on enlarging their sphere of influence. They belonged to a secret society which had been founded in Toledo in 1420 and was called "Confraternita della Guardugna" (robbery fraternity). Its statutes consisted of nine articles of which the most important was: "All brothers should die rather than confess, under pain of being excluded and degraded." In Naples, branches were set up in the twelve boroughs, and a hierarchy was established which included those in charge of each zone. These in turn elected the *capointesa*, or head of the entire organization in the city. New camorristi were admitted with a special ceremony, which still exists. This involved sucking blood from the wrist of the person who proposed you, and included a special ritual dialogue. When Tore De Francesco, the first *capointesa* of renown, was admitted the dialogue went like this:

HEAD: Who are you looking for?
TORE: I'm looking for my companions.
HEAD: Who are your companions?
TORE: The Camorristi.
HEAD: And what does Camorrista mean?
TORE: A man with one foot on the earth and another in a ditch.

The Camorra, then, was in the tradition of secret societies like the Freemasons, or the Carbonari. However, while the latter was a revolutionary society whose object was the unification of Italy, to which Louis Napoleon – the future Napoleon III – belonged, the main object of the Camorra was power and wealth through extortion money, and the control of brothels and gambling houses.

Like the Mafia, the Camorra early assumed the role of intermediary. When De Francesco was imprisoned for stabbing and killing three men with whom he had quarrelled, he soon took over the prison he was sent to, and established his own rules. There was the daily contribution of a *carlino*, a coin of the time, by each of the prisoners every morning. Disputes were settled, often with blood. A regular market was set up in the food and clothes with which the prisoners were issued. These were then sold back at a profit to the prison suppliers.

When the King departed in 1861, De Francesco and his men took over the policing of Naples before Garibaldi arrived. They thus fulfilled the traditional role of both Camorra and Mafia in arranging some kind of order when government could not supply it.

When Naples became part of United Italy, the Camorra continued to consolidate itself until, like the Mafia, it was contained by Mussolini. It too was helped by the Allied invasion in 1943. In Francesco Rosi's film *Lucky Luciano*, there is a realistic illustration of the American/Italian criminal, Vito Genovese, "helping" the Americans when the general in command arranges to send lorries to fetch food and equipment from the army dumps for sale on the black market by the re-established Camorra. In return, the general gets a new car.

After the war, the Americans returned two thousand of their worst criminals to their countries of origin – which in most cases was Italy. In 1961, the closure of Tangier as a free port, when it became part of the kingdom of Morocco, knocked out a competitor in cigarette smuggling. This is one of the biggest of the Camorra's sources of income, estimated in 1981 at 300 billion lire (120 million dollars) per year.

Every day, depending on the weather, about twenty to thirty motor boats furnished with powerful Mercury engines go out. They load up from tramp steamers about fifty miles from the coast. The State manages to intercept only about 10 per cent of the total. Why, one asks, does this happen principally in Italy? After all, tax on cigarettes is just as high in Britain and yet there are no fleets of motor boats at Dover, shooting out to meet tramp steamers in the English Channel.

In Naples it is estimated that thousands of people live from cigarette smuggling. Although the loss of customs duty on all contraband amounts to some four hundred and seventy billion lire ($310 million) a year, there are, paradoxically, ways in which the Camorra supports the society in which it exists. From a secret place after an accusation of murder, Michele Zaza, *mammasantissima* of Portici, boasted about the importance of contraband:

At least seven hundred thousand people live off contraband, which is for Naples what Fiat is to Turin. They have called me the Agnelli of Naples.... Yes – it could all be eliminated in thirty minutes. And then those who work would be finished. They'd all become thieves, robbers, muggers. Naples would become the worst city in the world. Instead, this city should thank the twenty, thirty men who arrange for ships laden with cigarettes to be discharged and thus stop crime!

Zaza could obviously be said to be biased! Nevertheless, one of the most dangerous aspects of both Mafia and Camorra is this economic dependence of so many people on their activities. What would happen to Palermo if the estimated 20 per cent of revenue which comes from heroin were removed? Even people who have no direct connection with the trade would be affected. One of the most unfortunate aspects of the commerce in both heroin and smuggled tobacco is that it is the poorest parts of Italy which earn money from it.

Like the Mafia, the Camorra is also involved in illegal building, and extortion. It is said to derive income from 26,000 shops and businesses in the Naples area, from match-sellers to supermarkets. With drugs, it seems to act more as an intermediary than in setting up heroin factories. Camorra members probably number about 10,000, with another 100,000 loosely connected. They are divided into two main groups: La Nuova Famiglia, or new family, and La Nuova Camorra Organizzata, or new organized Camorra.

La Nuova Camorra Organizzata is based inland, round the town of Ottaviano. Its undisputed head is Raffaele Cutolo, the *mammasantissima*, revered by his members who call him "Prince" and kiss his left hand as if he were a bishop. His headquarters used to be a vast palace, bought from the Princess of Miranda, where Gabriele d'Annunzio lived for some time. It is a sixteenth-century building with 365 rooms, one for every day of the year, and a large park with tennis courts and swimming pool.

As Cutolo spends much of his time in prison from where he sends out instructions to his camorristi, the everyday running of the "business" was until recently entrusted to his sister Rosa and her son Robert. Cutolo himself has pretensions to prophecy and has announced that he is Jesus Christ come to earth again with the power of life and death. He has also forecast that he will die at the age of forty-nine, in 1990.

He fancies himself too as a poet. When he had his lieutenant, Antonio Cuomo, stabbed in prison because he felt he might be a rival, he also had Cuomo's wife shot as she was driving to the Carabinieri to reveal everything she knew. When Cutolo heard that she was dead, he sat down and wrote a poem to their orphan boy which goes like this:

Death has taken first your father, then your mother.
A lot of time will pass before you realize this cruel destiny
And the tragic reality
Of a child alone, unique witness of a crime of the Camorra.
The law of the Camorra,
Ruthless and cruel,
Does not pardon traitors.
Child! Innocent witness, grow beautiful
Healthy and different.
Forget everything and everyone
For a better life.

La Nuova Famiglia also has its personalities but no absolute boss like Cutolo. One of the best known is a woman, Pupetta Maresca, who was born in 1935 in one of the coastal towns near Naples, Castellamare. Every year, on the day of the Madonna of Pompeii, her mother used to give a great festa, with a banquet for a hundred people, with fireworks and street dancing, to thank the Virgin for having helped her husband escape from prison!

At one of these festas, Pupetta got engaged to Pasqualone, a member of the local Camorra. Three months after their wedding, Pasqualone was shot. He was rushed to hospital, and Pupetta managed to conceal herself under his bed, although six months pregnant. Keeping to the Camorra code, Pasqualone said nothing to the Carabinieri, who also came to the bedside, but told Pupetta just before he died that a local *mammasantissima*, Antonio Esposito, was responsible.

So, a month or two later Pupetta took a taxi to a bar in Naples frequented by Esposito and, leaning out of the taxi window, shot him dead. She then escaped and declared to the press that she would only surrender when she had had her child, as she didn't want to give birth in prison.

She was, however, tracked down and sent to prison for ten years. When she came out, she lived with Umberto Ammaturo who was known as "the king of drugs", and with whom her brother, Ciro, was also working. They had two children, and in addition there was Pupetta's first child, Pascalotto, who had grown into a gigantic youth like his father. When he was eighteen, Pascalotto disappeared and Pupetta became convinced that it was the work of Cutolo's Nuova Camorra Organizzata. At a press conference she said: "If Cutolo touches one of my family I'll kill all his. I'll cut them into pieces, his assassins, his women, and even the children in their cradles." Later in front of a tribunal, in February 1982, she added: "Campania is suffocated by a power that is hidden but present at all levels. It is that of Raffaele Cutolo and his men.... They want the command of everything at all costs. You are either with them or against them. Cutolo wants to become Emperor of Naples...." Finally, she and her lover, Ammaturo, were arrested for the suspected murder of one of Cutolo's men, and for the murder and dismemberment of his psychiatrist, who with various pleas of insanity had got him off about ten years in prison.

Adriano Baglivo in his fascinating book *Camorra S.P.A.*, calls Pupetta *la pasionaria* of the Camorra. At one time she was so well known that two films, *Crime at Naples* and *London calls Naples*, were made about her adventures. In contrast to the Mafia, the Camorra does allow women to have prominent roles. Perhaps this is another difference between Neapolitan and Sicilian attitudes. In the Nuova Camorra Organizzata, Cutolo could hardly have done anything without his sister Rosa. Older than he is, she looked after him when he was a boy, and ran all his affairs when he was in prison.

War between the factions broke out openly in January 1980, a little earlier than in Palermo. The reason would seem to be the same: the fact that as both organizations become more international, they tend to expand beyond their territorial base at each other's expense. Unlike normal businessmen, their members react to strong competition with a gun. This means the start of vendettas, which in Campania has led to 650 murders between 1980 and 1983. Occasional truces have taken place, although as a Neapolitan explained to me these could be described as pauses for identifying new enemies. As one person is killed, another takes his place, and if a lot of these killings occur, there is not enough time for the opposing clan to find out who is now trying to assassinate them!

As a colonel of Carabinieri, Roberto Conforti, said, there are also the internal fights: "The clans themselves strike at those who breach their own rules, or who want to rise to the top too quickly." In fact the penalties for crimes within the Camorra are laid down as specifically as the ritual for those who wish to be new members. If, for instance, the "traitor" is a "blood brother" of a boss, he will be killed "violently" and his body will be subjected to violations such as decapitation or quartering and disembowelling, or having his heart torn out.

As in Palermo, the strain must be enormous. Adriano Baglivo describes the plight of a camorrista, Giovanni Mormone, who killed the brother of future Camorra leader Antonio Spavone. "I've killed a man," he said to his friends, "and every day when I get up, another man gets up too – a brother or a son of the dead man – and goes out armed, and sooner or later will try and kill me."

In the end, Mormone was killed by Antonio Spavone. "It's not me who is killing you but my brother!" Spavone is said to have shouted as he stabbed him to death. Some of the events are so bloodthirsty that it is amazing that people responsible for them still walk the streets. Antonio Spavone, who is called in the Neapolitan style *o malommo*, was for a long time a semi-retired "professional", with his telephone tapped but free to go where he wished, in spite of all he had done. One camorrista, returning from fishing, met a whole family on the stairs and massacred them with a boat hook because one of them flicked ash in his eye. He was let off on the grounds of self-defence! Another pursued someone he thought had insulted him to a fashionable hotel, shot him several times and killed him in front of several hundred people, for which he was imprisoned for only eight months.

It is extraordinary, too, the way prisons have become the headquarters of crime. Inside them, you can lead a comfortable existence, like the old days in Britain when a gentleman could have his supper brought in from a neighbouring restaurant, and the tailor would be admitted to measure him for a suit. In the Neapolitan prison of Poggioreale, where on average there are twenty-five prisoners to a cell, Cutolo managed to get a room to himself with a shower, while his own personal cook occupied the cell next door so that he could serve up dishes on request. Cutolo referred to the prison as "The State of Poggioreale" – of which he undoubtedly considered himself president. As a prisoner, he dresses impeccably with ties and shirts signed by their designers, a gold watch and shoes of crocodile skin.

Prison is also a great opportunity for rival gangs to obtain new recruits and consolidate old loyalties. Cutolo built up much of his organization in jail, through distributing clothes he received as presents, ensuring that the families of prisoners were paid regularly, and even providing drugs to those who wanted them.

When Cutolo was transferred to another prison, Salvatore Giuliano, of the Nuova Famiglia, opposed to Cutolo, wrote to his brother-in-law about his own successes in prison: "I myself have recruited about twenty members of the Neapolitan Brotherhood. The money is useful to keep them loyal. Here Cutolo no longer counts for anything. Here, we are the only ones who matter, the only ones."

The prison guards themselves are inevitably under threat, particularly with their families living outside. They are also dealing with criminals who have access to a great deal of money. A combination of threats and bribery ensures that they are amenable to bringing messages and even weapons in and out. In one sudden search by police inspectors, dynamite was discovered in holes in the floor, and bullets and revolvers under mattresses and in drawers. Certainly, murders seem to occur almost as frequently in prison as outside, both in Palermo and Naples. When the earthquake of 23rd November 1980 occurred in Naples, prisoners were allowed out of their cells and the camorristi of Cutolo's clan took advantage of the crowds and the chaos to kill nine of their rivals.

Another aid to the spread of the Camorra is the practice of exiling criminals to towns where they have to report to the police once a day. In Assisi, I asked the director of tourism whether there was any problem with drugs: "Well, there is now," he said. "There are two men from the Camorra exiled in a neighbouring small town who are setting up a whole structure for its distribution." Exile to towns near Rome has also meant expansion for the Camorra. Extortion money is now being demanded in Tivoli and Velletri, and the province of Romagna is the region of Italy most afflicted by drugs, with over 20,000 addicts.

How do you ensure that with their enormous resources, which can so easily corrupt opposition, the Mafia and Camorra do not infiltrate even further all over Italy? There has been evidence that Mafia money is behind casinos as far north as the Ligurian coast. Arrests were made in Milan on St Valentine's Day 1983 of what is called the "white-collar Mafia", in other words financiers, businessmen and those who have become rich through property deals, backed by money believed to have come from drugs. A cartoon in *La Repubblica* in January 1984 showed Italy as a violin case with two compartments. One was stuffed with bank notes, and the other contained a revolver.

Another cartoon in the same paper showed a Mafia boss asking himself why Italy was "our only enterprise that runs at a loss". How in fact do you fight when the problem – as always in Italy – is that the forces of the government are so often subordinate to the interests of families, regions and local concerns?

To what extent, also, are servants of the State involved in the very activities which officially they wish to stamp out? Two weeks before his assassination, General Dalla Chiesa summoned a well-known journalist, Giorgio La Bocca, for an interview, and told him very deliberately: "I am even more interested in the network that controls the Mafia which may be in hands above suspicion and which, having placed itself in key positions, controls political power."

If Orlando, Italy's representative at Versailles at the end of the First

World War, could be sponsored by the Mafia when there was presumably very little financial inducement, how much greater is the temptation today when both Camorra and Mafia hold the key to such an immense treasure chest!

GOVERNMENT MEASURES

Dalla Chiesa was appointed prefect of Palermo partly because of the assassination of the Communist deputy, La Torre, who had proposed a law in Parliament to confer the power to inspect bank accounts which had been so successful against criminals in the United States. La Torre also established lenient terms for "penitents" similar to those which were so successful against the Red Brigades.

These measures were passed within nine days of the Dalla Chiesas' murder, and now Italians will tell you that they are weapons which will bring the Mafia and Camorra to their knees. Yet the bank director I saw in Bologna was more cynical. He felt the law was difficult to apply because bank clients have a "Libretto al Portatore", an account book, in which they are not necessarily named. It is easy anyway to have an account under a pseudonym. In the end, it is a battle between the investigating financial police (the Guardia di Finanza) and the Mafia. How skilled anyway are the financial police? There is a shortage in Italy of real experts of this kind. That is why Ambrosoli, the man investigating the affairs of the banker Sindona, was shot outside his house in July 1979 – he was one of the few people skilful enough to follow up an investigation of this sort and could probably not be replaced. If the Mafia are able to transport tons of morphine to Sicily, turn it into heroin and then send it to the United States, Europe and other parts of the world, surely they are capable of concealing the money they get for it. Most of it originates from abroad, anyway. Given that the Mafia-ridden town of Trapani with 70,000 inhabitants has more banks than Milan itself, it is likely that the Mafia have their own banks, as well as everything else.

Certainly some mafiosi have been caught because of the new law, but it is probable that they will get over the initial surprise and cover their tracks. Meanwhile, no new heroin factories have been discovered since 1980, and supplies have been increasing everywhere. True, many "families" have decimated each other, and a few bosses who fled Sicily because of the war between the gangs have been arrested with the help of other governments: Giovanni Badalamenti in Spain and Buscetta in Brazil. However, despite the decimating war between different *cosche*, new recruits are not difficult to get. When there are 70,000 applicants for 300 vacancies for caretakers in Palermo, there can be little difficulty in enrolling new recruits for the Mafia.

Another problem is the pressure on judges and magistrates. Apart from Chinnici, a number have been assassinated in the last few years. Gaetano Costa, the Procurator of the Republic in Palermo, was assassinated in 1980 after he had signed thirty-three orders of arrest. Then, in January 1983, a couple of killers were sent out from the Cosa Nostra in the United States to eliminate Giangiacomo Ciacco Montalto, a judge who was researching into links between business and the Mafia in Trapani near Palermo. Montalto was also interested in relations between the Cosa Nostra in America and the Mafia in Sicily, and as the order to kill him came from New York it can be presumed that his researches were developing well.

Montalto gave an interesting interview on television before his murder in which he said that there was no magistrate in Trapani who dealt exclusively with research into the Mafia, and that there were no information banks on the spot. All records were held in Rome and were difficult to get hold of. When asked what happened to the research when a magistrate changed jobs, he said: "The historical memory of the research is lost."

Fifteen months after his death, in August 1984, another judge who shared his office, Antonio Costa, was arrested for "allowing himself to be corrupted by the Mafia". How far he was involved in Montalto's murder remains to be seen.

One person who is very critical of the difficulty magistrates have in dealing with the Mafia is Sebastian Patané, Procurator of the Republic in Caltanisetta, a big town in the centre of the island. One thing he complains of is that magistrates have to research into cases by themselves. If there were two of them, they would avoid the isolation which is usually their lot. Indeed, it is awesome to think of the agony of being a magistrate in Sicily, with the thought of a gun around every corner, and reservations about condemning a prisoner in case revenge is taken. In his film *Three Brothers*, Francesco Rosi has portrayed the terror of a judge involved with the Red Brigade trials: the fear when anyone comes to the door of the flat, the worries about the safety of wife and children, the recurrent nightmare in which he dreams he is being killed in a bus and left on the floor, bleeding, with a sack over him. For magistrates investigating the Mafia it must be the same.

Often, too, judges are from other parts of Italy and the isolation in a strange, hostile town, where even the dialect spoken is incomprehensible, must be even more disturbing. While if they are from Mafia or Camorra country, there are always the divided loyalties, the family alliances, the personal friendships to obscure everything.

Patané also condemns the lack of involvement of some magistrates: "A judge's profession can be done honestly without provoking criticism, but also without doing anything against the Mafia. We all know that there are some who stop everything at the first shiver of fear." He has also attacked the government, even saying: "The State is not in a condition to fight effectively against the Mafia."

Nevertheless, it is important to remember the bravery of many of those fighting the Mafia and the Camorra, and often succeeding. A breakthrough was made when the police arrested a thousand suspected members of Cutolo's Nuova Camorra Organizzata between June 16th and 19th 1983. These included a nun accused of being postwoman between different jails and a well-known television personality, Enzo Tortora, presenter of a weekly show called *Portobello* which had an enormous following.

The immediate cause for this was the confession of one of Cutolo's most loyal lieutenants, Pasquale Barra, known justifiably as *o animale*. Barra had known Cutolo when they were children in their home town of Ottaviano, and was called his "avenging angel". Among the various barbarous actions done for his chief was the murder of another camorrista, Francisco Turatello, by tearing out his bowels in the courtyard of a Sardinian jail and masticating them before throwing them away.

The reason for *o animale*'s change of loyalty was typical of the way a strong sense of morality, of law, can accompany the most murderous acts. In this case, *o animale* objected to the fact that Cutolo had had the wife of Antonio Cuomo killed in order to ensure she didn't tell the Carabinieri everything she knew (p. 201). It was against the law of the Camorra to kill women, he protested. "Now *o animale* wants to lay down the law!" was Cutolo's sarcastic reply. "Tell him to keep his place." Because of this and further disagreements, *o animale* called a magistrate to his cell and said: "Dotto', if you want to know everything, I am ready. I've got a thousand names and I am ready to serve them up to you on a silver platter."

Some commentators said, optimistically, at the time that this was the end of the Camorra. However, the thousand names belonged only to Cutolo's Nuova Camorra Organizzata and the rival Nuova Famiglia were hardly touched.

We drove out of Naples to Acerra to see Bishop Riboldi. We skirted Vesuvius and speeded over flat country, past empty fields under a cloudy sky in December. We passed untidy villages with the metal and concrete of factories on the outskirts. "Here the soil produces everything," wrote Goethe in 1787, "and one can expect three to five harvests a year. In a really good year, I am told, they can grow maize three times in the same fields."

Acerra is a crowded town and groups of boys strolled about the streets on a Sunday morning. We parked in the small piazza and went into the cathedral, where Mass had already begun. We had difficulty getting a seat. There was a large proportion of young people and the choir was accompanied by a guitarist. Members of the congregation read the lesson. After Mass, everyone shook hands with those nearest to them. Two girls in front turned round and extended their hands, and we in turn greeted some venerable looking ladies sitting behind us. When the collection was taken, change was given for thousand lire notes if requested. Afterwards, the bishop, a tall, strong man with a resounding voice, announced that a girl from Acerra with an eye disease had gone to Japan for an operation paid for by funds raised in the Church.

Then we accompanied the bishop and several other people who wanted to see him to his palace. The stone on one side of the staircase was misted with damp. As we went up, the bishop drew his finger along it. We sat in a dark reception room with simple chairs and tables and splodgy religious paintings around the walls. Outside, a bare field stretched out, surrounded by houses with cracked walls and black, stained surfaces. A fig tree and two orange trees stood in the middle, drooping slightly under the December sky.

Bishop Riboldi is well known in Italy, largely for his work in combating the Camorra. He is a Northerner from Milan and was a priest in Belice in western Sicily for twenty years. The situation there was difficult, he told us when we started talking. The peasants neglected the land because they dreamed of working in an industry that had not yet been set up. "They were neither peasants nor workmen," he said.

Here in Acerra there were other problems. "Most people don't know if the State is Italian or if the State is Camorra," he said. The climax of the civil war between the clans had been in 1982, with more than three hundred deaths. At this stage, Acerra had been frozen as a community, as if under an invisible dictatorship. It was, after all, only a few miles from Cutolo's town of Ottaviano. No one trusted anyone. Because of this no one talked about anything serious, even within the family.

In September 1982, Riboldi had decided that something must be done. At a festa, he denounced the Camorra. Everyone was stunned by his boldness. It was rather like a Greek legend in which youths and maidens are sacrificed to a monster every year. When someone says the monster should be killed, there is terror at the thought of fighting it, and yet hope is also born.

Later in 1982, a lawyer was shot in Acerra. People were so afraid of the Camorra that in the press it was called "a premature death". At the lawyer's funeral, Riboldi said, "We are the masters of the country. From now on we will fight the Camorra!" He also denounced everyone for accepting their own slavery. "What is the point of extending your life to eighty if you are a slave?" he asked.

That December, he organized a demonstration of five hundred students and young people in Ottaviano against the Camorra. As the town was Cutolo's headquarters, described by Camilla Cederna in her *Casa Nostra* as "the town of daily death", it was quite a test of courage, which fortunately did not lead to any disasters. There were further marches between December and February and the country was gradually mobilized until in February there was a march of 100,000 students in Naples, and the shopkeepers closed for two days as a protest against extortion.

After June 1983, when 1,000 suspected members of La Nuova Camorra Organizzata were arrested, people became more detached. The recruiting ground among the young was reduced. The Camorra was no longer regarded as invincible and, as it weakened, there were fewer new drug takers.

In addition to the marches and the sermons, Riboldi also gives lectures. The previous day he had given two, one of them attended by a thousand people in a cinema, where it was possible to be personal and talk directly to everyone.

"Aren't you afraid of assassination?" I asked.

"Danger is our profession!"

The Church, thought Riboldi, had a great advantage in taking this kind of approach because it was outside the State. A strong link with the young had been established which a political party, or the government itself, could not achieve because it represented other policies which the young might not support. However, it was now important to create a structure which could take the place of the Camorra and provide direct personal government and jobs. Otherwise, the Camorra would be able to re-form.

This indeed is the great problem, whether in Sicily or the Naples

region. As long ago as 1911 Norman Douglas in his *Old Calabria* quoted a
Professor Colajanni who said: "To heal the South, we require an
honest, intelligent and sagacious government, which we have not got."
Douglas also mentioned "the unseen hand at Rome – a hand which is
held out for blackmail, and not vainly, from the highest ministerial
benches".

Today, in 1985, there is not even any effective local government in
Palermo or Naples. In Palermo there is continual bickering within the
ruling Christian Democrat Party. In Naples the deadlock between the
parties was confirmed by the elections of December 1983, which
reduced the Communist vote slightly but otherwise left the situation
much as it was. Indeed for some time the only solution was to appoint a
Government Commissary with four assistants to take the place of the
mayor and councillors.

The prefect Riccardo Boccia, himself a Neapolitan, quoted
Boccaccio's description of Naples as "the city of misfortune". He told
me that when he arrived in September 1981, he feared that Naples
would turn into another Beirut with civil war between the clans. The
well-known archaeologist, the late Professor Raffaele della Causa, also
told me that he had advised his sons to get out of Naples and make their
careers elsewhere.

"Because of the effects of the earthquake?" I asked.

"Earthquake!" he said. "We've had earthquakes throughout our
history. No! This city is being ruined by political in-fighting. It has
wonderful theatre and music, an excellent university, exceptional
writers. It is Naples! But it is being throttled by those who should be
administering it. And people run down the Bourbons!"

In Sicily, Dalla Chiesa's immediate successor, De Francesco, said that
the Mafia will only disappear by the year 2005. By this, he meant that
the only way the Mafia will be eliminated is by a change in public
opinion; as Bishop Riboldi has shown, the same goes for the Camorra.
Before he was killed, Dalla Chiesa himself recognized this, and toured
schools and workshops denouncing the evils of the Mafia and its baneful
influence on the life of the citizen.

From an economic point of view, the difficulty is how to effect the
change-over from a corrupt economy to a healthy, flourishing one. In
Rome, I spoke about this to Luigi Spaventa, a well-known economist
and until recently an independent deputy on the list of the Communist
Party. Both he and Pino Arlacchi feel that the Mafia and Camorra do
more harm to the economy than is compensated by what are called
narco-lire – although the Minister of the Interior in August 1984 did

admit that hundreds of billion lire invested in the stock exchange came from the profits of drug-dealing and kidnapping.

Few businesses invest in the South because their directors may be kidnapped, they may have to pay extortion money and the cost of this has to be added to prices. Anyway, who wants to live in a chaotic society of marauding bands and robber barons in the twentieth century? For, rightly or wrongly, that is the way the South appears to Italians north of Rome, and to many foreigners.

As it is, many of the industries set up by the Cassa per il Mezzogiorno have folded. There are successful firms, like a branch of Fiat near Palermo, or Aer Italia near Naples. But few foreign firms are tempted, and tourism, so I was told in Palermo, is in decline. Between 1982 and 1983 there was a massive reduction by 80 per cent of British visitors. This, said the director of tourism in Palermo, was because there had been a series of almost simultaneous articles on the Mafia in the *Sunday Times*, the *Observer* and the *Sunday Express*. The overall fall for all nationalities was 10 per cent, which was also alarming, and this was repeated in 1984.

In Naples, a number of hotels were still being used recently by homeless refugees from the earthquake and, so I am told, for some time Naples has not been regarded as a stopping place for tourism.

Indeed, until there is faith in government in the South, a strong flourishing economy which reduces unemployment, and an administration which has no vested interest in corruption, the Mafia, Camorra and 'Ndrangheta will not disappear. This, though, is a vicious circle: none of these necessary conditions can exist if the three societies continue – and yet you cannot get rid of the societies until these conditions exist!

Unfortunately, in the South economic aid tends to enrich the wrong people. A pathetic example of this was the help sent during the earthquake in November 1980. Collected by schoolchildren and through appeals all over the world, a lot of it was stolen by the Camorra. Lorries laden with tents, bedding and food were simply driven off to hidden lairs and then "sold". It was like the old days in 1943 when Anglo-American military supplies were deflected to the black market. The effect of this was not only to prevent people who needed these things from receiving them as quickly as possible. It also disillusioned people in other countries and made them less likely to raise money for catastrophes in future – particularly in Italy.

In late September 1984, Tommaso Buscetta, one of the leading Mafia leaders, was extradited from Brazil to Italy, and "squealed". He was the first Mafia leader ever to do this. His motivation was not only that he was one of the "losers" in the Mafia war in Palermo, but also that his own sons, Antonio and Benedetto, had disappeared in August 1982, that his son-in-law was shot in his pizza shop shortly afterwards, and that his brother and nephew were also murdered. As a result of Buscetta's confessions, 366 warrants for Mafia members were issued in Italy and 29 in the United States.

As happened in Cutolo's gang in the summer of 1983, *omertà*, the refusal to speak to the authorities, had at last broken down. This showed that both the Mafia and the Camorra have outgrown themselves and become organizations in which rivalry and the development of a vast international structure have begun to destroy the loyalty and sense of family unity that were once their greatest strength. However, even with these devastating blows, any organization can reorganize so long as it has the prospect of so much wealth. A week after the arrests, following Buscetta's denunciations, the Mafia showed itself to be still in the killing business with the murder of a Mafia chief, Salvatore Piscotta, in a field outside Palermo. In Naples, the killing still goes on: on a Sunday at the beginning of September 1984, a bus stopped in the town of Torre Annunziata, near Naples. Gunmen emerged, and eight members of the local Camorra clan were left dead in the street.

Not till the poppy fields of Afghanistan and Thailand are eliminated will the temptations that keep the Mafia and Camorra alive be destroyed. Even then, there are so many problems going back to history, to the memory of grievances, the justification of wrongs, the unwillingness to understand the point of view of old enemies. Indeed, it is significant that it is the two old capitals of the Bourbon kingdom, Palermo and Naples, which are the centres of, respectively, the Mafia and the Camorra. Here is what Eugenio Scalfari, the editor of the Roman newspaper *La Repubblica*, wrote when asking Italians on holiday to reflect, in August 1984:

> You are surprised that contracts are fraudulent, that funds for earthquake victims, contributions to the EEC, and the moneys set apart by special laws end up in the pockets of organized crime.
>
> But why are you surprised? Did you really think that for over a hundred years it would be possible to impose on almost a third of the poor, the desperate, the inhabitants of ghettos, using them perhaps for a boom if there is a boom, for war when there is a war, to redirect the subsidies made to the South back to the North again ... without the wound becoming septic, without the whole organism becoming polluted, without the ruling class

catching the vices of arrogance and indifference, without criminal organizations themselves becoming institutions?

The Italian term *dietrologia*, translated literally into English, means "behindology". It refers to the belief that behind every event there are sinister, powerful personalities, or organizations, manipulating everything. Their true secrets will never be found out, so their identity is an endless source of discussion.

In his book *The Italians*, Barzini describes what foreign diplomats often feel in Rome. "Italy is the opposite of Russia. In Rome, everything is public, there are no secrets, everybody talks, yet one understands nothing." Understanding nothing creates a desire to speculate, often wildly.

When I discussed this with an Italian friend, he said: "Of course! You must remember we've always had so many different concentrations of power in Italy. And we've still got them: the biggest Communist party in Europe, the Vatican, the Mafia, big industrial interests in the North, the polarization of regions and of North and South. They're all related, too, to international forces, whether America or Russia, World Catholicism or Cosa Nostra. Even the Red Brigades were linked to the German Baader-Meinhof group and, probably, to the Palestinians, the Libyans, and every other terrorist organization under the sun. As these forces can't work openly through our political system, they have to intrigue, or work through secret groupings. We know that, so we spend our time worrying about what they're up to!"

As we have seen, the Mafia and the Camorra can be said to represent the Italian family structure directed to criminal ends. These hidden links of *clientelismo*, "friends of friends", favour for favour, personal contacts, operate to some extent in all societies. In Italy, however, they tend to be a norm in any walk of life.

As a result, a "tower of painted smoke" surrounds many dramatic events. Who, for example, were responsible for the bomb which in August 1980 killed eighty-five passengers and bystanders at Bologna railway station? Was the banker, Calvi, murdered or did he commit suicide under Blackfriars Bridge in London in July 1982? How much influence did the Masonic lodge, P2, really have, and how did its Venerable Master, Licio Gelli, escape from his Swiss prison in August 1983? Why, in 1979, did a bankrupt Italian banker, Sindona, who was to spend several years in an American prison, pretend he had been kidnapped and then turn up in Sicily? Who planted the bomb which blew up on a train between Firenze and Bologna killing twenty-nine people in December 1984?

When you ask these questions and perhaps half a dozen more, you begin to realize how far this undergrowth, this *sotto bosco,* extends in Italy. Does it, though, really have a great effect on the way Italy develops? Or is it all exaggerated by the press and by conspiracy theories into a kind of folk drama – partly because it seems to represent what people fear is true of Italy today? Certainly, it gives the impression to both natives and foreigners that Italians are more corrupt than they really are.

The possible involvement of political parties in intrigue is another subject for speculation. An example of this is the case of Ciro Cirillo, the regional president of Campania – the area of which Naples is the capital.

Cirillo, who is a Christian Democrat, was abducted by the Red Brigades in April 1981. He was released within three months because, so rumour has it, the Christian Democrats paid Cutolo, the Camorra leader, somewhere between $750,000 and double that sum to use his influence with the Red Brigades. In return, Cutolo is also said to have asked for a slackening of police activities against the Camorra, for control over the tendering for building contracts in Naples and for a reduction of his own sentence – as well as a new psychiatric test to show that he is not responsible for his actions. Both these last concessions were granted.

If true, it is scandalous that the largest party in government should have connived with the Red Brigades and Camorra to obtain the release of one of their politicians because the police were not effective enough. However, it would be strange if the Christian Democrats were flexible over the release of one of their minor officials, and yet refused so rigidly to compromise with the Red Brigades over the murder of their leading statesman, Moro.

This characteristic intertwining of interests and uncertainties is even more intricate in the whole drama of Calvi, the P2, and the Vatican. The main characters in this incredibly complicated story are, first, Sindona, a Sicilian banker who made a fortune under the Allied military government after the war when he was illegally trading in grain. This was the beginning of his American contacts and career. Later, his expertise was used by the IOR, the Vatican bank, when in the late 1960s they decided to move their investments from Italian industry into financial shareholdings, often in other countries. Sindona has great charm and a love of accounts: as he told Enzo Biagi in an interview, he has friends who bring him balance sheets to work out to calm him down whenever he seems nervous. His real objective, he said, has been to put creative ideas into practice and be of help to other people. In fact, though, one of his most obvious aims seems to have been to circumvent laws in order to further his own interests.

Because of the spread of bankruptcies in the 1930s, the Italian government of the time laid down that banks were not allowed to buy non-banking interests. That law still exists. To get round it, Sindona set up a number of foreign front companies. Once he managed to export money to these from his banks, he could speculate and buy and sell whatever he wished in Italy itself. Other companies were bought and sold at excessive prices, thus increasing their nominal value. If necessary, Sindona increased the value of their shares by buying more himself on the tiny Milan Stock Exchange. A kind of "puff organization" was thus created, using other people's money to speculate all over the world for personal gain. In this "game" the link with the Vatican bank, the IOR, was particularly useful. As part of a sovereign State, separate from Italy, it had no need to get permission to export currency abroad, and it also gave an immaculate aura to all transactions.

However, Sindona's empire collapsed in September 1974, largely because the Vietnamese war and the sudden rise in the price of oil produced unexpected fluctuations in the currencies in which he was speculating. Fearing arrest, he departed rapidly to the United States where he kept extradition at bay by continual reference to his list of 500 well-known and influential Italians who were guilty of major currency offences!

During the early '70s Sindona worked with Calvi, chairman and managing director of the Ambrosiano bank, which was one of the first banks in Italy, founded by a priest in 1896. Calvi learnt from Sindona: he too created front companies abroad. In addition, he worked with the Vatican in the person of Archbishop Marcinkus, an American of Latvian origin who directed the IOR.

Calvi's secret object was to acquire personal, financial control of the Ambrosiano bank through buying a majority of shares. This he hoped to do by using money exported to the complicated web of companies abroad which he controlled. This money was re-imported to buy the shares, or put into the San Gothardo bank which Ambrosiano owned in Switzerland. From there, it was deflected to the coffers of political parties, or of any groups or individuals who could be of use. In this he was helped by the head of the Vatican bank, Archbishop Marcinkus, who once remarked that the Church could not be financed by Hail Marys alone. Marcinkus himself was on the board of various companies abroad, controlled by Calvi, some of which the Vatican actually owned, and according to David Yallop in his book *In God's Name* was one of the principal villains of the piece.

The Calvi empire, in turn, went the way of Sindona's – partly as a result of the latter's bitterness when Calvi was reluctant to bail him out in his hour of crisis. On November 13th 1977, streets in the centre of Milan were covered with posters accusing Calvi of misappropriating millions of dollars and transferring them to banks in Switzerland. However, before this happened one of Sindona's allies had written to the Bank of Italy, threatening to sue them for failing to carry out their legal duties if Calvi was not investigated.

As a result, twelve inspectors arrived at the Banco Ambrosiano. This led to Calvi's arrest in May 1981. At his trial, he was condemned to four years' jail and a fine of 16 billion lire. However, as his lawyer then appealed to a higher court, he was allowed out on bail and for a short time resumed his position of chairman and managing director of Ambrosiano.

Meanwhile, his position and reputation had been further threatened by the revelation that he was a member of the Masonic lodge Propaganda 2, or as it is better known, P2. It may well be asked why the revelation of names belonging to a Masonic lodge should affect anything or anyone. Yet I remember arriving in Arezzo in February 1983 to find everyone shocked by the suicide of Mario Lebole, the man who, by starting a textile factory in Arezzo after the war, had done more than anyone else to encourage the industrial development of the town. His firm, Gio-Le, had gone from strength to strength in difficult times partly because it also manufactured clothes in Rumania, which were then imported into Europe at extremely competitive prices. Lebole, though, had been greatly affected by the revelation that he was a member of P2 and that the founder, Licio Gelli, was also on his board. Banks would not give him credit and other companies were reluctant to trade with him. After achieving so much, he now collapsed under the strain, and shot himself in his office.

The real significance of P2 was the fact that its members included thirty-eight deputies and senators, two serving cabinet ministers, fifty generals, admirals and secret service chiefs – not to mention prominent journalists, industrialists and bankers, including both Sindona and Calvi. It has been described as an alternative establishment, while the likelihood of it mounting a coup was only discounted because, as Gelli himself is reputed to have said, it controlled Italy anyway and therefore had no reason to.

It must also be remembered that the Masonic movement has always been more significant politically in Catholic countries, where it has often been an active, secret, revolutionary society. It was in fact banned by Pope Clement XII in 1738, only a few years after its foundation, because he feared it as an alternative religion with competing authority.

As a result of these revelations, the Christian Democrat government resigned and its place was taken for the first time since the war by a premier, Spadolini, who was not from the Christian Democrats but from the tiny Republican party.

Licio Gelli, the Venerable Master, or *il venerabile* as Italian newspapers love to describe him, had fought for Mussolini in Spain and Albania and had saved his skin by helping Communists in 1944 (see p. 9). Since then, his real achievement had been the wide range of contacts he managed to set up all over Italy and South America, where he had been a close personal friend of President Peron's.

Three afternoons a week, he would appear in hired rooms at Rome's Excelsior hotel and induct new, important members into his lodge, wearing a blue apron lined with red. Politically, most of his recruits had Right-wing tendencies. In fact, the only parties not represented were the Communists and Radicals.

Typical of how everything seemed to inter-relate was the way the list of 962 names was discovered, through the investigation by two magistrates from Milan into the events leading to Sindona's bankruptcy. Because one of the accused admitted going to Arezzo to see Licio Gelli, two Guardie di Finanza searched Gelli's villa in Arezzo. Finding nothing, they went to Gelli's office in Gio-Le. There, in a wall safe and in a brown suitcase beside it, they found not only the names of the members of the P2, but also dossiers which showed that Gelli had informers everywhere.

Before this, Sindona had been brought to trial in Manhattan for perjury and misappropriation of funds, connected with the bankruptcy of his American bank, the Franklin National. He was also sentenced to thirty months for pretending that he had been kidnapped: on August 2nd 1979, he had suddenly disappeared from his apartment in New York and reappeared, wounded, in a telephone box on October 16th.

What was he doing during this time? A theory, which like so many others might or might not be true, was expounded to me by a prominent leader of the Communist party in Palermo, who wrote an article about it in *Rinascita*, the Communist party journal. According to him, Sindona was in Sicily for 55 days without anyone interfering, although he was a wanted man. The reason he was not arrested was because he had been sent by the Americans to arrange the settlement of terms with the Mafia over the proposed Cruise missile base at Comiso. In his pocket, it was alleged, he had a letter from an American admiral, vouching for him.

As so often happens in Italy, what may be fantasy does have a certain logic. After all, to set up a missile base on the fringe of Mafia country would seem foolhardy unless some kind of agreement were made. Whatever the security arrangements, it might be difficult to prevent obstruction or sabotage. It would not be hard to find some kind of compromise with the Mafia, involving, perhaps, the allotment of building contracts. Sindona was an ideal intermediary, a native of Sicily, who during the war had probably also mediated between Mafia and Americans. At the same time, with a prison sentence in the offing he had a lot to gain from the Americans if he was successful.

Another version asserts that Sindona was trying to organize support through influence, bribery and cajolery prior to his possible trial in Italy. He was particularly worried by the allegation that he was responsible for the murder of Giorgio Ambrosoli who, appointed by the Central Bank in Rome to look into Sindona's Italian interests, had made some alarming discoveries.

Ambrosoli was a noble figure who was well aware of the risks he was running. "Whatever happens, I'll certainly pay a high price for taking on this job," he wrote to his wife. "I've worked only in the country's interests, obviously making enemies for myself." On July 11th 1979, he was dropped by friends at his home late at night, when a group of men stepped out of the shadows, asked him who he was, and when he told them, shot him.

Mystery also shrouds the death of Calvi. Forced by the Bank of Italy to reveal to his fellow directors that the Ambrosiano's lending to unspecified entities amounted to the huge sum of $1,400 million, he fled to London in June 1982, just four days before his second trial was due to take place in Milan. On June 18th at 7.30 a.m. a horrified city clerk walking to work noticed his body hanging from scaffolding under Blackfriars Bridge. The body was suspended by a three-foot length of nylon rope. In his trousers were bricks and stones weighing over ten pounds.

The first inquest, in London five weeks later, gave a verdict of suicide. This, however, produced an immediate uproar, particularly from Italy. What real evidence was there against the possibility of murder? Why had an open verdict not been given? This surely indicated a cover-up. Were there not many people and organizations with an interest in Calvi's elimination? It was even said that he had advanced fifty million dollars to Solidarity in Poland on behalf of the Vatican. A revelation of this sort could start a Third World War! And what of all those political figures whose parties were supposed to have received subsidies earlier on? And other financiers? And P2 members? Strong protests also came from his wife and family. It was inconceivable, psychologically, that Calvi would commit suicide when he knew that this meant his life policy would probably not be paid.

As a result, a new inquest was ordered. On March 29th 1983, the first verdict was quashed, and later in the year an open verdict was pronounced. On the face of it, though, suicide seems just as probable as murder. In 1983, three Italian forensic experts came to the conclusion on the basis of the post mortem that Calvi had probably taken his own life. It might seem absurd for Calvi to walk miles to hang himself uncomfortably under a bridge, obtaining nylon rope and bricks from somewhere in the middle of the night, when there were enough drugs and sleeping pills in his room in Chelsea to finish his life more peacefully. However, suicides are not particularly noted for logic. As strange, for that matter, was the theory of a boat taking the victim down river and professional criminals hanging a thirteen-stone man on intricate scaffolding, without leaving a mark of violence or a sign of drugging.

Why Blackfriars? It was supposed to have significance in Masonic lore – a sign, some said, that the P2 was behind Calvi's murder. Given, however, that Calvi himself belonged to the P2, the choice of place might as well have been made symbolically by him as a last sign of loyalty, or for that matter of defiance.

Certain it is that Calvi was intensely depressed just before his death and seemed to be afraid – although of what he didn't say. His thirty-five years' work in Ambrosiano bank had come to a dramatic end with dismissal by his own board. There were sixteen charges against him if he returned to Italy, and the virtual certainty of years of imprisonment. The day before his death, his secretary jumped out of the window of her office, leaving behind a vitriolic note attacking her boss. If Calvi was afraid of being killed by unknown people, this also could have pushed him to suicide.

With most of these questions, though, we are in the realm of the *Marie Celeste* or of speculation on the identity of Jack the Ripper.

Meanwhile, the P2 issue lingers on. A Christian Democrat deputy,

Tina Anselmi, published an official report in May 1984 which vouched for the validity of the papers found in Arezzo and for most of the names of P2 members listed. As a result, Longo, a Social Democrat finance minister, who was often seen in magazine photographs twirling in folk-dances at festas, was forced to resign.

Meanwhile, Gelli, who had fled abroad, presented himself in September 1982 at a bank in Geneva with a false name, dyed hair, a newly-brown moustache and spectacles, an Argentinian passport, and a voucher for $120 million from a numbered account. Circumstances seemed suspicious, so he was asked to return in the afternoon and police met him when he reappeared. As a result, he was held at the maximum security prison of Champ Dillon, which has a ratio of one guard to two prisoners. Meanwhile, the Italians tried to have him extradited for political espionage, fraud, extortion, and criminal conspiracy. The case was due to be heard on August 19th 1983.

However, as the nature of this saga might lead one to expect, Gelli escaped spectacularly on August 10th. The authorities had expected an attempt to get Gelli out with helicopters and the seizing of warders as hostages and what the prison governor described as "all the usual stunts surrounding these Italian-style operations".

In fact, all that happened was that Gelli bribed a warder with the equivalent of four months' salary, escaped through a hole in the fence, concealed himself in the warder's Renault van, and was then driven over the French frontier next morning. A helicopter then brought him to Monaco, since when he has not been seen again – although the German magazine *Quick* published a picture of someone they presumed to be him, with a straw gardening hat on his head, in the improbable disguise of a monk at the monastery of St Honorat!

Since then, Gelli has written several letters to the Italian people. The last one was rather touching. In it Gelli declared himself tired and old. As he was sixty-five he wanted to come back to Italy. There was a law stating that people over pensionable age could not be imprisoned but only held under surveillance at home, unless they had committed monstrous crimes none of which he had been accused of. So he wanted to take advantage of this and return to his beloved Tuscany.

Whether he succeeds or not, the last act seems to have been played of this extraordinary drama which in a few years has included a hanging in London, a prison escape in Switzerland, pretended kidnapping in New York, deception in the Vatican and the disappearance all over the world of almost one and a half billion dollars. Financially, Calvi's old bank has been reconstituted under the name New Ambrosian Bank, and the

Vatican have agreed to contribute some 250 million dollars to the losses; while, politically, hundreds of eminent people have had to resign.

One interesting conclusion is the way all the main actors have failed. As Barzini wrote more than twenty years ago, "Something always prevents an Italian from achieving a lasting, world-wide, stupendous swindle. He is usually the victim of his own machinations." As with the Mafia and the Camorra, a mistake foreigners make too easily is believing that spectacular criminal feats really are representative of Italy and that most Italians are involved with them, in one way or another. This indeed is one of the depressing things about the image of the South. There is so much that is beautiful, that is civilized, that is untouched by crime, and yet to Northern Italians or foreigners there seems to be very little except men with dark glasses and blue shirts, with sinister black hats and a bulging pocket.

Sadly, it does need to be said that Italians are not all thieves or fraudulent just because of an elderly, reserved Milanese banker who had fought in Russia in the Italian cavalry during the war, nor on account of a Sicilian grain dealer, nor because a miller's son from Tuscany managed to compile an address-book of some of the most influential people in Italy.

Although an intelligent civil servant I know said that in his opinion scandals only come to light when it is in the interests of one group of parties to attack their rivals, it is a sign of increased efficiency and integrity that the government, the Bank of Italy and the various police forces have managed to probe and reveal these aspects of "behindology".

VII
EVERYDAY CHALLENGES

Housing – Schools – Universities –
Law and Order – Medicine

HOUSING

Mortgages at cheap rates and for a reasonable time are difficult to obtain in Italy as there is no equivalent of building societies. Loans compete with government bonds (BOTT and CCT) which pay interest just above inflation and are not taxed. The situation was neatly summed up by a cartoon in *La Repubblica* in June 1983. It shows the Minister of the Treasury, Goria, and the 82-year-old President of the Building Association, Francesco Perri, as naked prostitutes in adjacent bowers. Goria is grinning as he gets smothered in bank notes for BOTT and CCT. Perri with a miniature house in his hands gets nothing.

Thus, if in Italy you want to buy a house, you can borrow perhaps a third of the price but at a rate of 12–13 per cent, repayable over five years. If you are buying a new house, you might also delay payment to the builder of another 20 per cent on the same terms.

People do band together in condominiums, a kind of co-operative in which no one makes a profit and therefore everything is cheaper. Even here, though, a considerable proportion of cash in hand is needed: a lady in Bologna told us that she had just bought a flat with three rooms and a loggia in a condominium at a cost of 45 million lire (about $20,000). Of this, she had to put down 25 million (about $11,000) and had to pay back the rest at an interest of 21 per cent over twenty years. As a result of such stiff terms, there were over 400 empty flats in Bologna for sale.

Leases do not exist either, because, I was told, owning your own house for a short time is incompatible with the Italian idea of *domus* which evokes solidity and permanence. If you have a house, you don't normally sell it to buy a better one as you get more prosperous with age. You keep it for your children, who were brought up in it, and add to it if you can when you need more room: in Bologna I saw a high-ceilinged room in an old medieval palazzo which had been extended tastefully with metal scaffolding, painted red, to add another tier and form a self-contained flat.

Rented accommodation is even more difficult. Ten years ago there was little problem renting a flat in Rome or in any major city. In 1978, though, the government stepped in. A law called the *equo canone* was introduced which divided tenants into two categories: those with an income above 8 million lire (about $3,500) a year, who paid an annual increase of rent equivalent to 75 per cent of the rate of inflation, and those below who paid only 25 per cent.* House owners thus found the rent they were receiving actually going down every year. As a result, in the census of 1981 no fewer than 25 per cent of living units were empty, with no fewer than 104,000 in Rome. One of the motives for new investment in housing had gone, with disastrous effects on employment.

One million seven hundred thousand families are involved as tenants under the *equo canone*, and the government now faces the real dilemma of what to do with a measure which harms almost everyone. The law was due to expire in 1982; but how could a large number of people suddenly be asked to pay rents which would be at least doubled with inflation – or else be evicted? In any case, the many illegal rents paid outside *equo canone* had set a costly norm which most tenants would find impossible to pay.

Equo canone was passed during the period of co-operation between the government and the Communists when so many measures which seemed morally right, but were not thought out in their wider context, were passed. Any attempt to make tenants pay more has been hotly opposed by the PCI, who defend the rights of the workers, of whom only a third, according to Berlinguer, occupy their own houses.

Because the measure now implies a clear class conflict of owners versus tenants, its termination has been postponed several times. There was talk of ending it in August 1983. However, this would have had to be announced in June, the month of the election – which few parties were prepared to risk. Since then there has been talk of increasing rent rises but maintaining the system in principle. Initially, the *equo canone* was restricted to towns with more than 3,000 inhabitants and there has been another proposal to limit this to towns with over 300,000, which would confine it to fourteen cities and only 20 per cent of the

---

* The figures were decided in 1978 when incomes were much lower and had not been increased artificially by inflation.

population. Another more forcible measure proposed by the
Communists is to fine those who keep flats empty.

It is unlikely that the market for houses will ever again be allowed
to find its own level, or for that matter that a proper system of
mortgages can be set up – given the number of opposing vested interests
involved.

An obvious answer would be to build more *case popolari* (the Italian
version of council houses). In 1981, the equivalent of about 350 million
dollars was invested, and it seems to have solved the problem in some of
the smaller towns. Thus, in Perugia there is no great problem because
the Commune is converting old convents into flats. Also, many people
who had flats in the centre have built themselves new houses in the
suburbs, leaving more space in the centre. Perugia is also exceptional in
that *case popolari* can be bought and sold. In many places, they also have
the excellent principle that *case popolari* should never form a separate
ghetto. In Viterbo, where 200 were built in 1983, the ratio was fixed at a
maximum of 70 per cent State housing on any estate.

In Bologna, *case popolari* have been used as a way of restoring the
historic centre. Those living in old flats were temporarily evacuated to
new communal housing in the suburbs. Meanwhile, under the
supervision of the well-known architect Pier Luigi Cervellati, their
original houses were done up and new modern conveniences were
combined with a high standard of historical restoration, thus achieving
two objects at once.

Another way out is the so-called "abusive" house. If you go to
Sardinia, or any part of the South, many towns seem to have a small
centre with town hall, church and piazza, while the rest consists of half-
built houses, most of them mere structures with a roof on, rather like a
skeleton with a hat and only bones below. Only occasionally is anyone
actually working on these houses, and along a coast like that of the Gulf
of Taranto, half-completed buildings straggle the shore like a
procession of fleshless prehistoric monsters. There is something desolate
and almost sinister about them.

These are the "illegal" buildings, and over seven million have been
built since the war. Many of them are put up by emigrants who return
to the South in the summer and invest their earnings in a home with the
help of families and friends. They will build the structure first and get
the roof on because, once that has been done, the building cannot be
bulldozed. Then they will equip it, floor by floor, according to their
resources. If they have a young son they may very well leave the top
floor until he grows up and gets married. The result is a strange house,

which looks like a box-kite for years, with one or two floors completed.

Recently, the government has been more vigilant in attempting to stop these illegal buildings. In Rome they actually have helicopters which scan the city. In August 1983, they swooped over a building site, scaring the owner who was working there, only to find that he did have permission. However, they did discover two "abusive" houses on the same day. Now, after a lot of trouble (see p. 67), Craxi's government has passed a law giving an amnesty on all these buildings so long as a fine is paid. This has helped government finance and, presumably, in future those building abusive houses will pay a fine on completion, and everyone will be satisfied.

The building urge, blocked by *equo canone*, has also expressed itself in the increased construction of second homes, and Italy is supposed to have more of these than any country in Europe. Some are ancient family houses deserted by emigrants to the city who, once they were earning well, returned to modernize their house and turn it into a summer resort. However, the enthusiasm for second homes has tended to deaden some small towns. In Assisi, I was told that many of the old houses are being bought by foreigners or rich Italians who occupy them only for a few weeks a year, with the result that the town is losing its identity and being turned simply into a tourist resort.

Some of these second homes are magnificent, although owned by people with relatively modest jobs. In Umbria, I went to a church and presbytery which had been bought for the equivalent of $5,000 by a university professor. Central heating had been installed, and bedrooms with bathrooms en suite, while a library-workroom had a wonderful view over the Umbrian countryside. Another, near Lake Bolsena, had a master-bed as big as a billiard table with an adjoining bath which you could almost swim in. At a restaurant we were invited to eat chestnuts and drink wine by a couple in the abandoned village they had restored in the Apennine forest, between Florence and Bologna. Most beautiful of all was a house in Positano with a terrace that served as a sitting room, overlooking the sea, with bougainvillea forming the walls. This was inherited, but it is often difficult to know where Italians get their money from. Perhaps it comes from accumulation during the boom, or through barter, *arrangiarsi*, or perhaps, with a peasant background, they save frugally for something they really want.

Certainly, there is a housing crisis in Italy, particularly among the poorer citizens in big cities. Sometimes one wonders how much of it is due to government interference. Italians have something of the triffid in them. If you try and confine them, their tentacles find unexpected

outlets and develop according to their true nature rather than
predetermined design.

Compulsory schooling in Italy started in the 1950s, later than in most
European countries. In 1951, five million people were illiterate. Even
those who were at school were often taken away again to help their
parents.

There is a moving scene in the Taviani brothers' film *Padre Padrone*, set
in the 1950s, when a shepherd comes to his son's school and tells the
teacher and the whole class that he can no longer look after his sheep
alone. His son stands there wetting his pants and leaving a little pool on
the floor, which is noticed by the boys when he departs with his father
to roars of laughter. The father hears, comes back, bangs his stick on the
table, and tells the class not to laugh because they too may soon be called
away to work.

In few other ways has Italy advanced more since the war than
progressing from this kind of situation to a relatively modern
educational system under which everyone goes to school. As always,
the quality of education depends on the social milieu in which it takes
place. You can go to a State school like Poggio Imperiale in a ducal
house near Florence which takes boys and girls from the age of five or
six, right up to the *maturità* exam at nineteen. Or you can go to the
extreme of an elementary school in Palermo, in the crumbling old city,
where some of the children have the faces of old people. "What good
does it do?" asked the caring yet sorrowful teacher, "when they live
with twelve brothers and sisters, and the mother is a prostitute, and the
father is a thief, and the children are trained to be pickpockets because
there is not enough money in the house? When I see reports of crimes in
the newspapers," she said sadly, "I look to see if any of my ex-pupils are
involved!"

As an Italian child, you may start at the *asilo nido* when you are only a
few months old. These are run either by the Commune or by private
bodies. Some of them are very good, offering nursery school facilities
from eight in the morning till six or six-thirty at night and a dormitory
with small beds for the siesta. When run by the Commune, they can be
expensive to support, because staff are numerous and well paid. In
Rome, costs work out at 830,000 lire ($350) per child per month,
whereas private *asili* can cost as little as 100,000 lire ($40), plus meals.
Children of mothers who have jobs are given preference and *asili* are in

short supply: in 1983, 26 per cent of the demand was unsatisfied in Rome and 34 per cent in Milan.

A child follows the *asilo* with kindergarten, called *la scuola di maternità*, until State education begins in the elementary school from the age of six till ten or eleven. Here, school is from 8.00 a.m. till 1.00 p.m. with no classes on Saturdays. These are then the normal hours for all schooling right through the system.

This timetable has three effects. First, it means that children are home every afternoon and the whole weekend. Second, it allows mothers to become teachers because they can be back in time to provide lunch. Third, it differentiates the rich from the poor. For the rich will arrange extra classes for their children in the afternoon in piano, English and other subjects, while the poor who cannot afford this will gradually fall behind.

Schools have always been mixed. I remember a friend describing the atmosphere at school in the 1950s when girls sat on one side of the classroom and boys on the other. "The teachers tried to keep us apart," he said, "because that was the morality of the time. You have no idea of the tension, the way we would peep at each other in class below our hands, laugh nervously when someone on the other side made a mistake, try to communicate when no one was looking." Things are different now. Uniforms have gone out, which means that everyone tries to be as well-groomed as possible from an early age.

Boarding schools are rare. They seem barbarous, like corporal punishment, to most Italians. Why should a poor little homesick kid be sent off to be looked after by others who do not belong to the family? Art, music, drama and games are out too. In fact, it is amazing that Italians are so proficient at football when they learn only in the streets or on a field which, usually, is near the church – it used to be the priest who looked after all social activities in the village or borough. However, football is now such a remunerative sport that impresarios look out for talent and will find ways of training any lad of thirteen who shows promise. Junior teams also compete nationally – I remember two of them playing each other for a whole hour in the main stadium before the Rome-Milan match in 1984.

At the age of ten or eleven, the child goes on to the *scuola media* until he is fourteen when, according to law, his compulsory period of education is over. However, most now continue at the *scuola superiore* until they are nineteen. Here they have a choice of different schools, or *licei*: *linguistico*, *artistico*, *classico*, *scientifico*, or professional courses in schools of tourism, accountancy, technical/commercial subjects, or hotel management.

Thus, everyone has a main specialization, but a broad range of different subjects is taught as well. If you go to a *liceo artistico* you spend twenty-four hours a week copying masterpieces and the anatomy of classical figures and, later, creating your own paintings and sculpture. However, you also have seventeen hours of mathematics, geography and chemistry, as well as some history of art.

The most prestigious of these alternatives is still the *liceo classico*. Thus, in Naples, the Umberto, which is *classico*, is sought after, while the Mario Pagano, which teaches general professional skills such as accounting, company law etc., is for students from a less educated background. Neapolitans go to the Pagano to get minor jobs in banks and offices. Those who go to the Umberto become lawyers, doctors and better paid professionals, or businessmen. Ever since the days of Gentile, Mussolini's education minister, the *classico* has produced an elite, and most of those now at the top have been to one. Some educationists criticize this system and also complain that it has been unchanged since 1929. "You have no idea of all the people who go to school and waste five years studying Greek and Latin, and another five studying philosophy, just because they don't know what to do," says a character in a modern novel by Andrea de Carlo. Nevertheless, there is widespread respect for the educated – as instanced by all the titles with which people are addressed: *dottore*, *professore* etc. I remember in a restaurant, in Bergamo, having a conversation with a lorry driver. When he asked me what I did, I told him I was an English teacher. "Oh! That means you are a *dottore!*" he looked embarrassed. "You shouldn't really be speaking to me!"

Languages tend to be taught as badly as they are everywhere, except in Scandinavia, Holland and Germany. Until 1971 you could teach languages with a degree in law. There is also the complaint that because studies are too classically orientated, students are not sufficiently prepared for the modern world, particularly where the sciences are concerned. "My son can learn more from television than being taught Latin and Greek at school by those old biddies!" exploded a trade union leader I met in Potenza.

During the whole course there are assessments every year by the teacher, on a scale from 1 to 10. If you get below 6, you do the year again. At the end, there is the final exam, the *maturità*. The only written subjects are a six-hour essay in Italian and one paper on your specialization, whether Latin at the *classico*, or mathematics at the *scientifico*. In theory, you can also be tested orally on any two of the other subjects you have studied, which should ensure the preparation of a wide variety of subjects. In practice, you choose one of the subjects yourself, and the school chooses the other on the night before the exam. However, many students are told which paper they are going to do months before, so in practice the *maturità* can be as narrow as A-levels. Moreover, cheating is not penalized and you can actually buy cribbing belts, with little compartments like a cowboy's ammunition belt. Perhaps this is why, throughout the whole educational system, including universities, exams are often oral. One teacher at Rome university felt these were better, anyway: "For one thing," he said, "you can cover more ground. Speaking is obviously so much faster than writing and if the student is woolly you can question more searchingly."

Given that personal communication is so prized in Italy, it is not surprising that there is also a saint of exams to pray to: San Giuseppe da Copertino. He lived in Assisi in the seventeenth century, and was capable of jumping into the air as high as thirty metres. Despite these miraculous powers, his weak spot was passing theology exams and he only succeeded with the intercession of the Virgin.

Schools today have also been affected by the events which followed the tumults of 1968–9. There was a demand for an end to competitive attitudes and a reduction in the power of authority. One result was to make the exam system absurdly easy, and about 96 per cent now pass the *maturità*. Another was to make teachers more diffident in front of their students. As a professor in Turin explained to me, it has made them feel they have little authority and therefore they also take less responsibility. Why should they work hard for children who don't respect them, who may easily go on strike, or take up school time in political demonstrations? It has also brought the divisions of party politics into school. The effects of this are difficult to determine, but one still hears complaints that students are favoured if they or their parents belong to the same political party as the teacher.

History teaching is probably the area where biased interpretations show themselves most clearly, so I decided to look at two history books on the modern period which are most used in secondary schools: one by Gabriele De Rosa, a well-known Catholic writer, and one by Antonio Desideri, who is more to the Left.

As might be expected, De Rosa's book is plusher, with colour illustrations and more expensive paper. It is shorter, with only 523 pages compared to Desideri's massive 1300. De Rosa's book is apparently the work of one man and seemed competent and fair, particularly in its account of the contemporary malaise, the role of the Church and the exposition of Socialist ideas. Desideri's format is quite different and, as might perhaps have been expected from a writer of the Left in Italy, is more challenging and "intellectual". It consists of a range of extracts from no fewer than 610 books, essays and speeches by authors and politicians. These cover an enormous range of opinion from Pope John XXIII to Imre Nagy – the Hungarian prime minister executed by the Russians in 1956 – from Tolstoy to Marx, from Bakunin to Mussolini.

Both books must be stimulating to history students. Desideri puts the Left-wing view: the last extract is an analysis of the way May 1968 could never have been as successful without the participation of the workers; but he also illustrates other attitudes through the authors he chooses. Neither book seems in any way dishonest; neither is propaganda.

Desideri represents the approach of many schools in the State sector, De Rosa those in the private, which is mainly Catholic. A survey published in July 1984 shows that only 8 per cent of children go to private schools and that among the parents who send them, 53.7 per cent think that the "social atmosphere" is preferable, and 82.1 per cent that there is more guarantee of order and discipline. Over 70 per cent also think that the general organization is more efficient. However, among those who have sent children to both kinds of school, opinions are much more equally divided and more (55.4 per cent) think that the teachers are better qualified in the public sector. Given that those who can afford it can always get extra classes for their kids in the afternoon – as already mentioned – there seems little reason for people to use the private sector, which may cost the equivalent of $1500 a year. Many of those attending obviously do so because it is a family tradition, or for religious reasons.

Teachers in the secondary school sector are divided sharply between the secure and insecure. The secure have a permanent post, a *cattedra* as it is called, from which they cannot be dismissed, where the basic salary in 1983 was a million lire a month ($450), and where there is a good pension scheme. Appropriately, the insecure are called *precarie*. For years they may take odd jobs here and there, both in the public and private sector, trying to accumulate enough points – which include some for having children – to become eligible for a special exam, which is called *abilitazione* and occurs irregularly every few years. Many of the *precarie* emigrate to parts of Italy where it is easier to get a permanent job. Once they have got their *cattedra*, they will do their best to transfer to a post near home.

Results in the *abilitazione* will probably depend greatly on *raccomandazione,* following the example of the Virgin's intercession on behalf of San Giuseppe da Copertino! Here is part of a description of an *abilitazione* exam for English teachers in Palermo in 1983:

> The system of favours is particularly widespread here in Sicily. Theoretically, an examiner who lets a candidate pass because he or she is strongly recommended may expect a similar favour in return in some future moment of need.... More than 600 candidates turned up at 8.30 and by 10.30, crammed into a dozen rooms, sometimes two to a desk, they were off. The exam lasted eight hours altogether, with a continual stream of candidates going to the toilet where they cribbed from pre-prepared model answers. But just to be on the safe side, a large proportion of candidates smuggled in English-Italian dictionaries. As the exam progressed, the noise level rose and one examinee said afterwards that there were times when the noise was so intense that she could hardly hear herself think.*

As yet there is little teacher training, although those wanting to teach in elementary schools go to a special college called *magistrale* as an alternative to the *liceo* when they are sixteen. However, a law of May 12th 1982 provides for a new *concorso* which will take place regularly every two years. Those who succeed will do a year of teacher training. But even where this has already got going there is very little concentration on actual teaching skills – more on a thorough knowledge of one's specialized subject. In the regions an organization called IRSAE is being set up. Presided over by a university professor, this aims to encourage teachers to keep up to date and to research into new materials. In English teaching much is done by independent voluntary bodies like LEND and by the British Council, which organizes a massive conference in Bologna in April, attended by over two thousand teachers.

"English is extremely fashionable!" said a friend of ours ironically when we saw "Fuck!" boldly inscribed on a wall in Trento. The number of private schools for adults is legion: in Turin there are over fifty; in Milan about seventy-five, and in Florence over twenty. Standards vary enormously, depending on whether the owner is interested purely in business or has a genuine desire to teach his students professionally.

In order to remedy this situation, the former British Council officer in Milan, Harley Brooks, recently started a new school association called AISLI, which organizes seminars and inspections, but also insists

* Janet Olearsky, *EFL Gazette.*

on all staff being legally employed. This has resulted in a typical Italian paradox, for legal employment includes paying taxes: 42 per cent of the teacher's salary by the employers and 8 per cent by the teacher. The result is that AISLI schools have priced themselves right at the top of the market, as most other schools remain illegal and can therefore charge much less. British teachers do not stay in a school for long, except in cities like Venice, Rome or Florence, and would be much better off making National Health payments in Britain. Legality, therefore, simply means penalizing poorer Italians, and driving them to worse schools. What do you do in a system that doesn't work? Perhaps you hope it soon will, and see the best schools going bankrupt in the meantime, or when in Rome....

Schooling reflects a country perhaps more faithfully than anything except the family structure, because it involves or has involved everyone: parents and children, teachers and government. As may be expected anywhere, quality varies. The system is highly centralized but because of this it presupposes exceptions. It is humane, and on the whole everyone from prince to waiter mixes in the same classes – although again there are exceptions because of the elitism of some private schools and of the *licei classici*. It generates enthusiasm, yet often lacks professionalism, particularly in teacher training. The structure is disordered yet its outline clearly defined. It has spontaneity generated by the student movements of the 1970s, yet because of this it is ineffective in not demanding high enough standards. It urgently needs reforms, yet this is difficult because of the criss-cross of parties, the weakness of the bureaucracy and the obstruction of personal favouritism.

Perhaps one could say the same about educational systems in many countries, but they are not populated by Italians.

UNIVERSITIES

Cosenza is a town of 140,000 people in Calabria. It lies in a valley between a ridge fronting the sea and the high table-land of the Sila, where black squirrels abound and hill lakes are misty in the fresh mornings.

In Cosenza, Alaric the Goth died and was buried with much of the plunder from the first sack of Rome in 410. A dam was constructed in the river Busento and the water was then allowed to flow over Alaric's body and his treasure. Those who built the dam were put to death, and the fabulous wealth of Ancient Rome must still lie buried somewhere in the river mud.

We had come to Cosenza to visit the university, which is one of the few in Italy with a restricted student entry and built as a campus. It was opened in 1972.

Professor Aurelio Sesso, whom we were going to meet, had told us that he was not free before 11.00 as he was teaching. In fact he was free at 10.30 when we arrived, because a strike had been declared, and a student picket prevented anyone from going in or out.

The university is built on a hill with a design of rough concrete similar to that of the National Theatre in London. The main building is a labyrinth of open stone balustrades from which corridors lead into offices and classrooms. Student accommodation climbs further up the hill in tiers of flats and maisonettes. The grey walls were defaced by the black, spray-paint scrawlings beloved in Italy by students and political extremists.

We went to the main entrance and talked with the student pickets. One problem was that of finance, they said. The university had spent more than its budget. This meant that only 900 of the 1300 students who had applied for entry this year would be admitted. Also, the university was unique in insisting that those who had failed their exams (who are called *fuori corso* in Italian) could only stay on for one year. This was unfair as some students only really developed after many years of study. A further problem was that not all the students could stay in the lodgings provided. Many had to live in Cosenza where a room with three others cost 180,000 lire ($80) each, a month. Also, the university was a "parking place", the strikers said, because it was small: teachers only stayed a year or two before going on to work somewhere else.

What were their politics? They were "Antagonists", which meant they were against all existing parties. But they were also Marxists.

We went up the hill to the accommodation. Rooms were pleasant, with bathroom attached, some with wonderful views over the Calabrian countryside. They were supposed to be for only two beds, but in most rooms there were three. The extra one, we were told, was for the *fuori corso*, who shouldn't officially be there; but in this way no one could do anything about it. We talked about the university. The trouble was that courses led nowhere. There were so few jobs. It made for restlessness and a sense of futility.

Did they have a university magazine, or a theatre club? No, that wasn't usual at Italian universities. People were too individualistic to get together like that – especially in Calabria where most people came from separate little communes. They didn't even have a student common room. Italian universities were conceived as places where you simply went to lectures. Often you do most of your work at home.

There was a small quota of students from abroad who paid only 770,000 lire ($300) a year for food and accommodation and tuition. Sixteen students had come from China, paid for by their government. Other Italian universities admitted any foreigners who wanted to enrol, so long as they had passed their final exam at secondary school – this represented the application of the principles of 1968. Many universities were full of Greeks and Americans who couldn't get into their own universities. However, at Cosenza this was restricted.

In fact, despite their strike, students at Cosenza are lucky. The ratio of teachers to students is 1 to 10 and, because entry is limited, classes are manageable. Whereas most universities give only free tuition, many of the students at Cosenza get free meals, accommodation and also free transport down to the town and back. At Bari, and some other universities, poorer students do get grants of from 250,000 to 500,000 lire ($100–200) a year for living expenses. However, there is so much form-filling and delay, and descriptions of the parents' income, that it is hardly worth it.

In Italy, there are forty-seven universities and a total student population of over a million compared with 250,000 in Britain. This is partly because, since the early '70s, anyone with the *maturità* can enrol for a course. One effect of the boom of the early '60s was that those who had made money so suddenly wanted their sons and daughters to have the same advantages as everyone else, whatever their educational background. This has meant not only crowded lectures but also many students unequipped for learning. Professor Fulvio Papi, head of the department of philosophy in the well respected University of Pavia, expressed his attitude to the whole educational revolution when he said: "Today, people come out of the *liceo* without the formation which in the last three hundred years called itself culture. The young people of my generation were in a hurry to become adults, to know everything, and be able to exercise their judgment. Now, instead, they don't want to leave the ghetto of their adolescence."

Many universities in Italy continue the breadth of learning which the *scuola superiore* encourages. Faculties, headed by a president, are divided into Institutes, each of which is responsible for the different subjects which a *laurea* (or degree) consists of. Thus English or French may be taught as an accompaniment of a main subject in different Institutes, as well as a principal one in the Faculty of Modern Languages. Some degrees consist of as many as twenty subjects, five being done per year over four years.

There is no control over attendance. A friend of mine in Naples has no less than five degrees, although he is a father of a family and a director of ENEL, the National Electricity Company. He has studied for them all at home as a hobby. Another friend, Bruno Menapace, from Riva, north of Garda, took an English degree at Verona without ever going there except for exams and the final degree ceremony. In the middle of the course in languages, students may spend months in France or Britain or Germany learning the spoken language which the university cannot really teach them because as many as two hundred students may attend lectures. In theory, it is possible to spend up to twenty-five years getting your degree, although in fact two thirds of the students never finish anyway.

As there are meagre living grants only to those whose parents' income is below six million lire ($2,500) a year, students have to work, or be supported by parents who are reasonably well off, even if tuition is free.

The same freedom applies to staff. Italian professors are known as "the barons" because of their prestige and influence, not only on university life. They may delegate their work, and stand for the European Parliament, or take up a post at another university as well. Forte, the Socialist Minister of Finance in Fanfani's government in 1982–3, was also a university professor on half pay.

"Efforts are being made to induce professors to devote less time to their private business affairs and more to their academic commitments," writes Andrew Bryant in his *The Italians*. "They are being urged to hold but one chair, to reside in, or at least visit, the cities of their chair, or chairs, and to teach and undertake research in their universities." However, parties find it prestigious to have candidates or ministers who are also *baroni*. Needless to say, most of these stem originally from the *licei classici*.

Originally, the teaching scale was modelled on the German *Privatdozent* system. You became an assistant by doing research for five or ten years and then, before becoming professor, passed an exam at national level on your publications and teaching ability.

This system was abolished in 1964 and nothing took its place till a law passed in 1980. This provided for the creation of 45,000 new posts, divided into three categories. The lowest is "researcher", appointed through an exam and assessment of publications. Three years' teaching experience is also a requisite but, as in most universities throughout the world, there are no tests on the actual ability to teach or lecture.

The next stage is assistant professor, which can lead to full professor.

Promotion is theoretically competitive, although seniority has always played an important role in advancement. In addition, two thousand PhD students are to be taken on every year, from 1983–5, to do a three to four-year research doctorate. This certainly produces some kind of system, although the complaint of many is that it really has little to do with students, or good teaching: students will remain a nuisance who interfere with research. However, particularly in the sciences, it should do much to increase the background knowledge which any industrial nation needs today.

As might be expected, there is variety not only in the buildings of Italian universities but also in their organization. Florence has the first European university, founded in 1973. In Milan, the Catholic university, with its graceful arched courtyard next to the church of St Ambrose which was founded in the fourth century, depends on the Church. Urbino, the home of Raphael, is almost a university in itself, with 16,000 inhabitants and 18,000 students. Founded by Duke Federico in the sixteenth century, it was given the opportunity to become part of the State system in 1978, but refused. The Bocconi in Milan was recently also private, but now has changed itself into what is virtually a business university.

Italy has the oldest university tradition in the world. Salerno was the first, founded in the ninth century (it is believed) by "four masters": a Jew, a Greek, a Saracen and a Latin. Famous as a centre of medical studies, it was closed by Napoleon in 1811, partly because it had become a source of bogus degrees. In the twelfth century, before any Oxford or Cambridge colleges were founded, Bologna university had ten thousand students. The university of Naples was founded in 1224, Rome in 1303, Turin in 1404.

Today there is a lot of controversy about what role a university should play. Should it be primarily for research or for teaching? Italian universities are certainly distinguished by the former rather than the latter. Should it teach for "culture" or for professional ends? On the whole, Italian universities emphasize culture, and the classical tradition is still strong. Should it teach an elite, or open its doors to a wide mass of the population? At present, it certainly favours the latter.

However, the over-production of graduates is recognized as a problem. In November 1984, the prefect of Rome suggested that all universities should limit enrolment in the medical faculties to 70 per cent of the present number. Whereas in most industrial countries, the ratio of doctors to citizens is about one to 600, in Italy it is one to 275. However, in *La Domenica del Corriere* Pierluigi Magnaschi argued that this request was only a sign of pressure from the medical community who are afraid of too many rivals. If an excess of graduates was the issue, what of those who get their *laurea* in the arts, when their outlet in teaching is being reduced by a falling birth-rate?

To limit places, as they have been able to do in Cosenza because it is a new university, is something no government could achieve without immense opposition. It could also be said that the Italian university system anticipates the time when, in all industrial countries, further education will probably be encouraged as an alternative to unemployment. A measure conceived at a time of prosperity may have produced disorganization, irregular attendance, unrest, but it also gives hundreds of thousands of young people a chance to educate themselves, and a sense of belonging to society. If many of them don't finish their courses, it may be because, after a long period of waiting and study, they have found themselves a job.

This, though, can never be an argument for not raising teaching standards.

LAW AND ORDER

Toni Negri was arrested in 1979, during "the years of lead" as they are called because the Red Brigades were terrorizing so many Italian cities with their bullets. Negri was a lecturer at Padua university and a specialist on Kant and Spinoza. He had also written several books expounding the principles of a Left-wing movement called "Autonomy" which, if not directly linked with the Red Brigades, was associated with them.

Negri was charged with master-minding the kidnapping and murder of Aldo Moro, but this charge was dropped after a year. He was then accused of armed insurrection against the State, which was also dropped. However, one of the Red Brigade followers, Fuoroni, named him as an accomplice in the murder of a friend and as "morally culpable" of another killing.

In the meantime, however, Pannella, the flamboyant leader of the Radical Party, invited Negri to stand as a candidate in the elections of June 1983. Pannella saw this as a protest against the law which had been introduced at the height of the Red Brigade activity whereby an accused person could be held in prison for a maximum of ten years and eight months without trial. Negri had been in prison for over four years without being sentenced, and was therefore a notable victim of this law. Even those who mistrusted him felt it was scandalous that he, along with 4,000 other political prisoners, had been imprisoned for so long when he might well be innocent.

Negri was elected. A member of Parliament has immunity so he was immediately set free. When he went to the Chamber, groups of deputies blocked his path and shouted abuse at him. It was the first time that someone had come straight from prison to take his seat.

In September, a decree was issued suspending Negri, but just before it was passed he escaped to France. In Paris, he said he didn't see the morality of returning to prison, probably to spend the rest of his life there. "I'm not a Samurai!" he said.

In 1983, Enzo Tortora, a well-known television personality, was arrested for drug-trafficking. He too became a Radical candidate for the European elections, and was elected, after a year in prison without trial.

In Poggioreale, in Naples, no fewer than 2,350 out of 2,540 detainees had not yet been sentenced in 1984, and 50 per cent of the entire prison population in Italy was alleged to be in the same situation.

Why does it take so long to bring people to trial in Italy? One reason is the shortage of magistrates. There should be 7,197 on the books but in 1984 there was a shortage of 959. New recruitment attracts an inadequate number of people of a high enough standard. Although there were four to five thousand applications for 200 posts in 1982, only 172 got through the exam.

The Supreme Council of Magistrates tried to analyse the reasons and came to the conclusion that judges were not as well paid as State lawyers and other professions, that the working conditions were bad and that there is still an element of danger, particularly in Sicily and the Naples area – although the Red Brigades have been quiescent since April 1983. Numbers are also reduced through illness and pregnancies – 37 per cent of magistrates are women – and strikes of lawyers, like those which affected three principal towns in Abruzzi in March 1983, produce further delay. Also, many magistrates are attached to ministries as advisers.

Furthermore, the use of judges in trials is extravagant: instead of a jury and one magistrate in a criminal court, there are three professional and six lay judges summing up the case together.

Although many magistrates are exceptional individuals, preparation for the profession is minimal, particularly in finance, which becomes more and more important when dealing with "modern" criminals.

In fact, the criteria for becoming a magistrate are limited to being a graduate in jurisprudence, passing the exam and being in good health.

Also, promotion is by seniority which means that many judges who are at the top of the tree are waiting lethargically for retirement.

An instance of the effects of all this was the virtual collapse of justice in Catania in Sicily in April 1984, where for fifteen months there was no President of the Court of Appeal, the Procurator had retired two months previously, and both his substitutes were leaving. Another four magistrates had asked to be transferred. The office administration, too, was understaffed, and yet 57,581 civil cases and 72,433 penal ones were pending.

Procedures are slow. If someone is arrested, the case goes first to a magistrate who interrogates. If he decides to continue, the accused goes to another magistrate who also interrogates. Then, if there is good cause, the case goes back to the first magistrate who brings the accused to court. If the accused is found guilty, there is the appeal, which sometimes results not in a decision but in the case being sent back to the first court for reconsideration. On average, this process takes 546 days for less serious offences and four years for more serious ones, but in mass trials such as those of the Mafia or Camorra this time can be doubled. In some cases, too, a judge who is convinced of the guilt of the accused will simply allow him to wait for up to two thirds of what his sentence is likely to be. As a result, an innocent man may spend up to a tenth of his life in prison, without compensation when he comes out, and without the magistrate, who has made an error, being in any way penalized. As always, everywhere, mistakes do happen: when 800 people were arrested on charges of belonging to the Camorra in 1983, it was discovered, some time later, that a hundred had been arrested by mistake because they had the same names as those who had been denounced.

Office procedures are also time-wasting. Minutes in court are taken down in longhand, and trials are based on long, written reports. When Carlo Palermo, a judge from Trento, completed his investigations into charges of corruption in the Socialist party, he sent his report down to the president of the Chamber of Deputies in a lorry because it was so bulky. Who, one wonders, had the time to read it? The investigations on Tommaso Buscetta, the first Mafia super-grass, ran to 700,000 pages. As a journalist, Domenica Bartoli, wrote in *Il Giornale*: "I have the impression that our tribunals will go on using the quill pen in the age of the computer for a long time!"

Magistrates also have the responsibility for charging malefactors. This gives them enormous power and allows the eternal *lottizzazione*, or fight between parties – not to mention private wars between individuals – to enter in. You will suddenly find that a cinema is no longer showing the film advertised because a case has been taken out against it, as happened to a film, *La Chiave*, which we wanted to see in Naples. From his refuge in South America, Ortolani, who was Gelli's right-hand man in the P2, persuaded a magistrate to ban four books which had just been published which contained inaccuracies such as that he was short and fat – which he didn't consider himself to be – or that he was born in Viterbo when he was born in Rome. The entire private television channel was suspended for several days because a magistrate was doubtful about the laws which allowed it to exist in the first place. Most extraordinary of all was the action taken by the public prosecutor of Rome, Achille Ballucci who, having dropped charges against a large number of people involved in P2, was afraid that action would be taken against him by the Left. So, to anticipate, he counter-attacked and charged the Supreme Council of Magistrates with including coffees and lunches at the office among their expenses. This became known as "the golden coffee-break scandal" and had in the end to be sorted out by President Pertini himself. Magistrates are independent and can only be disciplined by the Supreme Council, but these internecine activities only take up more of their sparse time.

Another problem is the complicated nature of Italian law, which is based on Roman and Napoleonic codes. "The trouble is that the law tries to cover every eventuality," said a lawyer friend of mine in Sicily. "As a result it becomes so complicated that it can't be applied to anything!" In hospitals "No Smoking" signs include the number of the law which justifies them and in Vigevano there is a notice, presumably legal, forbidding people to ride bicycles inside the cathedral!

Criminal law is more straightforward, based on Mussolini's code which in turn was drawn from Rocco's before the First World War. A list of crimes is drawn up with the appropriate sentences for each, none of which now include the death penalty which was abolished in 1946, or women's adultery, which was taken out in the '70s, or crimes against honour which were removed in 1982.

The civil law, though, is a maze and alternative ways are used to disentangle it. About 80 per cent of cases end up with a Conciliating Judge (*giudice conciliatore*) whose role is to bring parties together rather than to deliver judgment. In cases between big firms, both sides can agree on an Arbitrator whose decision actually becomes legal.

In August 1984, the maximum term of preventive detention was reduced from ten years and eight months to six years, which produced an uproar. Many welcomed it as a return to normality after the "years of lead". Others felt it would mean the release of dangerous criminals still awaiting trial. In fact, the new measure may have beneficial effects on the whole system, especially as Italians are often galvanized only by emergencies. Reforms have been talked about for years. The stumbling block is lack of additional money which could allow the recruitment of more, better paid magistrates and the proper staffing and equipping of courts of law. Italians, as is well known, are past masters of bargaining, and additional pay for legal staff could doubtless be used by the government to obtain agreement on a better distribution of magistrates and simpler procedures.

What, though, of the people who have to carry out the law? Perhaps the best known Italian figure abroad is the Carabiniere because of his picturesque three-cornered hat, black uniform and white shoulder belt. In Italy, he, more than the police, seems to be the butt of jokes about stupidity:

QUESTION: "Why is Carabinieri marked on the door of their cars?"
ANSWER: "So that they know where to get in!"

QUESTION: "Why do the Carabinieri go about in pairs?"
ANSWER: "Because one can read and the other can write!"

CARAB: "What have you got in the boot of your car?"
DRIVER: "Half a pig."
CARAB: "Dead or alive?"

This derogatory humour may be part of the old antagonism between North and South as, like the bureaucracy, 80 per cent of Carabinieri are from the South. Nevertheless, they originated from Piedmont where they were founded in 1814 on the 13th of July, as if in anticipation of revolutionary Bastille celebrations! In 1820 they became the Royal Guards, and now form the presidential escort in Rome. Without them, the unification of Italy would have been difficult as they were largely responsible for suppressing the bandits and guerrillas in the South after enthusiasm for Garibaldi and the Savoys had waned. They have always been a part of the army and in war-time their force of 82,000 can be swollen to a quarter of a million men. In the first war, they acted as military police to stop mass flight after the defeat of Caporetto, and in the second they fought in Africa and Russia.

A sergeant major in Seregno told me that recruits have nine months' training. This may be as an electrician, or for drug control, or as a pilot, for the Carabinieri also have helicopters, motor-boats, aeroplanes and mechanized units. When a recruit applies, an investigation is made to ensure that no direct ancestor in the previous two generations has been in prison. And party politics? "After three years," said the sergeant major, "their loyalty is to the Carabinieri, neither to black nor to red!"

In a land of plurality it is perhaps not surprising that there are three other forces. One of them is the police who are under the Ministry of the Interior, while the Carabinieri are responsible to the Ministry of Defence. They operate only in large towns, while the Carabinieri are everywhere. They keep order in the streets, and there are also railway and postal police. Their ratio is 1:500 inhabitants.

Then there is the Guardia di Finanza which also originated in the Piedmontese army and was responsible for defending frontiers. They too have fought through all the wars since 1774, when they were founded. Their function is to stop contraband and for this reason they are also equipped with speed-boats and helicopters. When I talked to a general in Florence he told me that their job was also to investigate corruption and fraud. Under the new La Torre law (see p. 205), they are also entitled to examine bank accounts suspected of being mafiosi. Their training consists of a four-year course in jurisprudence and economics in their institute in Rome, which is the equivalent of a degree.

Unfortunately, their involvement with finance has led to a reputation for corruption. Someone I know had the Guardia di Finanza inspecting the systems in his warehouse. They threatened to stay there all summer, keeping his staff on through their holidays, unless he paid them to go away. The head of the entire organization, General Giudice, was arrested for making millions out of importing oil on a low tax quota and selling it as if it had been on a higher one.

The forces of law and order also have what are called "Vigili Urbani" which originate in the old police forces which each separate town or region had when they were independent. All are employed in their own towns, in contrast to the Carabinieri, who always post members away from where they might be influenced by friends and relatives.

Vigili Urbani are occupied as traffic police, and ensure that local regulations are obeyed. They are responsible to the mayor of the town and have purely local responsibilities. Thus they cannot arrest people outside their own commune, and in cases of serious crime such as drug offences, they inform the Carabinieri rather than intervening themselves.

One would have thought that this multiplicity would produce confusion. When I talked to the *questore* (head of police) in Naples about this, he said that the reason was historical. These powerful forces of order remain divided to prevent them from mounting a coup. There was in fact no real confusion because in each region all three national police forces are responsible to the *questore*, who ensures there is no duplication.

As always, though, the personal enters into the whole system. "With friends we interpret the law," runs an Italian saying; "with others, we apply it."

MEDICINE

"The system used to be all right, although we had our crises," said Dr Fossi. "We simply had a private medical insurance system which was compulsory. If there were deficits, the government usually made them up. This scheme started with the textile workers in the 1920s and spread to everyone after the war. The great thing was that it wasn't organized by government. Government is the hand of chaos in Italy.

"Then of course in the 1970s, with all that idealism which so rarely works in practice, it was decided to have a health service modelled on the British system, and everyone was financed from social security payments instead. The regions were given the responsibility and the whole country was split into areas averaging 150,000 inhabitants. Each was controlled by what we call USL (Unità di Sanità Locale). This is an assembly of 50 people, appointed by the region. They elect a committee of nine, who are responsible for every hospital in the district. They aren't specialists but they nevertheless make all the financial decisions: appointing staff, ordering new equipment, deciding how to allot the money which is provided by the government.

"With this, the usual Italian bureaucracy grew up: impenetrable, convoluted, slow. This was the excuse for the political parties to move in. Over the whole country, the DC took about 40 per cent of these committees, the Socialists 20 per cent and the Communists 14 per cent, with the rest split between the smaller parties."

I remembered a newspaper article in which a journalist, Mauro Bartolo, compared the parties invading the USLs to "marines come to conquer the appetising wealth of contracts, jobs and control of the whole medical system".

"Who did the hospitals belong to before?" I asked.

"Oh, they were public, and about a fifth were private, or under the wing of the Church. They were financed by patients' insurance money, or by donations from companies and rich people, which now are rarely given. They had, of course, to conform to the general government regulations about qualifications of staff, or hygienic conditions, but each unit was master of its own destiny. Now, doctors are civil servants, with a thirty-eight hour week. In theory, they can stop in the middle of an operation if they've completed their full working hours!"

In Seregno, near Milan, another doctor felt that the USLs worked if there were the right people on the committee, as in his region. "Any kind of organization works," he said optimistically, "as long as the people are good and the parties don't fight."

In parallel, a large private hospital system still exists, and in 1983 the government contributed 70,000 lire per day to patients who chose this. Many people still take out private insurance and in 1984 you could get basic medical cover for about 100,000 lire ($60) a month. Now, though, you have to pay for it in addition to social security contributions.

In Perugia I was told that when the health scheme started, doctors could opt for full- or part-time which meant being employed in the private sector when they weren't working for the State. Most had decided on full-time because of the extra security and pensions. Now, however, these salaries are lagging behind those in the private sector. It is difficult to change course at this stage because there is an excess of doctors and most of the good posts are occupied. As a result, there is a lot of discontent and morale is low.

One of the big problems is the lack of training for nurses: nursing is still not taken seriously as a profession. As in Spain, it is your family who are expected to look after you. When an English friend of mine was in hospital, it virtually shut down over Easter, with only two cleaning ladies in attendance, because families fed and looked after their relatives. If some local friends had not adopted him, my friend would have been hungry and solitary.

As so often, there is a serious money problem because the State now has to pay vast sums for the system it has annexed. No less than 72 per cent of the gross regional budget in 1981 was spent on the equivalent of National Health. There are also subsidized prescriptions. Medicines are divided into three categories: "unnecessary" medicaments which you pay for; more necessary things on which you pay 1,000 lire and 10–20 per cent of the price; then, the urgent, on which you pay just 1,000 lire.

Unfortunately, as in Britain, cutbacks tend to concentrate on this area. In 1983, Deagan, the Minister of Health, proposed abolishing free prescriptions, specialist services and every form of subsidy, except for stays in hospital, for all those earning more than 25 million lire ($11,000) a year. This would, as a trade union leader, Donatella Turturà, said, "destroy the fundamental lines of our medical reforms". In any case, doctors and chemists have to wait months for payment. A chemist I talked to in San Gimignano told me she hadn't been paid for three months, and had now been told that she would have to wait another five.

Another problem is that those from the South, where hospitals are not so good, come North for treatment at the expense of regions which are not their own. This also applies to tourists, and in the spring of 1983 doctors in Liguria decided to charge tourists for visits, prescriptions and medical analyses. "Liguria loses 100 to 150 billion lire [45–80 million dollars] in order to cover the requirements of the medical services," said Dr Eolo Parodi, head of the national federation of doctors.

Doctors often go on strike, or simply give their own prescriptions, instead of those of the State, so that patients have to pay for them at the chemists. "For two days, it is forbidden to be ill!" announced *Il Giornale* in anticipation of a two-day strike in Rome at the beginning of April 1984.

Nevertheless, some hospitals are magnificent. It all depends on whether they have benefited from what the Italians call *la pioggia*, or shower of money, which descends suddenly and unevenly throughout the whole system. In Bologna, I visited the university hospital which was built in the early '70s, when the university had funds. I talked to Dr Gunella in his department for training specialists in respiratory diseases and he told me that his equipment was among the best in Europe. He had fifty beds and each was equipped with a respiratory aid machine, while there were seven big ventilation machines for crises. The objective of his department was first to teach, then to do research and, third, to look after patients. For this, he had a staff of one professor, ten assistant professors, eighty nurses, technicians and secretaries, and twenty specialist doctors – all for thirty students and fifty patients. In a newly built hospital in Potenza, the head of the cardiac unit, Dr Tesler, had planned his department with an architect. In the hospital at Varese, there are two thousand employees to a thousand beds.

An interesting experiment has recently been made with the mentally ill. In 1978, asylums were abolished by what is known as law 180 (laws in Italy are all numbered). Under this law, many mental patients were to be sent back to their families, and others would live together in specially built homes as part of society. They were no longer to be what Italians call *emarginati* – literally "marginized". Fifteen beds were to be kept in each hospital to form a special ward for those who really needed specialized treatment. The rest were to be helped by clinics to which they could go whenever they wanted. This move followed the theories of Franco Basaglia, a professor of psychiatry, who believed that mental illness is caused largely by social pressures and perpetuated by the authoritarian nature of mental homes.

In London, I found it interesting to go to lectures and discussions on what was called "The Italian Experience", arranged by the British organization Mind. Among the lecturers, Dr Cecchini from Arezzo described how people had once regarded the mental home in his city as a remote, frightening place. When the new law was applied and patients were let out, there was panic. How would one deal with these strange, "abnormal" beings when one met them? Surely they couldn't work! Wouldn't the crime rate go up? It was necessary to protect one's children!

As criminal lunatics are still kept in special homes, fears were groundless and ex-patients were absorbed without great problems. The sense of shame and embarrassment which went with lunacy evaporated when these people were shown to be no more eccentric than some of those who were outside. Also, the ex-patients appealed to people's better instincts, needing help as they did after being shut up for so long. So also did families faced with welcoming those they had rejected before. In a special ceremony, the bars at the gate of the mental home were pulled down, and there was no longer a sense of a remote, eerie building in the town, which people referred to with an embarrassed laugh.

One Sunday, we came by chance on an open air dance in Spoleto for old-age pensioners who whirled happily in waltzes, fox-trots and quick-steps. On the edge of the dance floor was a young man giggling and clapping his hands to the music. People went up and talked to him and, although he was strange he didn't seem to feel alienated, or to disturb in any way.

In Rome, I visited one of the clinics which has been set up under Law 180 for mental patients, going out a long way by tram to a district of high buildings where Dr Antonuchi, who was in charge, told me there was a lot of poverty and violence. The clinic was in a small building next to a primary school. There were two dormitories with three beds in each, a ping-pong room, a kitchen, and various offices.

Dr Antonuchi told me that they usually had about three people staying overnight. Patients could do what they liked, go home during the day and come back in the evening, or vice-versa. Each patient had his or her psychiatrist. On average, those who stayed were there from a fortnight to six weeks.

We talked about Law 180, and the way hospital wards only took fifteen patients by law. "What happens if there are more?"

"We have corridors!"

I attended a discussion on patients who bore out Basaglia's theories. One was a worker from the Abruzzi who was difficult to deal with because of his different background and dialect. He had had a breakdown because his sister, with her husband and two children, had been turned out of their flat and had taken refuge with him. Another patient had married her uncle, with a dispensation from the Church. Extraordinarily enough, she hadn't known her relationship to him and now was afflicted with guilt. She had had a dead baby which she regarded as punishment. Both patients seemed disturbed because of circumstances, or the social situation, rather than from any inherent mental trouble.

Later, I read a report on how four middle-aged ex-patients had moved into an empty flat and now led a normal life together. They shared the chores and neighbours had helped them get furniture. A bed in a psychiatric hospital costs about a hundred thousand lire ($45) per patient per day. Supporting these ex-patients costs a seventh of that sum.

The real trouble, however, is that although Law 180 was passed in 1978, it is working only in Trieste, Gorizia – where Basaglia started his experiments – and Arezzo. The clinics have not been set up widely enough and, as a result, many of the original mental hospitals are not empty but contain people who are worse off than they were before. Two Englishwomen, Kathleen Jones and Alison Poletti, toured Italy to visit hospitals and wrote a horrifying report for *New Society*. Referring to one hospital, they described the psychiatric graffiti, the iron bars at the top of the stairs, the bare flexes, "doors off their hinges, walls half plastered, windows out". Only later did they discover that in 1978 there had been some up-grading, but when the new law was passed, the builders had left. South of Salerno, they found that the law hadn't been applied at all.

Partly because Law 180 is supported so strongly by the Communists, other groups of psychiatrists are opposed. Also, there is a lot of argument about Basaglia's system. It may be effective for certain patients, like those I saw in Rome, but there is doubt about its suitability for schizophrenics, who make up half the number of mental patients.

Certainly, it is asking too much of families to look after mentally ill patients if there are not enough clinics to give professional help. I remember an amazing scene in a Carabinieri station in north Italy where a man came in and shouted abuse at everyone. "He comes in and insults us like that every day," said one of them. "He's one of the 'liberated' patients. His two daughters have to look after him. It's almost sending them mad."

A result has been that the number of private hospitals has increased. Jones and Poletti give an example of one with a brochure which represents it almost as a five-star hotel. The reality is very different: "Bleak bare rooms with urine-stained floor. No activities. Locked wards (against the law for private Homes). Patients sit staring vacantly, or shuffle about aimlessly. Poor staffing. The outer gates are kept locked. A dumping ground for inconvenient relatives."

I went to one in Potenza in the South, which was private but lodged in an appropriate building and staffed by nuns. It was grim, as most mental homes are: one listens to animal noises, glances at unseeing eyes, sees faces which may resemble those of people one knows. However, whereas Law 180 treats all mental patients as if they were the same, there was a distinction here between those who were senile, those who were very ill and those on the border line. The border-line cases had been making cribs for Christmas in a big workshop where others were also working on ceramics and painting. Many of them, the director told us, went out to work, like those in the Rome clinic, and came back in the evenings. They did all their own cleaning and cooking.

The director himself felt that Law 180 was outrageous: "It may work for some but really it's just a theory!" He told us it was particularly inappropriate in Basilicata where many people lived in the mountains in tiny villages, and it was difficult to establish enough clinics as communications were bad.

Sometimes I wonder if the Italians' historical religious sense doesn't affect their attitude to planning and to organization, whatever party they may belong to. Often it just seems enough to have humane sentiments and fight for them.

It is certainly daring to try to create a substitute for the mental hospital at one blow, but the overall effect has been a lot of suffering. Of course, it is more complicated: there is also the ineffectiveness of government, the lure of private interests, perpetual interference from the "tribal" political parties, and the difficulty of legislating uniformly for a country which is so varied. The whole new health system is also an example of the difference in Italy between passing laws and actually carrying them out. As far as the hospital reforms are concerned, USL had still not been established in many regions in 1983.

The sentiments behind both the reformed hospital system and Law

180 are admirable. But as there is neither the structure nor the finance to support either of them, they have produced a crisis which is damaging not to the rich or the powerful but to the families who have been asked to bear the burden of relatives who are mentally ill, and to the patients and medical staff who, above all, they are designed to help.

VIII
THE CHURCH

*Decline? – Lay Movements and Reform – The Italian Church –
The Church's Role in Society*

In a pub in London, I talked to a Northern Irish Protestant. When he heard I was writing a book about Italy, he said he hoped I would do justice to the Roman Church.

"Justice?" I asked.

"Yes – show her up for the sink of iniquity she is," he said with dark hatred. He twisted his mouth. "Rome!" he spat out.

I said nothing and remembered the names by which the Church used to be known, and probably still is: "The Great Whore", "The Scarlet Woman".

It seemed strange to hear sentiments which might have been expressed by the old fanatics of the Reformation: John Knox, Calvin, Cromwell. On reflection, though, I realized that before living in Spain, before exploring Italy, I too had my simplistic assumptions: associations of the Inquisition and the Massacre of Saint Bartholomew; a Protestant antipathy to religion being expressed through a rich, powerful institution, in which unctuous priests call you "My son", and judge you at Confession, impinging on privacy and independence because sure they know what Truth is.

In Franco's Spain, however, I was surprised to find priests among the most balanced and intelligent people I met. In Italy, I came to admire the Catholic Church for its integrity and its concern for human beings – virtues shared, paradoxically, by the Communist Party.

Zorzone is a little village among the Bergamesque Alps which looks down on a deep valley, with snowy hollows between the rocks at the tops of the surrounding mountains. If you go out beyond the village, you walk along narrow paths cut into bare, steep hills where you can only stand with one foot behind another. If you kick a stone, it goes down faster and faster until it reaches the bed of a stream, far below, and you wonder if the same thing would happen to you if you fell. You can see another human being miles away, a moving splinter on the hills.

Zorzone is poor. Until 1980, three hundred men in the village mined zinc in the vicinity. There is a piazza called after those who have died at work: "Piazza dei Defunti del Lavoro". Many workers had silicosis until employers found it cheaper to import the zinc from Bolivia. Now, the men take a bus early in the morning and go to Bergamo or Milan where they work in the building trade.

In the main piazza, Gui Caspani and I stood outside the village church waiting for the Palm Sunday procession. Singing sounded from down the street and a group wended its slow way, carrying olive branches, with the priest and two girls singing at the back. The church was full. St Matthew's account of the Passion was read: a girl took the role of Judas, a boy that of Jesus while the priest was the narrator. In the middle, the priest, who was square set like a boxer, interrupted and said that he thought everyone should go on standing unless they were too old or exhausted – which meant that no one sat down. After Communion, everyone shook hands with those near them and filed out, greeting each other, kissing cheeks, shaking hands, embracing one another, or chatting.

Later, we went to see the priest in his presbytery by the church as Gui wanted to give him a present of embroidery from her mother. He was wearing a black polo-necked sweater and grey trousers, looking more than ever like a boxer, and he invited us into his parlour. A family was sitting round a table covered with an oilcloth: a girl with her baby who was only a few months younger than his uncle, another baby which an older woman was carrying. The priest said something about making sure the babies were well fed, and the younger woman answered that a diet of Ave Marias would make them grow strong. We were served grappa and coffee by a white-haired lady in black who in the course of conversation said she was seventy-five and would soon be "going over there".

We started talking about the Church. The priest said there had been a full congregation that morning but it was only because it was a special festa. People either worked very hard for the Church or they did nothing. This was partly because the generation which followed the convulsions of 1968–9 regarded the Church as a negative force. The referenda on divorce and abortion had been a shattering blow. Most people between twenty-seven and thirty-five were opposed or indifferent to the Church.

All this materialism was worrying, too. The only thing young people cared about was getting a new car: they thought that buying one was a great achievement. Drugs were terrible too. I told him about our visit to Comunità Incontro in Palermo. Of course, the Church did what it could, he said, but what were the efforts of a few hundred people compared to the thousands who took heroin?

It was very difficult, also, to recruit new priests. A priest was no longer the centre of the community as he once had been. Some years ago, he had been lawyer, adviser, teacher. If people were sick, they asked to see him. He knew and was accepted by everyone, and was an essential part of the fabric of the community. Now, in a society in which roles were more diverse, he could easily be lonely and isolated.

And politics? The Church was no longer as involved as it had been. It had been active a few years ago because of the fear of Communism. Now, however, that was no longer a real menace.

In fact, there has rarely been a time when there was not a crisis in the Church in Italy. Only 1 per cent of the population are Protestants so the division has rarely been a theological one. As the priest in Zorzone implied, it is today more of a struggle between faith and apathy in an increasingly urban society. "Suddenly, as the city grows," said Pope John XXIII in the early 1960s, "the cement enters the soul and any such scene as the Transfiguration departs, not to the realms of unlikelihood but to a place light years away." An article in the Jesuit magazine *Civiltà Cattolica* at the end of September 1983 announced that Catholics in Italy were now a minority. Ninety-seven per cent of new babies were baptized but the number of practising Catholics had gone down to only 30 per cent.

"Apart from the small, anachronistic fringe of the old anti-clerical core," the same article goes on, "the worrying thing is the lack of interest in religious problems, the rejection of Christ and the Gospels by those who are already familiar with them, and have perhaps also followed them, but now assert that neither Gospels nor Christ have anything to say to them."

Father Sorge, the director of *Civiltà Cattolica* whom I met in Rome, believes that mankind is in a state of "disappointment" because so many successive illusions have been shattered in the last two hundred years: first, the eighteenth-century faith in Reason, then in Progress, then in Nationalism, and now in Development, which has created tyrannical regimes and has abetted ecological disaster. Marxism too is a God that has failed and the decay in the number of practising Christians is perhaps a sign of this general sense of disappointment. It is necessary now, believes Sorge, for the Church to show that justice is an essential element of the Christian outlook, and to ensure that the disillusioned return to the fold. Religion, after all, does not offer the easy inducements which bring disappointment in this world.

Other Italian priests I have met have not been so concerned with the decline in congregations. The headmaster of a Catholic school in Seregno (Milan) said that, before 1968, lots of people went to church, but they didn't really know what it meant. There had always been a proportion of fashionable church-goers and habitués. Now only the genuine and the sincere remained, who thought things out more thoroughly and intelligently.

Franciscans are actually increasing in number, largely, I was told in Assisi, because they are more "of this world". Their fraternity, simplicity and democratic organization appeal to the youth of today. Franciscans are also missionaries and the image of St Francis himself is particularly attractive because of the saint's gentleness and love of peace in a tempestuous age. The criteria the friars rely on do not so much form a "bank" of doctrine but are based on whether St Francis would have approved.

In Assisi, I was taken round the labyrinth of rooms and friars' cells underneath the actual Cathedral by a Spanish friar from Santander who had decided to be a priest when he was fourteen. He had been in Assisi for six months and had written a potted history of the Franciscans, which he showed me. Although in his forties, he was still full of enthusiasm and betrayed no traditional prejudices. Napoleon had cleared all the friars out when he invaded Italy, he told me. Just as well, as they were venal then. The trouble was that people had given them lands and castles and jewellery throughout the centuries. By his action, Napoleon had in fact reformed them.

Together we walked round a complex of corridors and enclosed courtyards which would have done justice to Mervyn Peake's vast labyrinths in *Titus Groan* or *Gormenghast*. There was something surrealist about the unexpected things we came across in the silence, under stone arches or in great vaulted rooms. On a platform, two men were clearing up after an antiquarian exhibition, silently wrapping the medieval statues of saints in polythene.

In the "temporary" theological college with rows of doors either side of a corridor, the friar lowered his voice to a whisper in case some of the students were meditating. Originally, the friars had let out their

college, which was in the town of Assisi itself, for a few months in the
summer. But the man who had rented it in order to lodge people during
the tourist season now refused to give it back. In the Middle Ages, he
would probably have been excommunicated and ejected by the civil
arm. But what could one do now except go to law, endlessly and
tediously, and meanwhile find lodging for the students here, under the
Cathedral itself?

We penetrated further in order to find the bearskin which San
Giuseppe da Copertino, the patron saint of examination students, had
slept on, for his rooms had also been in this extraordinary complex.
However, we only discovered his hair shirt.

Everything was bizarre, but the outside world was never far away.
Thieves had even stolen articles from the friars' cells, particularly radio
cassette recorders. When Fray Elias, St Francis's successor, built all this
in only two years, just after the founder's death, there had been
opposition from other friars: it was too large and institutional; St
Francis would not have liked it, they said. But they had been wrong. It
was not set apart. Five million visitors were drawn to it every year.

As we emerged, the friar waved to a Spanish group which had been
waiting for him outside the gate, and which he was going to take round
the Cathedral. I thanked him warmly, and wished him luck.

It is significant that although the number of practising Catholics is
declining, the interest in Church festivals, whether at Assisi, Gubbio
(see p. 47) or anywhere else, is increasing. Ten years ago many of the
festas appeared to be dying out. However, the increase in cars and the
contrast between the celebrations and the drabness of modern life have
made a lot of difference.

There are more canonized saints in Italy than in any other country.
Umberto Eco in his widely read, recent novel, *The Name of the Rose*, set
in the fourteenth century, implies that veneration of images has been
strong for a long time. He puts scurrilous remarks about Italians into the
mouth of his main character, an English priest: "They are more afraid
of Saint Sebastian or Saint Anthony than of Christ. If you wish to keep a
place clean here, to prevent anyone from pissing onto it which the
Italians do as freely as dogs do, you paint on it an image of Saint
Anthony ... and this will drive away those about to piss."

LAY MOVEMENTS AND REFORMS

In Reggio Calabria, opposite Sicily, Luisa Catanosa, an English teacher,
explained that in a society which is dominated by *auto-consumo*, where

everyone is obsessed by their earnings and what they can buy, the Church is the one place where all can rally together. Pilgrimages are social events and can, in the neighbouring mountains of Aspromonte, involve as many as a million people who travel at night, mainly on foot, to a shrine. "These festas are more important than Christmas," said Luisa.

One Saturday evening we went together to Mass in Reggio. The service was held in the modern cathedral which was rebuilt after the devastating earthquake of 1908. The whole church was crowded out, with people moving continually as if in a piazza. One lady, followed by her son, climbed up behind the altar to put gladioli she had brought into a vase, and slipped, almost tumbling down. Then she went to kiss the hand of the archbishop who had just finished saying Mass. In the middle of all the movement was an enormous painting of the Madonna della Consolazione, standing head-high on the floor in an elaborate silver frame. The painting had been discovered in a hut sometime in the sixteenth century and brought to the cathedral. However, one night, just before the Madonna's festa, it disappeared and was found again in the original hut. Now, therefore, it was brought down to the cathedral for a brief period and returned, with 300 people carrying it in shifts. Many women went barefoot.

At Palermo university, Professor Buttita told us there was now more resistance to change among those he called the *sotto proletariato*. Many religious festivals had been revived and more young people took part in the Confratelli (lay brotherhoods) which organized them. Part of the drive for this had come from emigrants who returned and were disappointed that festas were not held as before.

In the north, I was told, religion was more "serious". Part of this was due to the better training of priests, which had its origin in the reform of seminaries by St Charles Borromeo, back in the sixteenth century. It is also in Lombardy and the Veneto that many of the lay movements which supplement and support the Church have developed. The oldest of these is "Accione Cattolica", formed of graduates whose object is to influence others at a cultural level. Under Fascism there was great hostility to this organization as it was regarded as a vocal alternative rather than as a support of the regime. Many leading Christian Democrats such as Moro, Fanfani and Andreotti were closely linked with it and had been pupils at one stage of Cardinal Montini who later became Pope Paul VI.

Another well-known lay group is "Comunione e Liberazione", founded by Don Luigi Giussani some thirty years ago. It has strong ecclesiastical links. A friend of mine who is a member tells me they often have exuberant singing sessions and discussions with the Pope in the Vatican. Their object is to relate closely to the Church, lead a Christian life, and persuade others to do the same: they are people who do not have vocations to be priests, but who want to be active Catholics and to disseminate their beliefs through example and Christian works.

Similar but more personal are the "Focolarini", literally the Hearth People, who form little groups of three or four for prayers, discussions and activities. Founded in Trento under bombardment during the war, this lay movement, started by a woman, Clara Lubich, has now spread to 150 countries with over a million members.

More active in the secular and political field is "Movimento Popolare", founded in 1976, which represents a more militantly political Catholic element, ready to oppose the Left, take part in demonstrations and heckle at Communist meetings. Their object, said Roberto Formigoni, their leader and an EEC deputy, is to "construct something in the socio-political field not in the ecclesiastical ... we've organized the list of Christians in schools and universities and today have got a majority everywhere in the elected student assemblies ... we have created cultural centres in more than a hundred Italian towns." In all, says Formigoni, Movimento Popolare has more than seventy thousand "militants" in Italy, and more than double that number who participate regularly in their activities. In Rimini every year they have a festival: in 1983 it celebrated the Friendship of Peoples, and more than 30,000 individuals of different nationalities attended. The discussion theme of the conference was "Man, the Monkey and the Robot".

Other less well-known lay organizations also flourish. One is described by Peter Nichols in his *The Pope's Divisions*. Named "Comunità St Egidio", it started during the troubles in 1968–9, with six people. It now has 2,500 adherents who meet regularly in an abandoned convent for prayers and discussions, do social work in the poorer suburbs of Rome, and run nursery schools and workshops for training apprentices. "Remember we are lay," said one of the leaders of this community to Peter Nichols. "We do not have a priest founder; our organization is that of an assembly. Everyone can come and say what they want." Of course they do have links with the Church and several members of the community spent an evening explaining to the Pope what they were doing. However, although fervent Christians, they are an independent community.

It is interesting, too, to hear of separatist groups: for instance, a heating salesman who says he has cured four thousand people through the laying on of hands, and claims to be St Peter. With an ex-priest, he has taken over an old church near Siena for his sect of three hundred people.

A more serious dissenter is Don Franzoni, who was once the Abbot of St Paul Without the Walls, one of the most important posts in the Italian Church which he was one of the youngest persons ever to fill.

I went to see him in his office, from which he now runs an independent religious organization. Copies of his paper *Nuovi Tempi* were stacked untidily on a table. On the wall, there were two large drawings. One showed Christ approaching a large stone replica of the Christian Democrat Party sign which has a cross in the middle. The next showed Christ who had torn out the Cross from the stone and was bearing it on his shoulders. The stone had cracked and fallen on top of a little figure who was guarding it.

"When did you leave the Church?" I asked Dr Franzoni.

"Leave – I've never left it," he said emphatically. "It's only that they don't recognize me any more. I'm still a priest. I'm celibate. I still celebrate Mass."

The rift, he said, had come in 1974 when he opposed the Church's campaign against divorce during the referendum. "I just didn't feel the Church should make divorce a religious issue," he said. "It is up to citizens to decide about their laws."

Then, in 1976, he joined the Communist Party as an Independent, which had stirred further fury. He is still on one of their advisory bodies. "Why shouldn't I?" he asked. "I think the Communists are the most humane political party we have. I disagree with much of their philosophy but what business of the Church is it how I vote?"

Now he has a centre near his former abbey and concerns himself with drug addicts and also non-European workers, mainly Tunisians and girls from the Philippines. "They are miserably treated," he said.

On the 26th of June he had arranged a meeting with a group of prostitutes. However, he had then been asked to a reconciliation meeting with Catholics on the same day. Of course, he refused to put off his original appointment. "That is the essence of what I mean," he said. "The most important people are the *emarginati* who normally don't count: the old, the handicapped, the unhappy. I have no temple. It isn't necessary. A few months ago I celebrated Mass in the Piazza Vecchia in Florence as a symbol of the Church entering the world, rather than always receiving worshippers in its gorgeous churches. Christ never had his own temple. I just have a place for people to come to if they want to. But we still have opposition in official circles: it's like the prodigal son – the person who objects is the brother."

Franzoni is also a believer in ecumenicalism, the free exchange between different Churches. One Sunday, his community worship with Waldensians in their church. The next, it is the Waldensians who come to his centre.

Ten years ago, he told me, it was all very difficult. The bishops were stiff and authoritative. Now, the younger ones are more flexible, although John Paul's rigidity of doctrine produces a certain severity. However, the distinction between the Vatican and the Italian Church has become more marked in the last few years, although not of course where dogma is concerned.

THE ITALIAN CHURCH

It is important to make clear the difference between the Vatican as the centre of a world organization and the Italian Church. In the past, this distinction hardly seemed to exist, and even a contemporary best-seller, *The Vatican Connection* by Richard Hammer, confuses the two. The ultimate head of the Italian Church is the Pope. However, it is Cardinal Ballestrero, the President of the Italian Episcopal Council, who runs the Italian Church. The Council meets several times a year and is composed of bishops who are heads of the sixteen clerical regions, with thirteen others who preside over various Commissions. Each of these Commissions deals with specific areas, among which are: "Doctrine and Faith", "Clergy and Liturgy", "The Family", "Education", "Social Problems and Work". The heads of these different Commissions and of the Administrative Council, to which they are responsible, are elected every three or six years.

The whole system is only about twenty years old, originating with John XXIII, and gives the Italian Church its own identity similar to the French, Spanish, German, or any other national Church.

Of course the Pope himself still has immense direct influence, both as Bishop of Rome and also because Italians still feel proud that their country has been the home of the Papacy for so long. Although it is officially a separate state, the Vatican is inextricably part of Rome and of Italy, and Popes have always played a major role in the country's history.

On the whole, a Polish Pope seems to be generally accepted by Italians. Inevitably, you hear chauvinistic criticisms that the Pope wastes money on his tours abroad which would be better given to developing countries, or that really he is only a salesman. However, among believing Catholics, the Pope is still the vicar of Christ on earth, whatever nationality he is, and John Paul II, or Papa Wojtila as the Italians call him, also has the gift of being human, personal and spontaneously witty. So much feeling in Italy is linked to the home-town or village, and when the Pope tours Italian towns he is doing honour to people's birth-places, the source of so much pride and devotion. I remember watching him in Viterbo, talking spontaneously from a balcony in the rain to a packed crowd holding umbrellas. Cheers punctuated his speech, particularly when he praised Viterbo, and even when he confused the name of the town's saint and called her Santa Rita instead of Santa Rosa, there were only mild protests. It would be difficult to imagine any other of the world's salient personalities making such an informal, human and bantering speech in a foreign language, as on that evening under the rain in the main piazza of Viterbo.

THE CHURCH'S ROLE IN SOCIETY

Those who judge Italian Catholicism as sinister or dominating often forget how human and informal it is. I have already described how much it does for drug addicts and homosexuals (see pp. 146 and 172). In many ways it tempers the weaknesses of the welfare state and is yet another example of that pluralism which makes the country so difficult to define and understand. It staffs hospitals, old people's homes, mental homes and schools, and runs universities in Milan, Rome and Piacenza, and a trade union (ACLI). The Movimento Popolare also finds work for its members and has centres where they sell cheap food to poorer people; while the parish priest, despite his loss of influence, is there to help his parishioners and regards the family as a particular cause for care.·

Wherever you go in Italy, you find priests directing some charitable operation, usually with specialist lay employees. One of the most moving examples of this was a home for handicapped children in Palermo. It was on one of the hills above the city, from which it was possible to see the ranks of tall buildings constructed with Mafia money. The home was built against a steep slope, on ground donated to it, and for the benefit of invalid chairs each floor was linked by slowly rising galleries, paved with black rubber.

A priest in civilian clothes, Padre Scaletta, was in charge, helped by lay organizers, teachers and medical staff. The money came mainly from the Banca di Sicilia and there were about thirty children attending during the day and another thirty who came to surgery in the morning and afternoon. There were few possibilities of permanent cures, Signora Orlando the organizer told me.

She explained that a few years ago a law had been passed giving extra grants to schools which took handicapped children into their general classes. On the whole the experiment had worked, stimulating the handicapped and encouraging normal children to help their unfortunate companions. However, none of the children in this home were healthy enough to benefit, and there was therefore a small school on the premises, supported by the government: in it, a smiling girl in a wheelchair was learning to write, and two other children passed a football back and forth to each other over their desks.

In contrast, the Church also organizes money-making activities, particularly in tourism and mass education. The rationale behind this is the need to protect young people from "pernicious" influences while they are away from their parents. Thus, to the discomfiture of other tourist organizations, Catholic firms send hundreds of young people abroad on summer courses. Because they can use the structure provided by Catholic schools and parishes, they can attract students who would otherwise go with independent agencies. In this sense, the Church arouses resentment because it enters the open market with advantages which come, not from better programmes or prices, but through an organization which has been built up for religious rather than commercial purposes. This, though, has been a dilemma since the early beginnings of Christianity. How far should the Church concern itself with earthly power, wealth and status? Can it rely simply on its "spirituality"? Should it keep aloof from the conflicts, intrigues and often the sordidness of the world about it?

In a sense, the history of the Church in Italy is of its gradual withdrawal from political power and status. It has come a long way since the days of warrior Popes and the direct administration of vast lands. Don Franzoni, although now excluded, represents a genuine feeling among Catholics that the Church's worldly role is mainly to help those in trouble, not to concern itself with voting for specific parties, or excluding other Churches. This also expresses itself in the work of hundreds of priests, who will help drug-addicts, prostitutes, the maimed and the ill, whether they are religious or not, in the hope perhaps of bringing them into the fold through the example they are setting.

One advantage of Church involvement is that it stirs an active conscience both in the individual and in society. An example is the recent movement in Palermo to create an alternative Catholic party because the DCs seem too interlinked in Sicily with Mafia interests. Another was the surprising outburst of Bishop Arnaldo Onisto in 1983 when he attacked Conte Marzotto, the head of the industrial association in Vicenza, which is both a highly industrialized region and strongly Catholic. The occasion was the refusal of Confindustria, the national employers' association, to renew the contracts of its workers, and the bishop wrote: "The economic, social and political system does not correspond with the way a man should live. It is necessary therefore to ensure that it be reformed, indeed it is necessary to reform the whole world of the working man." Of course the Communists and trade union leaders were delighted, while the head of the industrial association in turn accused the episcopal organization of being "a Marxist-Leninist society at the service of the trade unions".

All these questions will not be "resolved" neatly, any more than they will be elsewhere. In Italy, the Church is as much a way of life as a creed, and therefore complicated and confusing in many ways.

Still, deep in the Italian consciousness is the realization that the Church has been the one consistent unifier of Italy as the successor of the Roman Empire. At the same time, it has been the great opponent of *political* unification: placed in the middle of Italy, it was always the biggest obstruction to the merging of South and North.

Nevertheless, it is the one element in Italy which has given it "glory", ruling the known world, provoking "just" wars, arranging truces, even apportioning South America between the Spanish and the Portuguese, responsible more than any other body for much of the immense artistic heritage of Italy.

Most Italians accept the fact that Church laws, like any other, are there to be broken. Just as Italians were among the first to practise usury with their banking system in the Middle Ages, so their declining birth-rate would indicate that they practise contraception; abortion is now legal; so is divorce. Yet, although fewer of them go to Mass, or wish to become priests, they are still strong in this presence which enables them to be consistently aware of rules of right and wrong, to view everyone as people with individual souls, to feel that there may, perhaps, be a purpose in this life because it leads to another one.

Because of this the Church has helped to give Italians much of their humanity, their communicativeness, their balance between spontaneity and restraint.

In villages, the Church is like the bell-tower which looks out above the roofs, as if a sentinel guaranteeing order and calm. In times of joy, it is a strong maypole, pointing towards the sky, round which everyone cavorts and dances and sings. In time of sorrow, it is a black hearse, followed by weeping relatives. It is the cross on the Christian Democrat shield, the wife of the Secretary-General of the Communist Party going to Mass, the beauty of Orvieto Cathedral. Or the brisk trade in rosaries in Assisi, the dark intimacy of confessional boxes, the flutter of nuns at railway stations.

It is also thousands of other things. The one thing it is not is a pale, questioning spirit. It has formed Italy over the centuries, and with Italy it will change.

IX

THE ARTS

Media – Novels – Theatre – Cinema – Music –
Visual Arts and Design

MEDIA

I switched on the television and there was a blonde girl, with brown eyes, continually jerking her head forward as she sang, so that her hair fell in front of her face – whereupon she would pull her head back so that she could see again.

The Minister of the Treasury, Goria, a youngish man with a beard, was sitting on a sofa, while nearby was a varied group of singers and performers, lounging about or moving casually from one place to another. The blonde girl ended her song, sat down, and proceeded to ask the Minister light-hearted questions about the economy, which he answered flippantly, with an evasive smile.

Then the girl got up and sang again, moving energetically from one side of the set to the other. When she had finished, she sat down and started a phone-in quiz programme with listeners who were supposed to guess the missing words in songs which were produced exuberantly by a group who had suddenly appeared. Goria, meanwhile, sat rather gloomily on the sofa until the quiz game ended, and the blonde girl asked him a few more questions on the economy which again he parried evasively.

She then introduced a choir of middle-aged people who sang traditional songs. When they had finished, she thanked them profusely and began to discard various dresses to reveal a Spanish dancer's polka dot dress with ruffles on the shoulders. This enabled her to do a dance *à l'espagnole*, at which everyone else (including Goria) shouted "Olè" and clapped their hands. With her warm, dazzling smile, she then turned to everyone on the set and poured out a stream of *molte grazie, auguri*, and said how *simpatici* everyone had been, including Goria, who smiled once more.

I tried to imagine this happening on the BBC with Sir Geoffrey Howe or Nigel Lawson. Who, though, would go through these multiple accompaniments? Joan Bakewell? Angela Rippon? Sir Robin Day in drag? Or Mrs Thatcher herself?

The blonde lady was Raffella Carrà, probably the most successful performer of all those who appear on innumerable Italian television programmes. Sometimes she has an audience of seven million. Now forty years old, La Carrà, as she is known, has been a television star for over twenty years. In 1984, she created a political furore because she accepted a contract for three years at a salary of four and a half billion lire (about one and a half million dollars) which was objected to by the prime minister – in vain.

Italy has three official television stations: RAI 1, dominated by the Christian Democrats; RAI 2, run mainly by the Socialists; RAI 3, created specially to give a channel to the Communists, but both its director and the director of the news programmes are Christian Democrats. They are not allowed to make political attacks on television, but you can see each station's bias, particularly in the news broadcasts, where, for instance, RAI 2 will give more coverage to the Socialist Party Congress, and there will be more concentration on what Craxi, the Socialist prime minister, does and says. All three channels are run by a board on which all the political parties, including the MSI, are represented. According to its rivals, it is grossly overstaffed with seventeen thousand employees compared to one thousand in Canale 5, its main private competitor, which has about the same audience. As a result, it lost 20 billion lire in 1983 ($8 million) and about 155 billions ($70 million) in 1984.

RAI licence fees are cheaper than in Britain: in 1984 you paid 78,910 lire ($31) for colour television and 42,680 lire ($20) for black and white. However, RAI is also allowed to have commercial advertising. All three RAI stations compete among themselves. At a football match you may see an aeroplane flying low with a trailer advertising only one of the RAI channels. They also tend to put on similar competing films at the same time.

Until the mid-1970s there was only one channel, dominated mainly by the Christian Democrats. With an old television set, you automatically get RAI 1 when you switch it on. However, as the majority party weakened, there was increased demand by the other parties for new channels which they could control, and RAI 2 and 3 were born.

Then, in 1978, the special Constitutional Commission announced that

that private channels were not against the constitution as long as they were only local. Therefore, the only programme they couldn't broadcast was international news bulletins, which remain a monopoly of RAI.

This ruling was not actually a law – it merely removed a barrier. It was taken, though, as a sign of encouragement, and there are now at least a hundred private television stations in Italy, owned by individuals, newspapers, magazines or companies. New ones arise, frequently. Others go bankrupt. One advantage is that local businesses advertise: you can see a short film about the shop next door, or an announcement of the films which are on at the local cinema. Standards can be good, with lively debates on contemporary problems where a dozen people contradict each other, defy a helpless chairman, gesticulate so wildly that they almost strike one another, yet somehow manage to make a number of interesting points. Impressive, too, is the continual enquiry into Italy itself, its regions and history, how it functions or doesn't function, its folklore and customs. This, perhaps more than anything else, is helping to establish a national consciousness.

RAI has also embarked on major projects: *Marco Polo* has already appeared on foreign screens although, according to one RAI employee I talked to, it was disappointing in quality and overspent its budget: three and a half billion lire ($1.5 million) were spent on re-creating the Piazza San Marco in Venice, but it was hardly used and was finally burnt in a vast conflagration because no other company wanted to buy it. However, work has already started on major epics such as *Columbus, Quo Vadis* and *Treasure Island*. Productive, too, is the co-operation with film companies to produce masterpieces like *Chaos*, directed by the Taviani brothers, which is based on four short stories by Pirandello and can be shown either as a long film, as it has been in London, or as a television series.

However, competition has also lowered standards. There are no programmes for schools, except on video, and no exclusively cultural channel. The struggle for advertising produces gimmicks like the sudden stopping of a film at the most exciting part in a bid to hold viewers: I remember seeing a girl being pursued by a "baddie" through a wood. She stumbled and fell, and immediately the film was cut and advertisements began. The fact that you can receive as many as fifteen stations on one set may mean that people spend a lot of time switching from one to another, and actually watch nothing. I recall an evening with an Italian family when Richard Burton in the film on Wagner was inextricably mixed up with advertisements, a pop programme, a few snatches of the news and occasional glimpses of Alec Guinness in *The Bridge on the River Kwai*.

Pornography, too, is used as a bait for advertising. An English friend of mine returning to his hotel in the small hours was amazed when he switched on to some close sexual sequences, interspersed with adverts for washing powder and garden brooms. In the initial stages of private television there was a profusion of strip-poker games played by housewives; one programme included a beautiful girl who promised to do anything she was asked by telephone callers, and the requests were accompanied increasingly by heavy breathing as the programme developed.

In Milan I went to see Paolo Berlusconi, the younger brother of the owner of the largest private television stations. Once it was possible to start private television, the brothers invested in a small station at Biella in North Italy and, in 1981, bought what is now the major private network in Italy: Canale 5. Later, they acquired another, Italia Uno, which within six months increased its audience from under two million to three million and a half. Now both channels have local stations which reach 90 per cent of Italy.

The real enemy was RAI, said Paolo Berlusconi. It was quite unfair that they should receive licence fees as well as the income from commercial advertising. This meant that they could outbid any private network, largely at tax-payers' expense. For instance, both Canale 5 and RAI had competed for *Gone with the Wind*, but RAI had won because it had doubled the fees offered by Canale 5. It was a pity, too, that the private stations had to agree to RAI's monopoly of the news. It meant that, as always, the political parties could give their own version of events.

"But wouldn't you be linked to some party?" I asked, knowing that Silvio Berlusconi, his brother, was a personal friend of Craxi's.

"Well – perhaps. But we'd try not to be – at least with the news. What we'd like to do is to provide a really professional private alternative to State television – like ITV in Britain."

In fact, the Berlusconis now seem well on their way to doing this. In 1984, they bought another television station, Rete 4, and, despite Paolo's complaints about RAI's increased resources, total revenue is about 800 billion lire ($320 million) – almost the same as RAI gets from its licence fees. At the same time, the Berlusconis have had to put up with a lot of opposition: accusations of seeking a monopoly, and magistrates closing down their networks for short periods twice during 1984, in Turin, Rome and Pescara. In January 1985, however, a law was passed making private television indisputably legal.

The same duality applies to radio, where the three channels in RAI have their corresponding radio stations and there are also a mass of private broadcasts. "In Britain you would call them 'pirate' radios," said a friend of mine who works for RAI. "There are so many that if you are driving with the radio on, you are switched automatically to a new station whenever you turn a corner!"

This multiplicity does not apply to newspapers. Whereas one in three Britons reads a daily newspaper, only one in every eleven Italians does so, and the total circulation is only five million. It is often said that there are no national newspapers in Italy: *La Stampa* comes from Turin, *Il Giornale* and *Corriere della Sera* from Milan, and *La Repubblica* from Rome. These, though, are sold all over Italy, particularly in the North, and also abroad. *La Stampa* is owned by Giovanni Agnelli although, according to his editor, he interferes very little.

Two of these newspapers depend very much on their editors. Indro Montanelli of *Il Giornale* has always maintained a fiercely independent line, a no-nonsense approach which many Italians dub Right wing. As one journalist from Rome said to me: "Montanelli ensured that *Il Giornale* was the only sensible newspaper when the modish Left wing was in full swing in the 1970s." He has said of himself: "I'm a heretic. It's just as well I was born in this century or I would have finished at the stake!" As far as politics are concerned, he calls himself an "Anarcho-Conservative".

La Repubblica is one of the few newspapers which is increasing its circulation, largely because it is edited by one of the most brilliant editors in Italy, La Scalfari. If you talk to Right-wing people they will tell you that *La Repubblica* is Left, but as a foreigner you don't notice it. Certainly, it criticizes the Socialists or Communists as much as the Christian Democrats. It is perhaps the most bulky newspaper in Italy with many long pieces and extensive cultural and financial sections, but it also publishes articles by many of the leading journalists: Levi, Ronchey, Bocca. Politicians also have an opportunity of expressing their views, or answering points made against them, and there are sometimes long forums on the ills Italy suffers from, like the one on the economy quoted on page 108.

Corriere della Sera used to be the leading paper in Italy and, with a daily circulation of 600,000, it is still the most widely distributed – apart from *Gazzetta dello Sport* which, as might be expected, sells a million copies. The *Corriere* was originally modelled on *The Times* but it was almost eliminated by the naiveté of Angelo Rizzoli who bought it in 1974. It is a pathetic story of an optimistic young man who put his father's firm, one of the major publishers in Italy, deeply in debt to buy the newspaper and then found that the *Corriere* itself was in debt, to the tune of 20 billion lire ($10 million). Finding it difficult to raise loans, he ultimately allied himself with Gelli, the Venerable Master of the P2, and with Calvi who eventually was found hanged under Blackfriars Bridge. In the 1970s he expanded, with dreams of a press-television tie-up, and bought up small newspapers which were making a loss. "We were convinced we could pay our debts with the inflation," he said later. Finally, with the discrediting of Calvi and of the P2, he was arrested for fraudulent transactions and the whole firm of Rizzoli was put into receivership. Now the *Corriere* still limps on, abandoned by many of its best journalists.

All these newspapers are much more wordy than their equivalents in the Anglo-Saxon press. They are also more serious and probably go into the news in greater depth than their British equivalents. There are no tabloids. Rizzoli tried to launch one called *L'Occhio* but it had to close after six months.

In addition, there are the party newspapers of which the only one worthy of note is *L'Unità*, the Communist newspaper, largely because it is a consistent and ruthless opponent of the government and particularly of the Christian Democrats. In international news it is fairly straightforward and factual, but otherwise full of attacks on corruption, possible government links with the Camorra and the Mafia, "abusive" housing, the scandals of the tax system and the malfunctioning of the Welfare State. Nevertheless it is a dull newspaper, and as one of its editors admitted to me doesn't really reflect the richness and variety of the Communist Party in Italy.

Started under Fascism in 1924, *L'Unità* was closed after two years and revived in 1944. Gramsci chose the title as a symbol of the desired unification of the workers of the North and the peasants of the South. After the war, Togliatti wanted it to be a proper newspaper and not just a propaganda organ like other party newspapers. Now it sells an average of 150,000 copies daily with 500,000 on Sunday when it is sold from door to door by volunteers, without whom the paper would collapse. There has been a lot of discussion recently about whether it should have the words "Organ of the Italian Communist Party" below its name on the front page. Certainly, its circulation seems to have little to do with the number of Communist sympathizers in an area. Thus sales in Parma, where 35 per cent of the population are Communist, are negligible, and in Turin, where Communists represent 40 per cent of the inhabitants, it sells only 4,000.

Undoubtedly the most successful newspapers are the local ones, as might be expected in Italy. One of the best known is the Bologna newspaper, *Il Resto del Carlino* – a name that comes from the days when the *carlino* was a coin and the newspaper was given instead of change when a packet of cigarettes was bought. Although it is published in a region where there has been a Communist majority since 1945, the owner's policy backs the five-party coalition government.

"The owner lays down the margins within which we can operate. They're very broad. Then he leaves us to get on with it," the editor told me. Nevertheless, there is no clash with the Communists. Indeed, nothing better illustrates the way in which the regionalism of a newspaper is more important than political differences. People buy it because it reflects their homeland, whatever the owner's political views. In Bologna *Il Resto del Carlino* sells 80,000 copies, while *L'Unità* has a circulation of only 6–7,000.

All these local newspapers have a fairly full coverage of international and national news. Thus, the relatively small *Quotidiano di Lecce*, which covers south Puglia, has twenty-four pages. Of these, on November 3rd 1983, the front page covered mainly international news, four were on Italian affairs, one on the economy, three on foreign news, one on education, one on opinions, one on the European Cup and there was a page article on Beirut. The remaining half of the newspaper covered local news: one page on the region, four on Lecce and the province, one on sport in Lecce, two on the province of Brindisi, further up the coast, and one on Taranto. Anyone reading the *Quotidiano* would be reasonably well-informed on local, national and international news. The same applies to larger local newspapers like *La Gazzetta del Mezzogiorno* from Bari or *Il Mattino* from Naples. Even newspapers which are read throughout Italy like *La Repubblica* or *L'Unità* will have a section on local news in the different areas where they are distributed. Thus *L'Unità* has twelve pages of local news in Bologna – almost as many as *Il Resto del Carlino*'s fourteen.

What it comes to, then, is that most newspapers have the same balance of local, national and international news. The basic difference lies, as so often, between North and South. Whereas the bigger papers of the North are sold all over Italy and abroad, those in the South do not have the structure which makes this possible. As so often, it is Northern points of view which predominate and this applies particularly abroad where only the papers from the North are well-known – particularly the Milanese *Corriere della Sera*.

One reason Italians do not read newspapers so much is that there are a large number of weekly magazines which are designed to appeal to everybody. One group follows the lines of the American *Time* Magazine or the French *L'Express*. The best known are *Panorama*, *L'Espresso*, and *Europeo*. They consist of articles on a wide range of subjects from politics to finance and cultural events. Their speciality is research in depth, usually on sensational subjects dealt with in a serious way: drugs, homosexuality, where Italians make love etc. But they also deal with recurrent national problems: the crises in justice, housing, the health service, the economy. In summer, nudes appear on their covers to represent research into subjects such as "Torrid Summer: Causes, Effects and Remedies", "Topless", "On Holiday with Eros", "Perfect Holidays". Inside there are no snickers and little suggestiveness. After all, the cover may be a way of selling more copies, but at the same time these are subjects which are interesting in themselves.

These magazines are full of advertisements and, as a journalist on *L'Espresso* told me, "It is a magazine which has to be written so that advertisements can be sold." *L'Espresso* sells about three hundred thousand copies a week. Because of this and because Italian is not a world language like English, this type of magazine does not sell internationally or have its own foreign correspondents – unlike *Time* or *Newsweek*. It gets its news items secondhand. *L'Espresso*'s contributors have to get their articles in by a Monday and the magazine is not printed until the following Monday, so while it remains topical, it is not always completely up to date. As it is more concerned with research projects and comment, this is not so important. However, it cannot compete with the wide-ranging topical surveys of the great American weeklies, or *The Economist*.

Another more homely type of magazine which is widely read is represented by *Oggi* and *Domenica del Corriere*. These magazines illustrate an important characteristic of the Italian press in general: the fact that they do not write for specific social groups but attempt in one publication to satisfy readers of every kind. There seems to be no differentiation between "lowbrow" and "highbrow" – perhaps because most Italians are not aware of this distinction themselves. In either of these magazines you may get a continuing obsession with the antics of Caroline of Monaco in the same edition as an interview with Prime Minister Craxi, or a serious analysis of the iniquities of the taxation system, along with a correspondence page, a horoscope and two or three opinion pages on topical issues, whether the P2 or the examination system. Both magazines are enlivened by photographs.

On the whole, then, the Italian press deals with any subject, even the possible embroilment of ministers – who are not named – in the Mafia or in train explosions. It is conservative in that it has nothing sensational like *The People* or the *News of the World*, has no tabloids, and displays on the whole a stolid format. It is rarely vulgar, and illustrates the general absence of divisions of class or of "intellectualism". It gives good coverage to foreign news. Much of the press is local, but it is rarely provincial. Perhaps for these reasons, it is not so widely read.

NOVELS

Twice since the war, the Italians have produced a novel which has swept the world. The first was *The Leopard* by Giuseppe Di Lampedusa in 1957. The second was *The Name of the Rose* by Umberto Eco in 1981. Eco is a professor of semiotics at Bologna university. He has written many academic works but this is his first novel. In a televised interview in New York, he was asked why he had written it. "I felt I wanted to kill off a monk," he said, flippantly. He had spent a year, as he put it, "creating his world" – that of a monastery in the foothills of the Alps in the fourteenth century. From that world, characters and events had then developed naturally. "I expected it to be a best seller," he said ironically. "You know, all those girls! Such a modern environment! No philosophy!"

The novel is a detective story. Investigations are carried out by William of Baskerville, a visiting Englishman who is a monk. Not only is his name reminiscent of Sherlock Holmes but he even has a Dr Watson in the shape of his companion, a young monk called Adso who is the narrator of the story. Gradually the mystery caused by seven monks who die in strange circumstances is unravelled: one found in a cask of pig's blood, another floating in a bath house, another battered at the foot of a cliff.

The novel is extraordinary in the way it maintains interest through long discussions on whether Christ laughed and whether prelates should be poor, the clashes between Emperor and Pope of those times, and lengthy descriptions of the monastery itself. The reader is sustained by the authenticity and, thus, the fascination of discovering life in a fourteenth-century monastery, almost, it seems, at first hand. Eco is also skilful at raising the "detective" issue whenever interest might wane, and he writes superbly. There are, for instance, no less than five pages describing the sculptured figures perceived by Adso when he enters the church of the Abbey. Some transfigure him with joy but then his eyes alight on the monsters:

I saw a voluptuous woman, naked and fleshless, gnawed by foul toads, sucked by serpents, coupled with a fat-bellied satyr whose gryphon legs were covered with wiry hairs, howling its own damnation from an obscene throat; and I saw a miser, stiff in the stiffness of death on his sumptuously columned bed, now helpless prey of a cohort of demons, one of whom tore from the dying man's mouth his soul in the form of an infant (alas never to be again born to eternal life).

Eco shows the relevance of these five pages to the main story when Adso begins to feel that these sculptures represent what the monks are actually going to live out in reality. The whole description is thus given significance and suspense.

A publisher who knows Eco told me he had constructed this novel as a form of intellectual exercise, which is possible. Certainly, he must have derived a lot of pleasure in designing the monastery and particularly the library which has an intricate plan of fifty-six rooms, arranged with letters which correspond to "the image of the terraqueous orb". Finally, we find out that the reason for this slaughter of monks is that those murdered have discovered a hitherto unknown book by Aristotle on "Laughter", which in the opinion of an Anti-Christ, as William of Baskerville calls him, could bring about the ultimate collapse of the Faith through irreverence and mockery.

Such intellectual exercises brought down to the level of the average reader are characteristic of other modern Italian novels. In *1934* (published in 1982) Alberto Moravia contrives a complicated plot, influenced by the German poet Kleist's suicide pact with his mistress, Henriette Vogel. After publication, Moravia said in an interview that during the years 1976–80 he had been obsessed with the idea of suicide every morning when he woke up, but felt better once he had had a shower!

The story is set in Capri and revolves round the identity of two sisters who both look the same. Lucio, a young Italian intellectual, falls in love with the first sister, Beate, who has come to Capri with her husband. He follows them about, even hiding behind rocks while her husband is taking nude photos of her. They pass each other notes and she promises to come to his room but then departs one morning, to be replaced at lunch by her sister, Trude, who is accompanied by a mannish woman, and is as forthcoming as Beate was cautious and restrained. At this stage, the reader is confronted by various dilemmas: Are the two sisters the same person? If so, why is she playing these different roles? Is this a real love story or simply an imposed replica of what happened to Kleist and his mistress? I found both plot and characterization "acrobatic" rather than significant.

Critical Italian friends of mine feel that Moravia is always producing the same novel, which I think is a little unfair. In 1983 he produced a book of erotic short stories called *La Cosa* which has such varied situations as two lesbians with a pony, or a nurse who always touches up patients as long as they are covered by a sheet. As he said in a recent interview, he writes a lot about sex because it is one of the foremost means of communication. If singing were as effective a way for human beings to relate with one another, he would, he said, write more about singing.

It is interesting how a number of Italian writers feel the need for some kind of trellis, as if they can only grow their vines once that has been provided. In *Solitudes*, a collection of short stories which won the Strega prize in 1982, Goffredo Parise finds it necessary for some reason to give abstract nouns in alphabetical order, from "Felicità" to "Solitudine", as titles of his stories. What advantage this arrangement has, apart from its irrelevant sense of method, is difficult to determine. In fact, some of the stories are very moving, a few going back to the war. Solitude can mean either strength or pathos. Both of these are exemplified, whether in the story of the German soldier with his Italian friends, watching a hundred American planes going over to bomb Verona, or in "Patriotism", a story about an old man who has lost a leg in the war and accuses a young boy of lack of national spirit for refusing to help an old war veteran unzip his trousers in a public lavatory. There is something surrealist about these stories, which are at the same time condensed, controlled and vivid.

How far, though, does contemporary literature reflect Italian social problems? In *Uccelli da gabbia e da voliera* (Birds in cages or on the wing), Andrea da Carlo tells the story of a young man who is persuaded by his father and brother to work for a soulless American firm in Milan. He falls in love with a girl who is involved with a member of the Red Brigades. The novel is written in the historic present, and the atmosphere is created by descriptions of a multitude of successive actions rather than by any account of what the characters feel. There is a sense of paranoia, and of mystery as the man in the Red Brigade is shot and the girl is afraid the police are after her.

Other novels deal with specific problems. Thus Anna Banti in *Il grido lacerante* (The shattering shout) tells the story of a woman who sacrifices her ambitions for the love of her husband. Ugo Pirro, in *Gli ultimi giorni di Magliano* (The last days of Magliano) depicts a psychiatrist who deplores the loneliness and despair of his mental patients who are ejected when his mental hospital closes down under Law 180 (see p. 245). Of a more general nature is Ferdinando Camon's *La malattia chiamata uomo* (The illness called man) which depicts the sense of emptiness of the older generation which is without belief in the Church or a political party, confronted by feminism, and obliged to abandon its dialects and speak Italian.

One interesting novelist, who is well-known in Italy and France, and has had many of his novels made into films, is Leonardo Sciascia, now over sixty. He writes mainly about Sicily, where he was born. When I talked to him in Palermo, he said he had been greatly influenced by French literature and his short, limpid books have much of the style of French novelists in the '40s and '50s, from Vercors to Camus. Interestingly enough, he also said that Spanish writers who analysed their country, like Ortega y Gasset, had helped him understand Sicily.

Many of his novels portray an individual pitted against the web of the Mafia, or of vested interests. In *A ciascuno il suo* (To everyone his own), a middle-aged schoolmaster who lives with his mother has suspicions about the murder of a doctor and a chemist on a hunting expedition. As he makes his way home one evening he is offered a lift, and disappears. In *Il giorno della civetta* (The day of the owl), a lieutenant in the Carabinieri from Parma in the North investigates the murder of a man who was shot in the early morning as he got onto a bus. Cleverly, he extracts confessions from the people he suspects, but a minister in Rome is involved and in the end his whole case collapses.

The novels are masterpieces of tense restraint. They are also full of literary allusions. In *A ciascuno il suo* there are references to Virgil, Dante, Pirandello and many novelists, including Verga and Brancati. Such allusions are also to be found in Alberto Bevilaqua, another modern novelist, and are yet another indication of the lack of division between "lowbrow" and "highbrow" in Italy. A novel is regarded as part of literature, and whatever its theme should have its cultural references.

In all these novels there are few sparks of humour and much serious criticism of Italians and Italy today. Satire and comedy are left to the theatre and particularly to Dario Fo, the actor and playwright. Life is serious now in Italy and has to be written about as it is. Creation is serious too, even when it is an intellectual game. The days of Don Camillo are over.

THEATRE

The actors are sweeping round the stage in long cloaks when there is a cry from the audience: "It's all wrong!" "Not like that!" A man with a long coloured nose comes on stage, shouting, and throws all the actors' cloaks into a tub full of water. The water is sloshed around the stage. Some of it splashes onto the audience. Fortunately, it is warm. The stage remains puddled for the rest of the performance, effectively creating the effect of discomfort and mess of a hall in a medieval castle.

Macbeth settles down in front of television and discusses with his wife the murder of Duncan·who, in a cap and dark glasses, plays Patience at a table in the background. Macbeth first tries to shoot him. Duncan cries out but continues playing Patience. Then Macbeth knifes him. There is the same reaction. Finally Macbeth succeeds, and Duncan is laid out on the table and photographed from every angle by reporters.

The new king watches his coronation on television, approves, salutes. The feast begins. The ghost of Banquo leans, dead, on the table and everyone ignores him, except of course Macbeth who howls at this bloody face grinning up at him. Banquo falls under the table which is laid with plastic plates and a silver dish-cover. Macbeth raises the dish-cover and there is Banquo's head. Macbeth goes into paroxysms. Someone raises the dish-cover once more, and a hunk of meat has taken the place of Banquo's head. Lady Macbeth, who has been smoking throughout, disappears and kills herself. Meanwhile, Macbeth is reading a version of the play which says that he won't be killed until a wood moves. An actor appears with a little, false Christmas tree. Then Macduff appears, and Macbeth shoots one of his soldiers with a water pistol. Macduff explains that he was born by Caesarian section. Macbeth succumbs and then gets up and makes a speech, telling the audience that the play is over. All the actors stand on stage to the accompaniment of bagpipe music, so that clapping continues for a long time, caught up in the rhythm.

This is the Collettivo di Parma, whose work, writes John Francis Lane in the *Guardian*, "has been justifiably hailed as one of the great stage events of recent years in Europe". The group started in 1971, although most of its participants had already been working in the theatre. They were influenced by the experience of going through the "hot years" after 1968, by the Living Theatre which was expelled from Italy in 1969 for nudity on the stage, and by the visits of Charles Marowitz. Their theatre programme describes their development: co-operation with Dario Fo and Eduardo de Filippo, the maintenance of a rich comic tradition, political theatre. Then, in 1977, when "the 'heroic' phase of Italian theatre comes to an end ... the aim is both to examine individual feelings and to explore the universal truths in great literature".

The Collettivo is a co-operative and has no director. I went to see Gigi Dall'Agio who is their spokesman and who said that the Collettivo believed that theatre should reflect what actors feel. Actors, indeed, should not just try to interpret the roles that have been given to them, but create and reflect their own world in what they are performing. The tradition comes from the Commedia dell'Arte where actors thought up a whole range of dialogue before coming on stage, and then expressed it at random. For the Collettivo, actors are not separate from the audience. They are just other human beings expressing their personal reactions to a play. In this way they bring the play up to date. To perform Shakespeare in modern dress, or in a modern environment, is artificial. But to have a contemporary actor expressing his own feelings about his role means re-interpreting the sixteenth century in terms of the twentieth – however varied the reactions of different actors might be. The important thing is to have at least four months' rehearsal on each play. This gives time virtually to re-create Shakespeare on stage which I, as an Englishman, might think arrogant – but then Shakespeare belongs to all of us.

Why, though, I asked, couldn't they write their own plays? It was extraordinary the way only foreign plays were performed at Italian drama festivals. Italian playwrights, it seemed, did not exist, apart from Eduardo de Filippo and Dario Fo.

There is no tradition of really Italian playwrights, said Gigi Dall'Agio. Goldoni was a Venetian, Pirandello a Sicilian; Eduardo de Filippo was Neapolitan. Although lots of young people are interested in the theatre and the government gives a bigger subsidy to Italian playwrights, they don't attract audiences as do established plays.

Perhaps, anyway, it is no bad thing to create new drama actually on the stage rather than in an attic. Dario Fo has written over thirty plays since 1953. Several have been shown in London recently: *Accidental Death of an Anarchist*, *Can't Pay! Won't Pay!* and, in 1984/5, *Trumpets and Raspberries*. These satires are continuously revised to keep the political comment up to date. *Death of an Anarchist*, Fo told me, originated in a public debate in the early '70s in which hundreds of people asked him to write a play attacking the police, and made suggestions, some of which were incorporated. This was at a time when the police were thought to be responsible for pushing the anarchist Pinelli out of a window during an interrogation on his role in the Piazza Fontana bomb explosion in Milan in 1969.

Apart from these plays, Fo's *Mistero Buffo* is a one-man show of mime and improvisation which relies very much on contact with the audience. Seeing it in London at the Riverside Theatre, I was interested to notice Dave Allen, the Irish television comedian, among the audience. For Dario Fo's show, like Allen's, is full of satire on the Catholic Church. It made me even more aware of what an issue the Church still is both in Ireland and in Italy. When shown on Italian television in 1977, *Mistero Buffo* outraged both Catholics and Communists. Catholics inevitably disliked the mimed sketch about Pope Boniface VIII who, as he is dressing up in all his robes, suddenly sees Jesus approach bearing his Cross.

"Who is that?" he asks a retainer.

"Jesus!"

"Jesus?" he is perplexed.

"Yes. Jesus Christ."

"Oh, of course. Confusion is inevitable with two names like that!"

"Who are you?" asks Christ.

"Your Pope."

"Pope?"

"You remember you made Peter your representative on Earth? I'm his heir."

"His heir? I never made Peter my representative!"

The sketch on the raising of Lazarus also drew complaints. It takes place in a cemetery as if it were a popular festival. Bets are taken on whether Jesus will succeed or not. And when the tomb is opened, there is an imitation of a horse race. "Yes, he's beginning to get up. Oh, he's staggering. No, he's all right. He's almost up. Yes – yes – he's on his feet now!" Bets are paid, reluctantly, and then the narrator realizes that his pocket has been picked.

The Communists objected because they felt that Fo had adopted a concept of culture framed by intellectuals, rather than a "dialect culture" arising from the people.

In fact, both Dario Fo and his wife Franca Rame have been consistently persecuted, mainly by the Right wing and the police, ever since they left the commercial circuit in 1968 and set up their own company. With *Accidental Death of an Anarchist*, the police did everything they could to stop the show, even declaring that there was a bomb in the theatre. In 1973, Franca Rame was assaulted and covered with cigarette burns by a Right-wing group. The most spectacular triumph against this kind of persecution was when Fo was arrested in Sassari in Sardinia, just before he was going to do a show, and the audience demonstrated outside the prison, with other people coming in bus loads from neighbouring towns. Franca Rame gave a performance on top of car roofs, the press soon turned up to report on this major political demonstration, and Dario Fo was released next morning.

In terms of popular acclaim the Fos have had immense success, playing on occasion to audiences of fifty thousand. They often give benefit shows in factories on strike, in market places, even once in a football stadium. The shows are full of that personal banter with the audience which Italians are so good at.

Fo told me that he first became interested in miming and stories when he was a boy and went to sit of an evening with the glass-blowers on the shores of Lake Maggiore. "The stories they told sometimes went back thousands of years," he said. Then at university in Milan he had acted in student shows and had gone on to become a designer in the theatre, which had almost given him a nervous breakdown. "You should do what you're really interested in," an intelligent doctor told him, and his full theatrical career began.

Politically, it is no easier to define Dario Fo than it is many Italians. Perhaps if Montanelli is an Anarcho-Conservative, Fo is an Anarcho-Communist. Indeed, he would make a good, irreverent jester if the Communists had a court. His first group, Nuova Scena, was under the aegis of the Communists, but the association lasted only two years as his shows were too critical of the Soviet Union and the party's "revisionism". Certainly, though, he is exuberantly Left-wing, in favour of striking workers and against the lies he believes hierarchies fabricate in order to keep power. Now, of course, when disillusionment with the '70s is so strong in Italy, he is perhaps less convinced. " We made many mistakes," he said when I met him in 1984, "but mistakes are, sadly, inevitable."

Franca Rame, Dario Fo's wife, is also a brilliant playwright, actress and director, with a strong feminist emphasis. Among her best work is *A Woman Alone* which describes the misery of being a woman who has a husband she is not interested in, an obsessive lover, a brother-in-law who lodges in her flat in a wheelchair, wrapped in bandages after an accident, whose only mobile member is a hand which grabs any woman who happens to go near him. There is also a heavy breather who phones her regularly, and a peeping tom who lives in a flat opposite. The one person she can confide in is a female neighbour who lives just below the peeping tom, and to whom she speaks through the window.

In the end, she goes berserk, shoots the peeping tom, wounds the hand of her lover which has got caught in the front door, propels her brother-in-law down the stairs where you can hear him go down landing by landing, until finally he crashes through a window: "Ah! the stained glass window on the mezzanine!"

With her awakened baby howling its head off, she waits for her husband to arrive, with the rifle on her knee.

In an interview with Jim Hiley in the *Observer*, Dario Fo talked about Italy: "... yes, we are in a serious crisis. But some intellectuals enjoy booing and shouting of catastrophe. What is the responsibility of someone in my position? As Brecht said, in dark times we must sing of dark times. Not to wallow in them. To get rid of them."

Another giant of the Italian theatre is Eduardo de Filippo, who died in 1984 at the age of eighty-three. He too was an actor, director and playwright who expressed the life and exuberance of Naples, where he was born, in countless plays. His father was an actor, as were his sister Titina and brother Peppino, and his plays deal with the eccentricities, miseries, humour and tricks of the Neapolitan family, with its need to survive, its closeness, its treacheries. In *Inner Voices*, set in Naples in 1948, the intricate plot revolves round the relationship between two brothers, the Saporitos, and their neighbours, the Cimmarutas. Alberto Saporito accuses the Cimmarutas of murdering a man and concealing the corpse in a wall. The police find nothing and it looks as though Alberto is going to be accused of bearing false witness, while the Cimmarutas, who include a possessive spinster aunt and a mother who spends a suspiciously long time telling men's fortunes, also accuse each other. In the end it becomes clear that the person who has betrayed Alberto is his brother Carlo, who hopes to inherit all the furniture once his brother is imprisoned.

Eduardo, as de Filippo was called simply by everyone, continued acting and writing right up to his death. In 1983, he put on a solo performance at the festa in Montalcino where he played out various roles of his play *Questi Fantasmi* (These ghosts), recited some of his poetry and showed a film he had made in 1935. In 1984, he gave another solo performance of his translation into Neapolitan dialect of *The Tempest*. Here, again, we find the tradition of the Commedia dell'Arte: of improvised performances, of the combination of director, playwright and actor in one person, of the interpretation of drama in one place and, often, in dialect.

Vittorio Gassman has been another major contributor to popular theatre. In the 1960s he toured with a steel tent which moved from place to place, with cheap tickets. Recently he has put on *Macbeth* and *Othello* and, like Eduardo, "An evening with Gassman" of improvised monologues. He too is so eminent in Italy that when the Hollywood film star Shelley Winters divorced him, she said: "I thought I had married an actor – not an Italian institution."

Of course, Italian theatre has other outstanding actors, like Rosella Falk and Anna Proclemer, brilliant directors like Giorgio Strehler of Il Piccolo Teatro of Milan, and Maurizio Scaparro who in 1984 directed an extraordinary *Don Quixote*. Usually, though, they confine themselves to foreign plays.

Beside them are those who draw on the regions where everything in Italy has its roots: Dario Fo starting his career listening to the glass-blowers of Lago Maggiore, Eduardo with the lower life of Naples. I remember a young mime artiste, Giovanna Rogante, telling me how when she was a student at Bologna university, she would go out with a group to the neighbouring villages and perform an old verse play, *La Gorilla Quattro Mani*. They acted it out in traditional rhyme, and the audience of older people would interrupt with improvisations. There were also rhyme competitions. One person would start with a line and another would cap it. The winner was the one who could go on the longest, and one man could improvise like this for three hours. One of the favourite subjects was the brigand Musolino, a kind of Robin Hood.

In Sicily you can still see the traditional puppet shows. I remember going to a performance of the Napoli brothers from Catania, whose group acted out the medieval Duel between Orlando and Agricane. The puppets are four and a half feet high, splendid knights, weighing as much as forty kilos. As a result, their movements are stiff. They are manipulated head first, dragging their feet after them, and when they prepare for battle, they stamp one leg forward. In the show there was a lot of "conversation" between the knights, provided from back stage, accompanied by the banging of sword on shield. Fights were "realistic": heads came off, or blood spurted out suddenly from the armour. A damsel, Angelica, was rescued and a dragon and a giant slain. "We do it all from love," Signora Napoli told me after the performance. "We have over a hundred and seventy puppets. Some of them are a hundred and twenty years old. All the armour and vestments are made by hand. It is all from love!"

CINEMA

We walked down the Via Rasella in Rome. Here, thirty-two Germans were killed by partisans with a bomb in 1943, which resulted in the massacre of over three hundred hostages in the Ardeatine caves. The bomb-splinter marks were still on the wall of a house on the right, half way down the street.

Ahead of us, a police car suddenly appeared, picked up a girl of about fifteen who was standing nearby, and drove off slowly. We followed them. They stopped about fifty yards away and all got out. They walked a few yards, with the policemen on either side of the girl, then went up some steps and disappeared down an alleyway. "What's happening?" I muttered. The steps were broad, ochre-coloured and slightly crumbling from centuries of use. We climbed them hesitantly. They led to an alleyway with high walls on either side. Round a corner, the policemen were talking with subdued voices to the girl. When we approached, they were all silent and stood motionless. As we passed them, I looked at the girl. She had calm brown eyes, without any expression of alarm. We walked on, and then looked back. The policemen were talking softly again; the girl had her head inclined. A few minutes later, we returned, and the alley was empty. From nearby, there was the soft noise of an engine as a car pulled away.

We never solved the mystery. The police didn't seem to be interrogating the girl as if she had committed a crime. Was she giving information? Perhaps she was the daughter of one of them. But why, then, were they so subdued, without the exuberance which normally accompanies the meeting of relatives in Italy? Perhaps she was a police spy, and they were giving her instructions.

Whatever it was, it made me realize why Italian films can be so absorbing. It was as though the policemen and the girl had been acting out a scene. There was the memory of the dead Germans. Also, the alleyway, the crumbling steps. There was the mystery. Most Italian cities, particularly Rome, are film sets. Italians are a dramatic people.

Nevertheless, sadly, the Italian film industry has been declining over recent years. Many of the great directors of the '60s and '70s are dead: Pasolini, De Sica, Visconti, Rossellini. Since private television stations were allowed in 1978, there has been strong competition. Many cinemas are closed: David Willey mentions in his *Italians* that there used to be four cinemas in L'Aquila, the capital of the Abruzzi. Now there is none. In its heyday in 1968, Italy produced 294 new films. In 1984, in produced about 30. Cinecittà, the Italian film city in Rome which almost rivalled Hollywood in the '60s, only survives because television studios still use it.

In Rome, Francesco Rosi, the director of *Giuliano* and *Excellent Corpses*, told me that the cost of making films had gone up so much that most make a loss. The government gives no subsidies, although it does to theatre. Young people, he said, were too interested in the symbols of wealth now to have much interest, and the Left which had once stimulated so many films had exchanged integrity for demagogy. He had just returned from Seville where he was working on his *Carmen* and had been impressed by the way Spain without Franco was similar in enthusiasm and drive to Italy after the war when, in films, the great surge for self-expression had led to the neo-realism of the '60s.

Saddest of all is seeing brilliant directors like Lina Wertmuller now producing vapid films. Wertmuller directed the widely acclaimed *Seven Beauties* which is a cruel satire on the Italians' ability to survive under any circumstances. However, in the '80s Wertmuller has restricted herself to spry comedies: *Scherzo* is an absurd, involved movie which starts with a minister who finds himself imprisoned in his car because the regulatory computer fails; *Sotto, Sotto* tells the story of a school-girlish, lesbian love affair between two wives, which ends with a farcical fracas with the husband of one of them. The most irritating part is the self-conscious way the characters talk.

The '80s, though, have produced some remarkable films in the grand tradition. The Taviani brothers, who were responsible for *Padre Padrone*, collaborated with RAI to release *Chaos* in 1984, based on four short stories by Pirandello, set inevitably in Sicily. This form is felicitous for a film/television combination, as length is adjustable simply by omitting a story. Some of the camerawork is breathtaking. The stories are linked by a crow to which peasants have attached a bell, which flies over stark mountains or scrub-covered hills on which perch small villages or castles, giving a sense of the countryside in which the action is set. One scene shows Garibaldi, gaunt on a horse, holding a banner. In another, a family of children dive down a steep, long slope of white pumice stone to the blue sea below. One story is about a mother, in despair because her son emigrated to America years before. In a field nearby is her illegitimate son who is a shepherd. But she cannot bear to speak to him because he looks just like his father, who raped her and killed her husband. Another, which is very funny, is about a potter who makes a great jar for a landowner, then breaks it and is imprisoned inside when he repairs it.

Rosi, too, has found new lyricism with his *Three Brothers*. In the film the brothers, who have emigrated to the North, are reunited at their home in Apulia when their mother dies. They take part in the mourning ceremonies of keening women in black. A little grand-daughter goes up to the big attic and finds it full of grain, which she has never seen before in industrial Turin where she lives. She takes off her clothes and "swims" delightedly in the corn. There are various flashbacks to their parents' life together. In one, on their honeymoon, their young mother loses her wedding ring in the sand on the beach. The father rushes off and brings a large sieve, and they find the ring at last in the remains of sifted sand. At the end of the film, the credits are shown against the background of the old man's hand wearing both his own ring and that of his wife.

Olmi, the director of *Tree of the Wooden Clogs*, produced a film *Cammina, Cammina* which was acclaimed at Cannes in 1983. In it Olmi goes back to the Journey of the Kings in the New Testament. A joyous group of pilgrims wend their way to Bethlehem, exuberant, humane, simple people with lively children.

Fellini, maestro of the old Italian cinema, devised a strange fantasy, released in 1984, called *E la Nave va* (And the ship sails off). Set in 1914, it is the story of a pilgrimage of opera singers, artistes, a portly young Habsburg duke and his blind sister, to spread the ashes of a diva who has died over the sea near an Adriatic island. The group are distinguished by their extraordinary ugliness and egocentricity. There is a scene of the furnaces of the ship with the artistes standing high up on a gallery, watching the stokers work. Suddenly, one of the singers trills an aria, going on as long as she can. Another artiste competes, and another – while the stokers, black with coal, look up in amazement. Then a group of Balkan refugees come aboard, fleeing from the war which has just broken out. They cluster on deck, staring curiously as the passengers eat their copious meals. An Austrian cruiser appears, a fantasy image, all enormous guns and steel walls. The refugees take to the boats and throw a bomb down one of the funnels. In the explosion, the cruiser's guns go off and sink the ship. One of the diva's fanatical admirers sits in his cabin, watching a film of her, while the water rises. The journalist who has acted as narrator rows off in a small boat on a contrived silver paper sea.

Political themes have now almost disappeared from the cinema, apart from a few like Bertolucci's *The Tragedy of a Ridiculous Man*, about the middle-aged owner of a cheese factory whose son is captured by the Red Brigades. Unfortunately, so many of the enigmas which arise are never resolved. At the end, the son, whom the father thought was dead, appears casually – almost as if he were just returning from a ski-ing holiday. Not even an indication of what happened to him is revealed.

There are nevertheless a number of young directors who give confidence for the future. Maurizio Nichetti's *Splash* is a highly original pantomime satirizing modern advertising. Nanni Moretti's *Bianca*, released in 1984, is an eccentric account of a teacher in a modern school. Moretti plays the main part and everything seems to depend on his irregular forceful moods, which exist in a vacuum of pointlessness as a reaction to the superficial educational approach at the school, the lack of any reason to make an effort, the fact that no one seems at all *simpatico* – except the inspector who finally arrests him for murder, and who, like the main character, wears odd shoes.

The absence of sentimentality in modern Italian cinema is interesting. In Massimo Troisi's *Starting from Three* a young Neapolitan wanderer is drawn into bed by a mental nurse, who gives him lodging without much ado, and so their casual relationship continues. In *The Hustlers (Io, Chiara e lo scuro)*, a young couple who quarrel on a tram are ultimately drawn together and co-operate so that he wins the Italian billiard championships, which is the most important part of the film. One cannot imagine an Italian *Love Story*. In most Italian films couples seem to take each other for granted, with affection but little apparent ardour. Exceptions involve less conventional approaches to love, like Franco Brogi Taviani's *Masoch*, which is an up-to-date interpretation of masochistic love, or Salvatore Piscelli's *Immacolata and Concetta: The Other Jealousy*, which depicts an affair between two women of different social classes, ending in the murder of the richer woman who has betrayed the other with a man.

Certainly the Italian cinema is still vital, despite its reduction in size. The link with television has been and will probably continue to be productive. Peter Bondanella sums up the customary Italian flaw when he writes in *Italian Cinema*: "As ever, the weakness of the film industry in Italy derives not from a dearth of individual talent, but, rather, from the relative instability of its economic structure, and its production, distribution, and financial system."

MUSIC

In Perugia, I talked to Andrew Starling, an Englishman who runs the "Amici della Musica", which operates not only in Perugia but also in Palermo, Rome, Turin and L'Aquila. The association originated with a private sponsor, Alba Buitone, but now gets the equivalent of $90,000 a year from the government, although when the money will arrive is always uncertain. As a result, they have to spend $10,000 a year on interest for loans.

The State has always subsidized music, emphasized Andrew, ever since the days of Papal patronage which was largely responsible for the outburst of Italian musical talent since the Renaissance. The advantage of State sponsorship is that it is possible to hold more concerts of modern music than in Britain, where private sponsors want to attract as many people as possible with better-known music.

Andrew Starling's immediate problem was to find a suitable concert hall. Ever since a disastrous fire in the antiques fair in neighbouring Todi killed thirty-five people, to be followed by a yet more catastrophic fire in a Turin cinema in 1982, security regulations have been tightened all over Italy. The San Carlo opera house in Naples was all right because it had broad corridors, but La Scala in Milan has lost 400 seats, while the opera house in Rome has been closed for months of rebuilding. Previously, Starling held his Perugian concerts in a large gallery in the museum, but that no longer satisfies the fire regulations.

A main problem with Italian music lies in the training. Music is not taught at school, but there are conservatoires which are blended in some cases with *scuola media* (starting at eleven) or in others with *licei* (starting at fourteen to fifteen). These are inadequate, as I was consistently told, throughout Italy. "Italians think they invented music and are not sure they have to learn" was one comment. "The teachers would not be there if they were good musicians" was another. "The trouble is that Italians are individualists. The conservatoires train them to be good soloists but not to play in an orchestra." Also, there are too many music students, so that premises are crowded. A big proportion concentrate on the piano with the result that performance in wind instruments is weak. As a result, there are very few good orchestras in Italy, apart from those of La Scala in Milan and Santa Cecilia in Rome.

Of course, as always, there are spontaneous attempts to remedy this by unofficial organizations. I found an interesting example in Testaccio, a workers' quarter near the pyramid of Cestius in Rome. Here, a co-operative, the Scuola di Musica, is "squatting" on the first floor of an old slaughter-house. Hooks where the dead animals used to hang still protrude from the walls. Although the Scuola is small, with about six studios and a big pavilion for the orchestra in a neighbouring garden, it has a four-year course in instrumental music from electric bass to the violoncello. Many of the teachers are also students. Thus an accomplished clarinettist who teaches may also be studying composition. Although they have no government subsidy, and are in constant fear of being ejected from their squat, they have a band of fifty musicians which plays everything from jazz to classical music, and have even produced an opera, *Il Regalo dell'Imperatore* by Giovanna Marini, which has been performed in Barcelona, Avignon and Paris. Like their chairman, Martin Joseph, most of the musicians earn their living elsewhere, but co-operate to teach and work on any project which may arise.

Opera, of course, is the musical form most closely associated with Italians. In Palermo, I visited Maestro Arrigo, the artistic director of opera, who has composed several operas himself, including *Addio Garibaldi* which was recently performed at La Scala. He had just been listening to new applicants for the choir, which was tedious, he said, because some had voices like old crows. The unions, however, insisted that everyone who applied be given a chance, and at least he had found three excellent sopranos. The trouble was that after a three-month trial, singers were there for life, however much their voices deteriorated.

In opera, he told me, most of the money came from government sources: only 10–15 per cent of income was from ticket sales. At Palermo, they had a hundred performances a year and eight thousand subscriptions. This meant that the building was full for most of the year, particularly as the gallery had now been closed because of fire regulations. Italians, he said, were not so addicted to ballet, but opera was in their blood: even the girls cleaning your window sang, and watching Italian plays, you sometimes felt they were going to take off into opera at any moment.

After the war, said Maestro Arrigo, intellectuals despised opera. Luigi Nono, one of the leading post-war composers, wrote oratorios instead. Eighty per cent of music was controlled by the Communists, partly because so much depended on backing from the Commune or Region which, as often as not, had a majority of the Left. He himself was non-political. "I am for a real democracy of the individual," he said, "not for parties." His opera house was a little island in this respect and, as it worked well, he wasn't interfered with.

Sicily was one of the most active music centres in Europe, said Maestro Pagano, the director of the orchestra, particularly with modern music. He had an enormous orchestra of eighty-three musicians but there were not many concert halls which could take them, so, as a full orchestra, they played mainly in ancient Greek theatres in summer. They were popular but the problem, as everywhere, was that music lovers tended to prefer records. Audiences were mainly teachers and students. There were lots of old people too, who gave abundant applause but few shouts for encores. Pagano, too, was critical of the conservatoires. They encouraged spontaneity, which was natural to Italians, rather than technical excellence.

Naples, as well as Palermo, has always been at the heart of Italian music in the South. On the sea front, Riviera di Chiaia, there is a villa drawn back from the road, with green lawns and elegant columns fronting a low classical building. This is the Villa Pignatelli which used to belong to General Acton, Prime Minister of Naples when Nelson was there. Now it is a concert hall, run by Dr Dino Eminente who invites good soloists from all over the world for chamber music concerts. They rehearse in the morning, and anyone can wander through the beautiful eighteenth-century rooms with their collections of porcelain, and listen to them. In May, they have a festival in co-operation with the opera house. There is also a theatre at the royal palace in Naples, and another in the palace at Caserta. Amidst the chaos of a town overrun with cars, these places seem refuges, going back to times before the turmoil, speculative building and overcrowding.

Dr Francesco Canessa, the director of the opera at San Carlo, told us that the financial situation is similar to that of the Amici della Musica in Perugia. The grant of about eight million dollars per year to the opera arrives every six months. But salaries have to be paid, so loans are made at interest 22–23 per cent. The debt thus mounts up, until every ten years or so the government eliminates it. A symptom of this situation is the way a union representative has been known to announce over a loudspeaker before the curtain goes up that they are allowing the performance to go ahead, even though they have not been paid their wages. Many other opera houses are in the same precarious position. The one in Rome receives about ten million dollars a year but in 1983 had debts of fifteen.

San Carlo, like La Scala and other opera houses in Italy, has a relatively short opera season and holds concerts for the rest of the year. One result is that it is very difficult for the visiting foreigner to get tickets unless he is staying long enough in a city to get a subscription, or has friends who will "arrange" tickets.

In Naples, they stage six or seven different operas in three months, with about twenty days' rehearsal for each of them. In Germany and at Covent Garden, on the other hand, eminent opera singers even move from one country to another to play different parts on successive evenings, because they are paid for each performance. The result, said Dr Canessa, is that in Naples they are much more professional. "I would not have the company from Covent Garden here," he said, "because there would be too much criticism."

Their present plans are to have six traditional Italian operas a season, and one eighteenth or nineteenth-century Neapolitan work. These latter are available partly because Naples has the biggest music library in the world. It was set up in the seventeenth century when a law made it compulsory for anyone publishing or performing music to place a copy there. Stravinsky discovered Pergolesi's *Il Flaminio* in the library, and based his ballet *Pulcinella* on it. You can still see the manuscript with his notations on it. To celebrate the centenary of Stravinsky's birth in 1983, *Il Flamino* was sent to Versailles where it was performed in the theatre to great applause.

A precursor of *Il Seraglio* by Nico Jomelli – who preceded Salieri, Mozart's rival, as master of music at the Imperial Court in Vienna – has been discovered in the library by Alan Curtis, an American. I was told it would soon be performed at Caserta by a baroque orchestra with old instruments. In 1984, they were to stage a nineteenth-century Neapolitan opera *Crispini e la Comare* (Crispin and the fairy godmother) by Ricci, composed in 1850.

There is still a lot of unclassified music in the library, so one never knows what new works may be discovered.

Now the San Carlo have come to an agreement with the Fenice in Venice to exchange an opera a year. Why not with Florence or La Scala? "They don't have the same great musical tradition," said Dr Canessa.

Certainly, the festas of central Italy and La Scala now rely much less on their own talent. In Spoleto, at the Festival of Two Worlds, sponsored for twenty-six years by the Italo-American composer Carlo Menotti, they even had Ken Russell's version of *Madame Butterfly*, in which she was transformed into a whore whose one aim was to marry Pinkerton so that she could become an American housewife.

What though of musicals? Here again, the only outstanding one comes from Naples, directed by Roberto De Simone, the artistic director of San Carlo. Originally staged in 1918, *La Festa di Pedigrotta* commemorates an old Neapolitan festival of dancing and song which took place every September 7th in a grotto of the Madonna, which was popularly believed to have been opened up by Virgil with the help of twenty devils.

Another musical appeared on film in 1980: Pupi Avati's *Help Me to Dream* which is about a girl, Gianna, who is star-struck by the pre-war films and songs of Hollywood. During the war, an American airman suddenly appears on her doorstep, as his aeroplane has had engine trouble. Inevitably, she falls in love with him: he is a jazz pianist and knows all the songs she loves. When peace comes, he goes away and, despite his promises, never returns.

Italian directors have also inspired much of the recent enthusiasm for filming opera. Zeffirelli released *Traviata* in 1983, and Rosi's *Carmen* was shown in 1984.

And modern composers? Luigi Nono and Luciano Berio are probably the best known. Berio is now in his sixties, and has opened up new forms of expression, particularly for the voice. His *Laborintus II*, one of his best known works, uses extracts from the *Divine Comedy* and from modern poets like Eliot, Pound and Sanguinetti as an essential part of his music, merging words with a diversity of sounds. Application is varied: *Laborintus II* is a stage work and can be expressed as a dance, or simply as an allegory, or as a story.

Luigi Nono used to be a Maoist and has tried, without much success, to bring his music into factories and workers' reunions. It might be thought that music is one of the arts which lends itself least to political application. Yet his *a floresta e jovem e cheja de vida* is a protest against the Americans in Vietnam. American phrases and Vietnamese voices, the shouts of soldiers and the sound of shots and bombs are set against dirge-like, wandering music. With later works like *Con Luigi Dallapiccola*, Nono produces what Bernas called "snapshots of sound" which tend to stand on their own, rather than merging into a central theme.

Modern music in Italy, as elsewhere, has been much influenced by Webern, Stockhausen and Schoenberg. Nono in fact married Schoenberg's daughter, and has also worked closely with music and musicians from the East. Popularity with the public depends partly on who the performer is. In Naples, I remember a concert hall completely crowded out to hear Stockhausen and Webern – and also Beethoven. But the pianist, Maurizio Pollini, was very well known.

Young composers have reacted now against atonality and produce work that is more romantic and melodious. But as Andrew Starling said to me in Perugia, is it possible to talk of national music except in opera? What makes Mozart Austrian, or Elgar British? Beethoven forged his music by breaking rules, but today there are no rules to break. For years, now, in every country, composers have been individuals in limbo, expressing sounds that fulfil them personally. As are painters, with form and colour.

VISUAL ARTS AND DESIGN

At an exhibition of modern Italian painting, there were large pieces of dirty white paper with revolutionary slogans on them, a poster of the Carabinieri with scrawlings underneath, abstract paintings with different lines and colours, a video show of a "happening". In one room there were fascinating machines: you pushed a button and small connected slabs "breathed"; or what looked like lead dust was projected onto the glass of a case, and fell slowly in different shapes, many of which looked like wintry, grey ducks. In one room, a large wooden Christ was stretched over the floor, and numerous music stands, arranged as if for an orchestra, held photographs of old movie stars instead of music. At the side, a small, shiny statue of Venus stood, sadly, looking at the wall, with the front of her body covered with a jumble of coloured rags.

The exhibition was lively, varied, inventive. Apart from the poster of the Carabinieri and the Italian names of the artists, I found it difficult to say how far it was uniquely Italian. Certainly, it was an "experience" and it focused attention on surfaces and a combination of colours which one might normally ignore, or not be aware of. I remembered an exhibition of Burri, one of the best-known Italian artists, when he was at the stage of exhibiting bits of sack in frames. I was aware it might be a fashionable "con", but at the same time realized I had never really examined a sack before and would have found it difficult to describe its surface accurately. Why should one want to do that, anyway? I suppose some modern art adds awareness of the world around one.

Burri has now left that phase behind. After selling millions of dollars worth of sacks to Americans, and experimenting with *Combustions*, which represented patterns of oxyhydrogen flames, in 1983 he mounted a display of colourful abstract paintings in an empty shed in the naval dockyard of Venice.

Milan, rather than Rome or Florence, is the centre of painting in Italy. Of the 121 artists at the exhibition of modern Italian art, over seventy came from Milan and only two from south of Rome.

In January 1984 in the magazine *L'Espresso*, the critic Renato Barilli wrote an article on the latest currents in Italian art. From the fashion of the early '70s of choosing and exhibiting everyday objects (a school called "ready made"), one natural, if unexpected development is a return to figurative art. "Given that all possibilities of inventing new forms have been tried and exhausted, the only alternative is to re-cycle the ready made" – in other words to paint more realistically. From this tendency, started by a painter called Salvo, who reproduced the angels of Carpaccio and Raphael in an almost childish way, three schools have now developed: the purely classical which includes versions of Renaissance paintings in a modern or unusual context; light ornamental but figurative sketches which look as if they were designed for ceramics; and more expressionist, colourful paintings with whirling lines and bright colours.

An art critic in Milan told me that in the '70s abstract paintings by Italian artists fetched such high prices that they were bought en masse without even being looked at, crated up and loaded onto lorries to be exported. That, he was glad to say, was no longer the case. "Paintings just became a product," he said, "like slabs of Carrara marble." Now, Milan has lost to London and New York. "In any case, we've never been able to compete with painters like Hockney or Bacon," he said. "Or sculptors like Henry Moore. Really apart from Guttuso, or De Chirico, we have no one with the same international reputation."

The art scene in Italy is probably plagued more than most by forgeries. In the summer of 1984 there was a scandal because some heads, found in a canal at Leghorn, were accepted as genuine by the director of the Modigliani exhibition. Later, it was discovered that they had been put there by three students who had sculpted them with a common hand-drill, as they proceeded to demonstrate on television. Since the war, when a special squad of Carabinieri was set up to investigate art frauds, no fewer than seven thousand forgeries have been discovered, and four hundred expert copyists have been arrested.

Although restaurants are full of modern paintings, often left there by artists who exchange them for meals, there is a certain cynicism about modern art in Italy: the feeling that the success or otherwise of contemporary painting depends as much on public relations as quality, which is often difficult to determine – or on the favour of a critic or reviewer, and whether you have friends who "persuade" the Commune to put on an exhibition of your works. As elsewhere, modern art tends to be a specialized taste, appealing to certain groups of individuals. Gone are the days of painting and sculpture for the people, or the times of new discoveries in approach or technique. This is sad when one considers the art that Italy once gave the world. But even talented painters – and there undoubtedly are such in Italy – are confined by the weight of their inheritance and by the contemporary fragmentation of expression and artistic values.

As Barilli wrote at the end of his article on the return to figurative forms: "The only thing this teaches us is that tendencies go in circles at a giddier and giddier rate, and that everything passes and comes back on the river of time." Like a merry-go-round rather than an autostrada.

In design, though, Italians have certainly found a wide public. Barzini in *From Caesar to the Mafia* tells of a morning when, strolling through New York, he saw in an antique shop an open pan used in his parents' kitchen, with the same dent he remembered, priced at thousands of dollars. Like other cultures which have not had an industrial revolution which produced utilitarian forms, squalor, and a sacrifice of personal taste and creativity to mass production, the Italians have retained the visual sense they had as artisans – in the same way as the Swedes, the Finns or the Danes. As Sally Brampton wrote in the *Observer* about dress design: "The Italians take fashion so seriously that they would rather have a new jacket than a colour television, a skirt than a spin drier."

The extraordinary rise of Milan as the present centre of dress design began when, in 1968–9, the stylist Missoni decided to present his collection in America. Then Cerruti opened a boutique in Paris. Then, so the story goes in Milan, Mariuca Mandelli, the founder of Krizia – a name she took from Plato – stamped her foot because she didn't see why the centre in Italy of ready-to-wear fashion should be Florence, when it was so difficult to get to, with no airport nearer than Pisa. In 1972 she and her husband Aldo Pinto put on a show in Milan with other Milanese designers.

In the following years, others abandoned Florence until it was confined to domestic and masculine ready-to-wear collections. By 1983, the fashion business was responsible for exports worth four and a half billion dollars, 17 per cent up on 1982, while at the Milanese collections in March 1984 there were 21,000 buyers in four days – an increase of 37 per cent on 1983.

This has been achieved through a combination of creativity and taste on one side and of good marketing and quality work on the other. In an amusing article in the *Guardian* called "The Great Italian Leg Show" Brenda Polan describes her increase in temperature and drop in objectivity when she first arrives at a collection. She compares herself to a child in a candy shop wanting to buy everything. "For the Italians," she writes, "clothes are very much about expressing sexuality. The very richness of the fabric is about tactility: the aura of expensiveness ... is sexy in the way the pungent smell of leather in the back of a Rolls Royce is sexy. Money (and its trappings) is the great aphrodisiac."

As can be imagined, there is little problem about marketing and publicity now that designers like Armani, Ferré, Versace and Valentino are well known all over the fashion world. Collections are held twice a year and for five days about thirty designers drape models in all their latest styles. Enterprises are, as so often, mainly family businesses.

Mario Valentino has his factory in a poor area of Naples and it is still run by his family, although he, his wife and two daughters are now millionaires – in dollars. Fendi is run by sisters, Krizia by husband and wife, as is Missoni. Benetton, outside Milan in the Veneto, which produces over thirty million garments a year for the young market, is managed by two brothers and two sisters.

It is small workshops which provide the quality, especially those in the north between Biella and Como where they have had years of experience in working with leather, silk and textiles. This also happens all over Italy. In Perugia, Ellesse, who make tasteful and expensive sports wear, employ 1,000 workers directly in the main factory, but 2,500 in small groups. In Positano, near Sorrento, an entrepreneur called Cinque transformed the fishermen's village into a centre for holiday wear. Now there are over 300 dress shops in this luxury holiday resort which has 3,500 inhabitants. An English girl I met there worked with an Italian partner who, she said, was really an interior designer but had plenty of ideas about styling clothes, which she puts into practice to produce sample models. These they would sell to one shop at a considerable price, with no bargaining. Then the style would be imitated by other shops. There was nothing they could do about this, she added, shrugging her shoulders, as she gave us tea on her little balcony.

Like the interior designer at Positano, few Italians train or specialize before launching themselves. They seem to have innate confidence in their taste, and feel it is an important part of their lives. Italian design is applied to many fields, whether it is the chassis of Cadillac cars, the form of a Ferrari, or shoes and leather goods, furniture or ceramics. Often a firm which started in one field will branch out into others. Ferragamo, in Florence, is a good example of this. It was started by Salvatore Ferragamo, born at the turn of the century in the village of Bonito near Naples. By the age of ten, Ferragamo had learnt everything his local cobbler could teach him. At eleven, he started his own business, and then emigrated to the United States where in the '20s he made shoes for the "greats" in Hollywood, until he returned to Italy. Now he is dead, but his family continue his work. His widow is in charge of the firm, his daughter Fiamma is responsible for the design of ladies' shoes and also handbags and small leather goods, while another daughter, Fulvia, designs scarves and ties and a third, Giovanna, looks after ladies' ready-to-wear fashions.

As David Willey tells us in *The Italians*, Giorgetto Giugiaro, who has designed aerodynamic shapes for twelve million cars, has just produced a new shape for pasta, commissioned by the Voiello spaghetti factory in Naples.

If Italians find modern painting frustrating, they can turn to what is around them, and produce something which everyone seems to find beautiful.

X
CONCLUSION

A professor at Urbino university told me that when he was in London as a youth, he was employed by an old, rich English couple to come to their house at nine o'clock every morning and wander around singing for an hour in order to wake them gently and musically. At ten o'clock, he brought tea to their bedroom, and his job for the day was over.

In doing this, he fulfilled an idea which many Northern Europeans have of the Italians: cheerful, full of song, prepared to help in any way, good-humoured. Also, perhaps, slightly ridiculous, particularly because of gesticulations.

I think, though, that Italians are, mysteriously, very complete beings. For one thing they are "pleasure people". They take care to make everything pleasant both for themselves and for others so long as the situation is personal. Whether it is food, or the way they arrange flowers, or fruit on stalls, or how they greet a customer in small personal shops, or the way they dress, there is always an attempt at style and beauty. In Palermo the mayor, Elda Pucci, countered my criticism of the dirty streets by saying that it was indeed strange, as Palermitanos cared a lot about the beauty of their homes. Italians make friends rapidly if they know you can speak their language, and ignore you if you can't – what good does a stumbling conversation do anyone? Indeed, Italians are very realistic, doing things if they lead to pleasure, and not worrying very much otherwise.

In order to enjoy things, they work hard – you can't imagine Bristow in the London *Standard*, whose one aim is to do nothing at work, appealing to Italians. Or that poster for a British building society with a man asleep on a sofa and the question beneath: "What is he doing?" "He's earning seven per cent with the — Building Society." An Italian earning 7 per cent would consider himself unfortunate as interest rates are much higher than that, but with a regular income he would certainly not expect to sleep it away. He would buy something which would increase his status and make him feel proud, or spend it on women, or go for an exotic trip to somewhere he had never been before, or buy a more expensive ticket for a football match.

A sign of their sense of proportion is the way Italians rarely get drunk – unless they are mountain people. You go to a football celebration, where cars full of shouting youths tear along the streets, with waving banners. Very rarely, amidst all the tumult and trumpeting, do you see anyone tottering about or slumped at the side of the street, as you do with football fans in any other European city. After all, drink does not express exuberance: it only deadens it, and produces awkward behaviour and a hangover.* Everything in its proper place. You drink when you are eating to improve the flavour of food. In Palermo, I met an English teacher who gave a party for his students with wine and peanuts in the English fashion. Unfortunately, many left after half an hour because there was no food. Realizing his mistake, he rushed out to get sandwiches, but when he came back there was nobody there. Because they are pleasure people, they will leave if it is not to their liking.

To foreigners, Italians often have extraordinary elegance and dignity. You look out of a car window and see a girl on a bicycle with whirring ear-rings, a trendy hair-style and a grey and black outfit if those colours happen to be in fashion. Even old ladies will probably wobble past on their sticks with bent figures, dressed in the latest style.

Bella figura, which is difficult to translate without a context, but means roughly giving a good impression, is one of the most important things in life. After all, it is a pleasure to be admired. If you are a middle-aged man, you may be surprised at the way girls glance at you in the street, until you become aware it is really because they are looking to see if you are admiring them, however uninterested they may be in you. Compliments are an essential part of a mutual admiration society. This partly explains the success of Italians with Northern women, and the disappointment which Italian women feel when they go to Northern Europe where compliments tend to be regarded either as insincere or as an unscrupulous way of playing on vanity to achieve one's ends.

Years ago, I remember showing my cheap, old watch to a Sicilian. "You were married when you got it?" he asked. "No." I answered.

---

* Significantly, there is no Italian word for "hangover", although the equivalent exists in every other European language.

"And you got your wife with that watch!" he exclaimed in amazement. I recall, too, an Italian friend who spent twelve years in Australia. "There we would dress anyhow," she said, "drive a second-hand car, drink beer at meals. Here, my friends go out and buy thousand-dollar dresses, make sure they always have a new car, eat like princes when they invite you to dinner. And yet Australia is, surely, wealthier than Italy."

Christopher Hibbert in his book on *The Medici* tells of an old peasant who approached Lorenzo de Medici because he had had some property stolen. "They tell me that taking other people's property is in fashion," he said. "In which case, that is all right. However, if it is not ... then perhaps something could be done."

This *bella figura*, and the slavery to fashion, can be irritating. But of course it is the surface of personal living. The relation of inner attitude to exterior appearances is still exemplified by the eighteenth-century story quoted in James Morris's *Venice*, where an Englishman at a service in St Mark's refuses to kneel: "I don't believe in Transubstantiation," he whispers to his companion who is protesting. "Neither do we," hisses the Venetian, "but get down on your knees, or get out." Underneath, when you get to know Italians, you find as many individualists as anywhere.

Much of the attitude to fashion and *bella figura* comes originally from village life where everything is personal, you know everyone, and the way you appear and behave is important. It is always interesting in Italy asking about people's parents and grandparents. The father of the plump man sitting in a Mercedes with an impeccably brushed coat was a forger of iron gates. Or that lady in a fur coat has a father who once worked on the land while her mother washed clothes in the river as a young girl.

An illusion that some foreigners have is that Italy is a country of cities: Florence, Venice, Rome and Milan, Turin and Palermo. Yet even today only 40 per cent of Italians live in towns of more than three hundred thousand inhabitants, and it is surprising how few of the inhabitants of bigger cities were actually born there. As Amendola, the late Communist leader, once said, Italy has changed more in thirty years than during the previous two thousand. Yet little can change at root in thirty years; all that happens is that two-thousand-year attitudes are applied to new situations.

Italians themselves will often deny this. Being modern and cosmopolitan is one of their dreams. They have over the centuries been dominated by foreigners and as many as twenty-five million of them

have emigrated to other countries. As a result, they are the least
chauvinistic of peoples. Now, change has brought wealth. They reject
the times of previous poverty and hardship when foreigners patronized
them and to be Italian was something almost shameful: "Thank God for
the Spaniards," wrote Rossini in the last century. "If there were no
Spaniards, the Italians would be the last people in Europe." Because
they have now adapted the qualities of their peasant culture to
contemporary life, they are as open to modern ideas as any country in
Europe.

Northern Italians, particularly, often deny the continuing strength of
family links because they feel there is something primitive about it, true
only of the South. "Oh, it's the foreigner's cliché about Italy," said a
lady from Trieste scornfully to me. "The Italian family! It's like pizza!
It's one of the things always associated with Italy." "Yes," I answered,
"but, like pizza, it does exist!"

As has been repeatedly stressed in this book, it is the unity of the
family as an economic unit that gives Italians their security, their
confidence and warmth, just as the Church, whether they believe or
not, takes care of their spiritual restlessness, allows them to get on with
the realistic quest for beauty, ease and pleasure which they have always
had, without endless soul-searching. Indeed, it is the family and the
Church which seem to give them that balance between restraint and
spontaneity, between self-interest and courtesy which is so characteristic. Without these set margins of behaviour the Italian would probably
deteriorate into a debauched, totally materialistic being. His realism
would become unprincipled. He might also feel the pointlessness of
struggling because he would not be working for those close to him, and
because he would not feel that perhaps there was an ultimate purpose to
living. Indeed, the tragedy of the two hundred thousand young heroin
addicts is just that.

However, the family, or clan, is the source of many of the ills of the
country. Without that unifying link, the Mafia would not be so
powerful, and government and the parties it contains would not be so
largely a collection of vested interests. Political parties are the family
writ large, with their endless intrigues for sectional benefit rather than
national improvement, which affect every walk of life – even the arts.
One could almost establish a law: the effectiveness of any national
government is in inverse proportion to the sense of unity among the
family. Or again, fairly obviously, but often forgotten: the stronger
local loyalties are, the weaker is central government. Hitherto the only
workable compromise in any strongly regionalized country such as

Germany or the United States has been a federal structure. Unfortunately, Italy was unified on the basis of central Piedmontese rule, followed by that of Mussolini. Now, this centralization is proving difficult to unscramble because so many vested interests have established themselves.

Indeed, the great menace to the future of Italy is a government that cannot be contained sufficiently. On the whole, the economy has been going well in the '80s, with inflation down to single figures in November 1984, an increase in exports of 5.8 per cent and an increase in labour costs, per unit of output, of only 5.3 per cent. Much of this is due to government policy and to negotiations between the large industrial organizations and the trade unions. However, the frightening thing is the way credit is increasingly being taken over by government, and the fact that the public debt has risen faster than other OECD countries since 1970. Simply paying the interest on this debt is now the equivalent of one in every ten units of everything produced in the country.

In Italy, many things have to be stood on their heads. To Socialists, nationalizing the means of production is still an aim, although this has ceased to mean much in many countries. In Italy, though, there is open opposition to it even from the Communists because nationalized industry, which even goes to the extent of owning 22 per cent of ice cream production, works so badly and loses so much money. One answer is to increase government income by ensuring that taxation is paid equitably by everyone, which is a worthy objective. However, this means hitting the black economy which in 1984 is believed to have "outboomed" the official figures. The obvious conclusion is that Italians themselves are doing fine, and that it is only government which is dragging them backwards, with its enormous debts, its parasitic parties, and its ineffective bureaucracy. Indeed, it is a strange thing that immediately an Italian becomes a bureaucrat he seems to lose his vitality, like someone very muscular who goes to fat more easily than a person less strongly built.

The essential problem today is how Italy can preserve the vitality of small family groups without at the same time being smothered by the effects these have on government, or on criminal organizations.

There is no doubt that in industry, firms like Olivetti, Fiat, Pirelli or Buitoni can outgrow family origins and yet remain efficient and successful. Perhaps it is because all the "fathers of a family going out to work" benefit by co-operating in modern management techniques. Therefore, they work hard and produce results. Indeed, it is the very acquisitiveness which makes for Italian economic success which simultaneously operates against it in government and in the organizations which make fortunes from heroin or cocaine.

How, in a relatively new country which as a nation has never really proved successful, do you develop the outstanding civil service or political nucleus which is willing to sacrifice its own short-term gain for the good of the country as a whole? Why should people pay taxes when they feel they are merely adding to the coffers of robber barons whose productivity for the nation, which they are entrusted to supervise, is scanty? If Marx were writing *Das Kapital* in Italy today, he would discover another economic class. Aristocracy he would probably leave out. The bourgeoisie would definitely be in, and also probably the proletariat. But the additional class would probably be government which, apart from a few individuals with integrity and the efficiency of some organizations like the Bank of Italy, often seems just another business enterprise.

Up to 1969, government inefficiency was almost an advantage: it allowed everyone to benefit from the boom, and distributed some of what it received to underprivileged areas like the South of Italy. However, the strenuous years which lasted from 1969 until the beginning of the 1980s overloaded it. The attempt to make Italy an ideal State incurred enormously expensive burdens like the health services, which now are limping, and encouraged political parties to compete for lucrative participation in government organizations. It also raised inflation to absurd levels, and strengthened the power of the trade unions as yet another "tribe" in a divided nation. At the same time it weakened those strange hybrids called the Communists, who might have had the public spirit to create a national government in co-operation with the Christian Democrats. But then would power have allowed them to go to an election with the slogan they used in 1978, "We have clean hands"? Would a government without a real opposition have been good for the country?

Napoleon called Italy "the most beautiful land on earth" although he was Emperor of the French. Among many outstanding examples, there are the coasts of the south and, further north, the Cinque Terre with their high vine-covered hills sweeping down between little fishing villages to the sea; the mountains of the Abruzzi; the flavour of ancient mysteries: the Etruscan tombs and in Sardinia the inexplicable shapes of the Bronze Age Nuraghi: structures like small medieval fortresses, standing often amidst green slopes, below an Aragonese castle on a hill.

Over the years, Italians have spoilt some of their country with speculative building, particularly in the South – although both Rome and Florence have kept high-rise buildings under control, unlike some British cities. Perhaps the main damage to the environment is from the unrestricted mania for cars. Go to the Piazza del Plebiscito in Naples, enclosed on one side by the royal palace and on the other by a colonnade and a church which is modelled on the Pantheon in Rome. In one corner of the square you can see Vesuvius, outlined against a corner of the palace in the blue sky. Yet if you want to examine the equestrian statues in the middle of the square, you have to edge your way through a mass of parked cars, and once you have reached your objective, you have to calculate the way out carefully, or you may not emerge till evening. Or go to Florence, where cars cluster round the Duomo like the eggs of an enormous queen-ant, and it is almost impossible to walk anywhere, particularly on the banks of the Arno.

Much has been achieved, though: at least pollution is not as bad as twenty years ago when swimming had to be forbidden at Ostia; the Red Brigades, it seems, have been smashed; North and South are closer together; prosperity continues to increase; mass arrests in the Mafia and the Camorra indicate that there is a chance of ultimately bringing them under control, particularly if their transformation into big business enterprises no longer makes them immune to the defence of *omertà* and the closeness of family communities.

Italy has had an industrial revolution which has transformed it in only thirty years. It is amazing that, given this, it has held together so well.

Most Italians you meet, though, seem depressed – particularly young people. If this book reproduced only the endless criticism of their country which one hears from them, it would be a gloomy document indeed. This is partly because they expect so much. Beside the humility about the more recent past there is always the pride which their long-term heritage has given them. For long, they were the cultural leaders of Europe, even when subjected to the rule of most major countries in Europe. Even after the war, they were leaders in taste, design, the cinema, admired as the museum and cradle of Europe. Their industrial success produced the proud saying in the '60s: "God made the world and Italy made everything in it." In some ways, they feel they are not now as successful as they ought to be, as it seemed they might be.

The early '80s, too, have been an empty period. A leading film critic, Fernaldo di Giamatteo, wrote in his *Universal Dictionary of the Cinema*, published in 1985: "Italian films have not been successful because, like society itself, they are empty, lost, superficial." The idealism and verve of the '70s are over, and that has left a sense of shock and bewilderment, and uncertainty about ideas. Just when Italians felt they were rich enough to afford greater equality, justice, better schools and universities, a reformed medical service, and better houses for everyone, the 1973 rise in oil prices made everything more difficult. In any case, these things cannot be created by the stroke of a pen, or as a result of strikes and endless demonstrations. Organizations are only as good as the government that creates and maintains them. The bitterest truth for an idealist in the 1980s is that Italy has reformed or created structures that do not work well, and is still dependent for its considerable prosperity on the enterprise of private industry, and on a vast black economy which is successful because it consists largely of family firms.

Like most other people, Italians would like to be what they are not: efficient in an evident sense. In fact they are effective in terms of achievement, but appear inefficient because they are impulsive, have too much humanity and tolerance, and personal relations are important. This was summed up by the indignant rebuke of a radio interviewer who asked a German in the summer of 1983 what he thought of the Italians.

"Disorganized," was the brief reply.

"Maybe," said the interviewer, stung. "But in our apparently disorganized way we have still achieved as much as you in the last thousand years."

Italians are in many ways the most adaptable Europeans: without the obstructive pride and moralizing about life of the Spanish; without the burden of past success and the sense of inflated status of the French or the British; without the rigidity of the Germans and Scandinavians. In so far as these broad generalizations are valid, Italians resemble the Americans, perhaps because their massive immigration has influenced that country. The difference is that Italians have a unique cultural heritage and a sophistication which comes from having experienced almost every conceivable disaster and regime in history.

The future depends very much on whether Italians with all their qualities can continue to survive side by side with a State which may have to become more arbitrary in order to untangle their many problems. The State has always been mistrusted. Back in 1935, in the remote village of Gagliano in Basilicata, Carlo Levi wrote about the peasants' view of the State: "Everyone knows that the fellows in Rome don't want us to live like human beings. There are hailstorms, landslides, droughts, malaria and the State. These are inescapable evils; such there always have been and always will be." Although this was fifty years ago in a primitive village in the South, the sentiments are still felt in much of Italy. Talking about his play *Questi Fantasmi*, Eduardo de Filippo said: "These political parties far from our view are ghosts, they too; perhaps they have now succeeded in turning us also into ghosts."

It is difficult to imagine Italians as pale ghosts. But their big revolution is their low birth-rate which is bound, shortly, to change the whole family structure and give more responsibility to the State for care of the increasing number of the aged. What will happen when there is no longer the spur of those who remember the poverty of the war and pre-war, which still makes hard work almost instinctive? Then there is the crisis of whether the State will go bankrupt and what it will do in terms of spreading its net yet wider to avoid it. It will be a very different Italy at the turn of the century. There is always the other strand in the Italian character: the desire to *sistemare*, to organize.

It would be tragic if Italians did gradually lose their vitality, their personal view of each other, their will to survive, and felt nothing underneath their *bella figura*; if they allowed themselves to be devoured by the "ghosts" who gnaw at everything because they have no flesh of their own; if they yielded to that great pressure for uniformity which affects us all.

On the brighter side, it is possible that Italy will find the political goals and the effective regionalism it needs in a developing Europe. Because they distrust their own government, Italians are more in favour of a federal Europe than any other members. Also, as the years go by, Italy will perhaps lose that feeling of inferiority which in some spheres has made her copy other nations too easily and inappropriately. "We have been like the man in the Bible who buried his talents," said a friend of mine in Spoleto. "Now we are beginning to realize that there is no reason why we shouldn't dig them up, and use them." Particularly in the Computer Age.

BIBLIOGRAPHY

Acton, Harold, *The Bourbons of Naples*, Methuen, 1956.

Acton, Harold, *The Last Bourbons of Naples*, Methuen, 1961.

Anderson, Burton, *Vino*, Papermac (Macmillan), 1982.

Andreotti, Giulio, *Visti da Vicino*, Rizzoli, 1982.

Angeli, Franco, *Gli Anni del Cambiamento*, Censis, 1982.

Antonucci, Piperno & Luoni, *Tra il Dire e il Fare*, Bulzoni, 1983.

Ardagh, John, *Tale of Five Cities*, Secker & Warburg, 1979.

Ardigo & Donato, *Famiglia e Industrializzazione*, Franco Angeli, 1976.

Arlacchi, Pino, *La Mafia Imprenditrice*, Il Mulino, 1983.

Baglivo, Adriano, *Camorra S.P.A.*, Rizzoli, 1983.

Bartlett, Vernon, *North Italy*, Batsford, 1973.

Barzini, Luigi, *The Italians*, Hamish Hamilton, 1964.

Barzini, Luigi, *From Caesar to the Mafia*, Hamish Hamilton, 1971.

Barzini, Luigi, *The Impossible Europeans*, Weidenfeld & Nicolson, 1983.

Bevilacqua, Alberto, *Il Curioso delle Donne*, Mondadori, 1983.

Biagi, Enzo, *Italia*, Rizzoli, 1980.

Biagi, Enzo, *Il Signor Fiat*, Rizzoli, 1976.

Bocca, Giorgio, *Italia Anno Uno*, Garzanti, 1984.

Bondanella, Peter, *Italian Cinema from Neorealism to the Present*, Frederick Ungar, 1983.

Bryant, Andrew, *The Italians*, Praeger (N.Y.), 1976.

Caizzi, Bruno, *Gli Olivetti*, Editrice Torinese, 1962.

Calvino, Italo, *Marcovaldo*, Secker & Warburg, 1983. (Trans. William Weaver.)

Casadio, Quinto, *Gli Ideali Pedagogici della Resistenza*, Edizioni Alfa, 1967.

Catarsi & Spini (Editors) *L'Esperienza Educativa e Politica di Bruno Ciari*, Nuova Italia, 1982.

Cederna, Camilla, Casa Nostra, Arnaldo Mondadori, 1983.

Chamberlain, Narcissa & Narcisse, *The Flavour of Italy*, Hastings House, 1965.

Chegaray, *Italie Insolite*, Les Presses de la Cité, 1971.

Ciment, Michel, *Le Dossier Rosi*, Editions Stock, 1976.

Cornwell, Rupert, *God's Banker*, Gollancz, 1983.

Correnti, Santi, *Canti D'Amore del Popolo Siciliano*, Longanesi, 1981.

Corsaro, Ignazio, *Disonestopoli*, Editrice Fiorentino, 1982.

Cronin, Vincent, *Napoleon*, Penguin 1971.

D'Antonio, Mario, *La Costituzione di Carta*, Mondadori, 1977.

Davidson, Alistair, *Antonio Gramsci: Towards an Intellectual Biography*, Merlin Press, 1977.

De Carlo, Andrea, *Uccelli da Gabbia e da Voliera*, Einaudi, 1982.

De Crescenzo, Luciano, *Napoli di Bellavista*, Mondadori, 1984.

Denti di Pirajno, *The Love Song of Maria Lumera*, Deutsch, 1965.

De Rosa, Gabriele, *Storia Contemporanea*, Minerva Italica, 1982.

Desideri, Antonio, *Storia e Storiografia*, vol. 3, G. D'Anna, 1982.

Di Fresco, Antonio Maria, *Sicilia: 30 Anni di Regione*, Vittorietti, 1976.

Donato, Pierpaolo, *La Donna nella Terza Italia*, A.V.E. 1978.

Douglas, Norman, *Old Calabria*, Century, 1983.

Douglas, Norman, *Siren Land*, Secker & Warburg, 1982.

Eco, Umberto, *The Name of the Rose*, Secker & Warburg, 1983. (Trans. William Weaver)

Falcioni, Giorgio, *La Macchina di Santa Rosa*, Edizione Quatrini, 1982.

Fava, Giuseppe, *I Siciliani*, Capelli, 1980.

Fernandez, Dominique, *Le Promeneur Amoureux*, Plon, 1980.

Fogoler, *T'al Dighi in Dialet*, Citem, 1983.

Ginzburg, Natalia, *Le Piccoli Virtù*, Einaudi, 1984.

Gismondi, Arturo, *Gli Anni Piu Difficili*, Il Renovamento, 1973.

Giussani, Luigi, *Comunione e Liberazione*, Jaca Books, 1980.

Gleijeses, Vittorio, *A Napoli Si Mangia Così*, Societa Editrice Napolitana, 1977.

Goethe, J. W., *Italian Journey*, Penguin Classics, 1982.

Grimal, Pierre, *Rome*, Arthaud, 1982.

Grindrod, Muriel, *Italy*, Benn, 1968.

Hammer, Richard, *The Vatican Connection*, Penguin, 1982.

Hibbert, Christopher, *The Rise and Fall of the House of Medici*, Allen Lane, 1974.

Hobsbawm, E. J., *Primitive Rebels*, Manchester University Press, 1978.

Hofmann, Paul, *Rome*, Harvill Press, 1983.

Hotchner, A. E., *Sophia*, Bantam, 1979.

Knox, Oliver, *From Rome to San Marino*, Collins, 1982.

Levi, Arrigo, *Un Idea dell'Italia*, Mondadori, 1979.

Levi, Arrigo, *Ipotesi sull'Italia*, Il Mulino, 1983.

Levi, Arrigo, *La DC Nell'Italia Che Cambia*, Laterza, 1984.

Levi, Carlo, *Christ Stopped at Eboli*, King Penguin, 1982 (Trans. Frances Frenaye).

Levi, Primo, *La Chiave a Stella*, Einaudi, 1978.

Lilliu, Giovanni, *La Sardegna*, Edizione della Torre, 1982.

McCormick, Colin & Julie Colacicchi, *Life in an Italian Town*, Harrap, 1982.

Mariotti, Giovanni, *Burotro*, Feltrinelli, 1984.

Martino, Maria Carla, *Viaggiatori inglesi in Sicilia nella prima metà dell'Ottocento*, Edizione e Ristampe Siciliane, 1977.

Massie, Alan, *The Death of Men*, Robin Clark, 1982.

Moravia, Alberto, *La Cosa*, Bompiani, 1983.

Moravia, Alberto, *34*, Secker & Warburg, 1983. (Trans. William Weaver)

Morris, Desmond, *Gestures*, Triad/Granada, 1982.

Morris, Jan, *The Venetian Empire*, Faber & Faber, 1980.

Morris, James, *Venice*, Faber & Faber, 1960.

Morton, H. V., *Traveller in Rome*, Methuen, 1957.

Mount, Ferdinand, *The Subversive Family*, Unwin, 1983.

Newby, Eric, *Love and War in the Apennines*, Picador, 1983.

Nichols, Peter, *Italia Italia*, Macmillan, 1973.

Nichols, Peter, *The Pope's Divisions*, Penguin, 1982.

Norwich, John Julius (Ed.), *The Italian World*, Thames and Hudson, 1983.

Origo, Iris, *The Merchant of Prato*, Penguin, 1955.

Parise, Goffredo, *Solitudes*, Dent, 1984. (Trans. Isabel Quigly)

Pomilio, Mario, *Il Natale del 1833*, Rusconi, 1983.

Price, David, *The Other Italy*, Olive Press, 1983.

Quartermaine, Luisa (Ed.), *Italy Today*, University of Exeter, 1985.

Ray, Cyril, *The New Book of Italian Wines*, Sidgwick & Jackson, 1982.

Riboldi, Antonio, *I miei Anni nel Belice*, Citadella, 1977.

Robert, Jean-Noel, *Les Plaisirs à Rome*, Les Belles Lettres, 1983.

Romano, Sergio, *Histoire de L'Italie du Risorgimento à nos Jours*, Seuil, 1977.

Saraceno, Pasquale, *L'Intervento Straordinario nel Mezzogiorno nella Nuova Fase Aperta dalla Crisi Industriale*, Svimez, 1983.

Seward, Desmond, *Naples*, Constable, 1984.

Sciascia, Leonardo, *A Ciascuno il Suo*, Einaudi, 1976.

Sciascia, Leonardo, *Candido*, Einaudi, 1977.

Sciascia, Leonardo, *Il Giorno della Civetta*, Einaudi, 1983.

Soldati, Mario, *La Busta Arancione*, Oscar Narrativa, 1984.

Sorge, Bartolomeo, *La "Ricomposizione" dell'Area Cattolica in Italia*, Citta Nuova, 1979.

Templeton, Edith, *The Surprise of Cremona*, Methuen, 1985.

Valenzi, *Sindaco a Napoli*, Riuniti, 1978.

Vittorini, Elio, *Conversazione in Sicilia*, Einaudi, 1966.

Willey, David, *Italians*, B.B.C. Publications, 1984.

Yallop, David, *In God's Name*, Jonathan Cape, 1984.

Institutional Books

Annuario Statistico Italiano, Roma, 1983.

L'Esercito Italiano, Ufficio Storico, Roma, 1982.

Quei Giorni delle Macerie della Paura e della Rabbia, Il Mattino, 1981.

INDEX

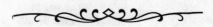